Clinical Management of Gastrointestinal Cancer

Cancer Treatment and Research

WILLIAM L MCGUIRE, *series editor*

Livingston RB (ed): Lung Cancer 1. 1981. ISBN 90-247-2394-9.

Bennett Humphrey G, Dehner LP, Grindey GB, Acton RT (eds): Pediatric Oncology 1. 1981. ISBN 90-247-2408-2.

DeCosse JJ, Sherlock P (eds): Gastrointestinal Cancer 1. 1981. ISBN 90-247-2461-9.

Bennett JM (ed): Lymphomas 1, including Hodgkin's Disease. 1981. ISBN 90-247-2479-1.

Bloomfield CD (ed): Adult Leukemias 1. 1982. ISBN 90-247-2478-3.

Paulson DF (ed): Genitourinary Cancer 1. 1982. ISBN 90-247-2480-5.

Muggia FM (ed): Cancer Chemotherapy 1. ISBN 90-247-2713-8.

Bennett Humphrey G, Grindey GB (eds): Pancreatic Tumors in Children. 1982. ISBN 90-247-2702-2.

Costanzi JJ (ed): Malignant Melanoma 1. 1983. ISBN 90-247-2706-5.

Griffiths CT, Fuller AF (eds): Gynecologic Oncology. 1983. ISBN 0-89838-555-5.

Greco AF (ed): Biology and Management of Lung Cancer. 1983. ISBN 0-89838-554-7.

Walker MD (ed): Oncology of the Nervous System. 1983. ISBN 0-89838-567-9.

Higby DJ (ed): Supportive Care in Cancer Therapy. 1983. ISBN 0-89838-569-5.

Herberman RB (ed): Basic and Clinical Tumor Immunology. 1983. ISBN 0-89838-579-2.

Baker LH (ed): Soft Tissue Sarcomas. 1983. ISBN 0-89838-584-9.

Bennett JM (ed): Controversies in the Management of Lymphomas. 1983. ISBN 0-89838-586-5.

Bennett Humphrey G, Grindey GB (eds): Adrenal and Endocrine Tumors in Children. 1983. ISBN 0-89838-590-3.

Clinical Management of Gastrointestinal Cancer

Edited by

JEROME J DECOSSE

and

PAUL SHERLOCK
Memorial Sloan-Kettering Cancer Center, New York

1984 **MARTINUS NIJHOFF PUBLISHERS**
a member of the KLUWER ACADEMIC PUBLISHERS GROUP
BOSTON / THE HAGUE / DORDRECHT / LANCASTER

Distributors

for the United States and Canada: Kluwer Boston, Inc., 190 Old Derby Street, Hingham, MA 02043, USA.
for all other countries: Kluwer Academic Publishers Group, Distribution Center, P.O.Box 322, 3300 AH Dordrecht, The Netherlands.

Library of Congress Cataloging in Publication Data

Main entry under title:

Clinical management of gastrointestinal cancer.

  (Cancer treatment and research)
  Includes index.
  1. Digestive organs--Cancer--Addresses, essays,
lectures. 2. Gastrointestinal system--Cancer--
Addresses, essays, lectures. I. DeCosse, Jerome J.
II. Sherlock, Paul. III. Series. [DNLM: 1. Gastro-
intestinal neoplasms--Therapy. W1 CA693 v. 18 /
WI 149 C6415]
RC280.D5C57 1984   616.99'433   83-17316
  ISBN 0-89838-601-2

ISBN 0-89838-601-2 (this volume)

Copyright

© 1984 by Martinus Nijhoff Publishers, Boston.

PRINTED IN THE NETHERLANDS.

Contents

List of contributors

ABE, Mitsuyuki, Department of Radiology, Faculty of Medicine, kyoto University, 54-Shogoin Kawahara-cho, Sakyo-ku, 606 Kyoto, Japan.

BEAHRS, Oliver H, Mayo Clinic, Rochester, Minnesota 55905, USA.

BLUMBERG, Baruch S, Institute for Cancer Research, Fox Chase Cancer Center, Philadelphia, Pennsylvania 19111, USA.

CLEMETT, Arthur R, St. Vincent's Hospital & Medical Center, 153 West 11th Street, New York, New York 10011, USA.

COOPER, Edward H, Unit for Cancer Research, The University of Leeds, School of Medicine, Leeds LS2 9NL, England.

DOSORETZ, Daniel E, Department of Radiation Therapy, Massachusetts General Hospital and Harvard Medical School, Boston, Massachusetts 02114, USA.

FOSTER, James H, Department of Surgery, University of Connecticut School of Medicine, Farmington, Connecticut 06032, USA.

GILES, Geoffrey R, Department of Surgery, St. James's University Hospital, Leeds LS9, England.

GOLDBERG, Stanley M, Division of Colon and Rectal Surgery, Department of Surgery, University of Minnesota, 516 Delaware Street, S.E., Minneapolis, Minnesota 55455, USA.

GOLDENBERG, David M. Div. of Experimental Pathology & Div. of Nuclear Med., Univ. of Kentucky & Veterans Administration Medical Centers, Lexington, Kentucky 40536, USA.

GUNDERSON, Leonard L, Mayo Medical School, Consultant in Therapeutic Radiology, Mayo Clinic, Rochester, Minnesota 55905, USA.

HOOKS, Vendie, Division of Colon and Rectal Surgery, Department of Surgery, University of Minnesota, 516 Delaware Street, S.E., Minneapolis, Minnesota 55455, USA.

HOSKINS, R. Bruce, Southern Illinois University Medical School, Department of Radiology, St. Johns Hospital, 800 East Carpenter St., Springfield, Illinois 62729, USA.

KELSEN, David, Solid Tumor Service, Department of Medicine, Memorial Sloan-Kettering Cancer Center, 1275 York Avenue, New York, New York 10021, USA.

KURTZ, Robert C, Gastroenterology Service, Memorial Sloan-kettering Cancer Center, 1275 York Avenue, New York, New York 10021, USA.

LONDON, Thomas W, Institute for Cancer Research, Fox Chase Cancer Center, Philadelphia, Pennsylvania 19111, USA.

MACMAHON, Brian, Department of Epidemiology, Harvard School of Public Health, 677 Huntington Avenue, Boston, Massachusetts 02115, USA.

MARTIN, J. Kirk, Mayo Clinic, Rochester, Minnesota 55905, USA.

MORTON, Donald L, Division of Surgical Oncology, Jonsson Comprehensive Cancer Center, UCLA School of Medicine, Los Angeles, California 90024, USA.

NIGRO, Norman D, Wayne State University, School of Medicine, Clinical Laboratories, 645 East Mullett Street, Detroit, Michigan 48226, USA.

NIVATVONGS, Santhat, Division of Colon and Rectal Surgery, Department of Surgery, University of Minnesota, 516 Delaware Street S.E., Minneapolis, Minnesota 55455, USA.

RICH, Tyvin W, Joint Center for Radiation Therapy, Harvard Medical School, 50 Binney Street, Boston, Massachusetts 02115, USA.

ROLFSMEYER, Eric S, Division of Colon and Rectal Surgery, Department of Surgery, University of Minnesota, 516 Delaware Street, S.E., Minneapolis, Minnesota 55455, USA.

ROTHENBERGER, David A, Division of Colon and Rectal Surgery, Department of Surgery, University of Minnesota, 516 Delaware Street S.E., Minneapolis, Minnesota 55455, USA.

RUSSELL, Anthony H, Department of Radiation Oncology, University of Washington, 1959 Pacific Street, N.E., Seattle, Washington 98195, USA.

SHILS, Maruice E, Memorial Sloan-Kettering Cancer Center and Cornell University Medical College, 1275 York Avenue, New York, New York 10021, USA.

STORM, F. Kristian, Division of Surgical Oncology, Jonsson Comprehensive Cancer Center, UCLA School of Medicine, Los Angeles, California 90024, USA.

TEPPER, Joel E, Massachusetts General Hospital and Harvard Medical School, Boston, Massachusetts 02114, USA.

ZIMMON, David S, St. Vincent's Hospital & Medical Center, VA Medical Center, New York, New York 10010, USA.

Cancer Treatment and Research

Foreword

Where do you begin to look for a recent, authoritative article on the diagnosis or management of a particular malignancy? The few general oncology textbooks are generally out of date. Single papers in specialized journals are informative but seldom comprehensive; these are more often preliminary reports on a very limited number of patients. Certain general journals frequently publish good indepth reviews of cancer topics, and published symposium lectures are often the best overviews available. Unfortunately, these reviews and supplements appear sporadically, and the reader can never be sure when a topic of special interest will be covered.

Cancer Treatment and Research is a series of authoritative volumes which aim to meet this need. It is an attempt to establish a critical mass of oncology literature covering virtually all oncology topics, revised frequently to keep the coverage up to date, easily available on a single library shelf or by a single personal subscription.

We have approached the problem in the following fashion. First, by dividing the oncology literature into specific subdivisions such as lung cancer, genitourinary cancer, pediatric oncology, etc. Second, by asking eminent authorities in each of these areas to edit a volume on the specific topic on an annual or biannual basis. Each topic and tumor type is covered in a volume appearing frequently and predictably, discussing current diagnosis, staging, markers, all forms of treatment modalities, basis biology, and more.

In Cancer Treatment and Research, we have an outstanding group of editors, each having made a major commitment to bring to this new series the very best literature in his or her field. Martinus Nijhoff Publishers has made an equally major commitment to the rapid publication of high quality books, and worldwide distribution.

Where can you go to find quickly a recent authoritative article on any major oncology problem? We hope that Cancer Treatment and Research provides an answer.

WILLIAM L. MCGUIRE
Series Editor

Preface

In this second volume on gastrointestinal cancer the editors have attempted in the 'Cancer Treatment and Research' series, to complement the first volume by including a set of different subjects which have recently attracted attention as newer concepts in the diagnosis and management of gastrointestinal malignancies.

As in the first volume, we have selected authors who have made major contributions in their field in the United States and abroad. Gastrointestinal cancer is a worldwide problem and research contributions know no geographic boundaries. The second volume emulates volume 1 in reporting advances in the biology of gastrointestinal cancer as it relates to diagnosis and management. Understanding of the basic biology of the disease is essential for optimal improvement in its outcome and its prevention.

The development of appropriate immunologic and biochemical markers is the goal for the early diagnosis of gastrointestinal cancer. Cooper and Giles from Leeds, England, present the current state of the art with markers and also give us a view to the future. Accurate staging of gastrointestinal cancer is essential for predicting prognosis and planning management. Martin and Beahrs from the Majo Clinic in Rochester, Minnesota review the current concepts regarding staging of gastrointestinal malignancies and make a plea for a uniform system based on the UICC and American Joint Committee's TNM system.

Pancreatic and hepatocellular carcinoma are major problems worldwide, the latter particularly troublesome in the less industrialized countries of the world. Both are difficult to manage and the great majority of patients afflicted with these diseases die. MacMahon from Harvard Medical School, Boston, discusses newer concepts regarding the epidemiology of pancreatic cancer. Because of the dismal prognosis of this disease and the difficulties with early diagnosis and management, understanding those at risk may be an important step towards the control of the disease. In regard to hepatocellular carcinoma, it has become evident that there is a relationship with this disease to hepatitis-B virus. Blumberg and London from Fox Chase, Philadelphia, discuss this relationship and postulate that the control of hepatitis-B would clearly dramatically aid in the control of hepatocellular carcinoma.

The management of both malignant disease of the liver and esophageal cancer has posed major problems with results that have not been satisfactory. Foster from the University of Connecticut places the management of primary and metastatic cancers involving the liver in perspective and stresses the indications for surgical management. Kelsen from the Memorial Sloan-Kettering Cancer

Center in New York discusses the combined multimodality treatment of carcinoma of the esophagus. Newer chemotherapeutic approaches in conjunction with surgery or radiation show promise in perhaps aiding in the management and improving survival with this cancer which generally has been resistant to therapy.

Although large bowel cancer has a reasonably good prognosis, the problem of low rectal cancer has created difficulties because of the need for colostomy. Rothenberger and his colleagues from the University of Minnesota discuss the options in rectal surgery and detail the major advances in restorative rectal surgery. Gunderson and colleagues from the Mayo Clinic outline the additive effects that radiation therapy may have in the management of rectal cancer. They discuss the preoperative, postoperative and 'sandwich' techniques. Nigro from Wayne State in Michigan describes the approaches in the management of squamous cancer of the anus with combined multimodality therapy.

Gastrointestinal bleeding, jaundice and malnutrition are major complications that may occur with cancer or its treatment. Supportive care of the patient with cancer is essential and needs to complement the primary treatment of the tumor. Kurtz from the Memorial Sloan-Kettering Cancer Center discusses management of gastrointestinal bleeding in patients with cancer and indicates that a vigorous diagnostic approach is necessary since not all bleeding is from tumor. Zimmon from the Veterans Administration Hospital and New York University in New York approaches the problem of the management of jaundice in selected patients with cancer by various non-surgical approaches including the endoscopic one. Shils from Memorial Sloan-Kettering Cancer Center discusses the nutritional management of patients with impaired or absent function of the various organs of the gastrointestinal tract.

The last three chapters encompass some newer approaches in the management of patients with gut cancer. Abe from Kyoto University, Japan outlines their excellent results utilizing intra-operative radiation therapy for gastrointestinal malignancies. Their preliminary results as well as some investigators in the United States are very encouraging in improving the situation in patients with very poor prognosis. Goldenberg from the University of Kentucky discusses the practical application of some of the newer concepts regarding antigen/antibody treatment of malignancies. Finally, Storm and Morton from the University of California, Los Angeles, outline their results with hyperthermia which show promise for managing some of the more resistant gastrointestinal cancers.

The editors wish to express their thanks to the authors who have contributed to this volume. It is evident that advances are occurring and with continued research hopefully many of our current problems in the management of gastrointestinal cancer will disappear.

Jerome J. DECOSSE, M.D.
Paul SHERLOCK, M.D.

1. Biochemical markers in gastrointestinal malignancies

EDWARD H.COOPER and GEOFFREY R. GILES

1. Introduction

There is a great wealth of experience of markers in gastrointestinal disease. Several tests such as those for alpha-fetoprotein (AFP) and carcinoembryonic antigen (CEA) have now moved firmly from the realms of experimental study into widespread clinical use. This transition from research to routine clinical chemistry, especially for CEA, has partially been justified by the scientific evidence that the measurement of the marker was helpful but has also been the result of astute advertising by the manufacturers of commercial kits and the economics of such tests. Indeed the cost effectiveness of the measurement of CEA is a matter of considerable debate with opinion leaders in major institutions sometimes taking diametrically opposed views.

In 1983 it is right that in an overview of the laboratory tests available for the investigation and monitoring of patients with gastrointestinal cancer, we try to restore some objectivity to the several pious hopes expressed in the literature for the last ten years concerning a wide range of analytes that might possibly be helpful clinically: alas so far few have fulfilled their promise. We will also attempt to integrate the results of laboratory tests into their true context of the sum of clinical information available to the physician or surgeon when the test is ordered. The essential question is how does the knowledge of the level of a particular analyte in the blood or urine add to the information available to the clinician and to what extent will this information influence his decision making?

Two main lines of research contribute to studies of biochemical and immunological markers in gastrointestinal cancer. First, there is a major effort to find markers that are tumour specific and have the sensitivity to identify early stage, asymptomatic, tumours. It will be seen that with a few exceptions we are still far short of this goal. Second, there is the use of markers once a diagnosis has been made, the aims being to stratify patients in terms of their survival probability, to detect recurrence and to monitor treatment. In this second set of tasks classical tumour markers can be reinforced by several types of non-specific tests that

J.J. DeCosse and P. Sherlock (eds), Clinical Management of Gastrointestinal Cancer.
© 1984, Martinus Nijhoff Publishers, Boston. ISBN 0-89838-601-2. Printed in The Netherlands.

reflect tumour burden and the reaction of the body to the general effects of invasion or the particular consequences of the damage to an organ system. In this secondary supportive role there has been considerable progress with many alternative tests available to the clinician. The problem now is to select the right combination of tests for the particular question that needs investigation at different stages in the evolution of the disease. There is a real risk of over investigating the patient for a trivial gain in information.

Those tests that are organ specific, for example associated with carcinoma of the pancreas, will be discussed in relation to the organ. The patterns of change of these analytes will then be examined in relation to the main sites of primary tumours in the gastrointestinal tract and their pattern of local and metastatic spread. Finally, we have added a brief appendix on the methods that are available to prove statistically whether the measurement of an analyte can add significantly to the information already available to the clinician. This statistical approach is obviously not essential for clinical practice but perhaps provides a way in which evidence should be critically examined prior to becoming overwhelmed by the pressures of commercial exploitation, or borne on the wave of false optimism.

2. Biochemical markers

2.1. Alpha fetoprotein (AFP)

AFP is a classical oncodevelopmental glycoprotein, it is synthesised early in foetal life by the liver and yolk sac, reaching its highest level in the foetus at the end of the first trimester with an AFP of 1–3 mg/ml [1]. The level of AFP then declines and in infants born at term, the concentration of the protein is between 2 and 17 ng/ml and it gradually falls to a normal adult level of <5 ng/ml [2]. Human AFP has a molecular weight of 64,600 daltons with a biological half life in the blood of 3 to 4 days [3]. Primary tumours of the liver and the yolk sac are often associated with the reactivation of the foetal genes for AFP production and a pronounced increase in the level of the protein in the blood.

Since the discovery of AFP in mice by Abelev et al. [4] in 1963, the identification of a similar protein in the serum of a patient with hepatocellular carcinoma by Tatarinov [5] an immense research effort has been put into the understanding of the physiology of AFP synthesis, its function and disturbance in disease. Several authors have reviewed the topic in recent years, among them Adinolfi [1], Sell [6, 7] and Hirai [8]. Reference to these extensive articles can provide the background of the experimental evidence of the structure and assay of the protein, its apparent function in animals. Measurement of the AFP concentration in amniotic fluid has given a method for the pre-natal diagnosis of certain developmental defects [1].

The AFP molecule shows a microheterogeneity which is associated with the carbohydrate side chains that contribute some 3 to 4% of its total weight. These sugar side chains exhibit varying degrees of affinity to plant lectins, in particular Concavalin A (Con A) and lens culinaris agglutinin (LCA) in a characteristic fashion which is related to the origin of the AFP.

The patterns of reactivity of foetal yolk sac AFP with LCA and with Con A closely resemble the pattern of AFP produced by germ cell tumours: whereas the reactivity of foetal liver AFP are similar to those produced by primary liver cancer [9]. These properties are an important basis of tests designed to aid the interpretation of the clinical significance of a raised AFP concentration in amniotic fluid. However within primary liver cancer there is considerable variation in the lectin binding patterns. These lectin affinity patterns provide further strong support for the concept that AFP synthesis in malignant tumours of the germ cells and hepatocytes is biochemically analogous to the AFP production in yolk sac endoderm and foetal liver cells respectively.

In the context of AFP as a tumour marker there are some broad generalisations that can help in the interpretation of the results of this assay. Partial hepatectomy in rats is a powerful stimulus for the proliferation of parenchymal and stromal elements of the liver which will grow until the liver is restored to normal size. AFP production is also stimulated by experimental partial hepatectomy but tends at tis maximum levels to be delayed as compared to the induction of the major waves of cell division [10]. On the other hand, no such elevation of serum AFP has been detectable in 11 adult patients who have undergone partial hepatectomy for benign disease but was elevated in 29% of patients with acute hepatitis, 34% of patients with chronic hepatitis and 75% with massive hepatic necrosis. This suggests the increased AFP in hepatitis is not a reflection of liver regeneration [11]. In tissue culture, hepatocytes of foetal and adult origin tend to show their maximum synthesis of AFP when they are in an active growth state whilst albumin is produced by the cells throughout their period in culture [10]. Study of the action of chemical carcinogens that are known to induce hepatic cancer in rodents have shown that in several such model systems there may be a transient activation of AFP synthesis soon after exposure to carcinogens to be followed by a massive upsurge of the level when the tumours arise in the liver [8]. Resection of the tumour in experimental animals and in man will be associated with a fall in the circulating AFP.

2.2. Carcinoembryonic antigen (CEA)

Carcinoembryonic antigen was discovered in 1965 by Gold and Freedman [12] and defined as a tumour-specific antigen of the digestive tract in man. The presence of CEA in foetal tissues and its absence in the corresponding adult tissues and the hypothesis that its synthesis was recommenced in bowel cancer cells was the reason why the protein was called the carcinoembryonic antigen.

The chemistry of CEA is the subject of numerous reviews (Fuks *et al.* [13]: Gold *et al.* [14]: and Shively and Todd [15]).

The major step forward was the development of sensitive immunological assays for CEA that are able to identify protein concentrations down to 0.5 ng/ml. Once these systems had become reliable a vast amount of data began to accumulate about this test. Some confusion occurred as various assay systems in the pioneer laboratories had widely differing levels for their normal and abnormal ranges that were unique to the particular assay. However, the great bulk of results during the past few years have come from use of the Roche radioimmunoassay and more recently Abbott commercial assays whose results are closely correlated to the Roche assay. Several other commercial CEA kits are now available in Europe and Japan. The results using different CEA assays are not interchangeable on the same patient, but the general trends are highly correlated.

In brief, CEA is a glycoprotein of molecular weight 175,000–200,000 daltons with 50–60% of its weight made of carbohydrate, which is responsible for the wide heterogeneity of molecular size. The high carbohydrate content makes the protein soluble in perchloric acid which is an extraction step used in some of the commercial assay systems for CEA. A number of CEA cross reacting antigens have been isolated and characterized (NCA and its closely related antigens). Antisera to CEA used for clinical assays are selected to keep this cross reactivity as low as possible.

2.3. Pancreatic tumour antigens

The discovery by Banwo *et al.* [16] in 1974 of an oncofetal antigen associated with human fetal pancreas and pancreatic tumours started a major search for putative markers of this type. The pancreatic oncofetal antigen (POA) now has emerged as the most promising antigen for the serological diagnosis of pancreatic cancer. The research has centred in London [17], Chicago [18, 19] and Roswell Park [20]. POA is a glycoprotein with a molecular weight of 40,000 daltons but tends to exist in the blood as an α_2 globulin with a molecular weight of 800,000 daltons. POA has been prepared from foetal pancreas and pancreatic cancer. Shimano [20] prepared pancreatic cancer associated antigen from the ascitic fluid of a patient with pancreatic cancer, this was later shown to be similar to pancreatic cancer associated antigen (PCAA).

Immunoperoxidase linked staining techniques have been used to examine the distribution of POA in tissues. Hobbs *et al.* [17] found POA in the secretory cells of adenocarcinoma of the pancreas, and the adenomatous parts of fetal pancreas, they found a very low frequency in other types of gastrointestinal cancer. Immunofluorescence microscopy has shown POA in the signet ring cells in gastric cancer [19].

The serum levels of POA (using a rocket immunoassay) and PCAA (using an enzyme immunoassay) have been measured in a variety of tumours and benign gastrointestinal diseases. In Hobbs's experience a level of 7 U/ml tends to discriminate pancreatic cancer from the moderate increases of POA in colon and stomach cancer and chronic pancreatitis. Hunter *et al.* [19] reported levels >14 standard units/ml (= 18–20 μg/ml) as discriminating. They found raised levels in moderately and well differentiated cancers; carcinoma of the pancreas had the highest incidence of raised levels. There appears to be some microheterogeneity of POA and PCAA that probably is due to differences in the carbohydrate content.

Tumour antigen tests with a limited data base. The interest in CEA, AFP and to a lesser extent POA have provided a firm data base so that their use in routine gastroenterology can be judged on solid evidence. There are some additional tests that may eventually find a place in clinical medicine, this section briefly introduces these tests.

2.4. Tennessee antigen

Tennessee antigen (Tennagen, TAG) is a glycoprotein extracted from a colon adenocarcinoma; it has some similarities to CEA but is antigenically distinct from CEA [21]. A commercial hemagglutination inhibition assay is available. Initial results indicated that more than 90% of patients with large bowel cancer had values greater than the upper limit of normal 5.5 ng/ml serum including Dukes stage A. Subsequent investigations have failed to confirm these first impressions. Sampson *et al.* [22] reported TAG has a sensitivity of 71% and a specificity of 77% for gastric cancer: however it was a less attractive test in colorectal cancer with a sensitivity of 76% but a specificity of only 44%. Pentycross [23] has cast doubt on the upper limit of normal, finding higher values than first reported and confirmed the low specificity of the test. In his series, although higher values were found in patients with active cancer, persistently raised levels were found in tumour-free patients. Gray *et al.* [24] reported that 29 out of 31 patients with resectable colorectal cancers had a raised serum level of TAG compared to only eight with a raised CEA. However, the lack of specificity and the persistent elevation after resection of all macroscopic cancer limits the clinical usefulness of TAG.

2.5. Tissue Polypeptide Antigen (TPA)

Tissue polypeptide antigen is a polymeric protein made up of units of 45,000–20,000 daltons, without sugar or lipid conjugates. TPA is found in most tumours and a haemagglutination inhibition assay and more recently a radioimmunoassay has been devised for its measurement in body fluids, see Björklund [25] for review.

There have been a few studies of TPA levels in colorectal cancer, Andrén-Sandberg and Isacson [26] studied 157 patients and found high pre-operative levels of TPA were associated with a bad prognosis. In monitoring TPA, levels rose several months before the detection of recurrence in 10 out of 13 patients. A comparative study of TPA and CEA in gastric and colorectal cancer has been made by Wagner *et al.* [27]; they concluded both TPA and CEA are not tumour specific markers, raised TPA levels occurring in inflammatory states. Thirty out of 39 (76.9%) cases of carcinoma of the stomach showed a raised TPA, compared to a raised CEA in only 18 out of 39 (46.1%). Tumour stage and TPA levels were related. In colorectal cancer, TPA was raised in 37 out ot 60 (61.6%) and CEA elevated in 38 out of 60 (63.6%).

2.6. Acute phase reactant proteins (APRP)

APRP are a group of plasma proteins predominantly synthesised by the liver whose levels in the blood are increased in response to a wide variety of non-specific inflammatory processes [28]. They consist of two groups, the fast reactants, which include C-reactive protein (C-RP), serum amyloid A(SAA) protein and a_1-antichymotrypsin (ACT) and the slower reactants, a_1-acid glycoprotein (AGP), a_1-antitrypsin (AT, haptoglobin (Hp), ceruloplasmin and fibrinogen. The fast reactants can rise within a few hours of a stimulus such as wounding; their half life is short, <2 days. C-RP and SAA can increase their concentration by as much as 100–1000 fold during the reaction [29,30]. Several other proteins such as complement factors exhibit a weak acute phase response.

The APRPs have tended to be overlooked as tumour markers as they lack specificity or the sensitivity required for the detection of small tumour masses. Nevertheless, evidence is growing which suggests that, in the context of prognostic assessment, patients with several forms of cancer, notably bladder, kidney, stomach and colorectal, a raised APRP tends to be associated with a downgrading of the chances of survival [28, 31]. The acute phase response in cancer of the stomach, colon and hepatic metastases cannot be ascribed to infection; it is more probable that it reflects the rate of extent of tissue destruction and release of the messenger molecules controlling the rate of hepatic synthesis of this cascade of proteins. The precise functions of the APRPs in inflammation are still uncertain. Some of the proteins have antiproteolytic activity (ACT and AT), haptoglobin binds haemoglobin, ceruloplasmin transports copper and removes free radicals. The action of AGP, C-RP and SAA are less well understood; all exhibit immunosuppressive activity and may be important in the modulation of other protein pathways involved in an inflammatory response, such as the coagulation and complement systems. See Pepys [29], Arnaud and Gianazza [32], Glenner [30] for reviews.

It has been argued that the erythrocyte sedimentation rate (ESR) can provide the same information as measuring acute phase reactants. In practice, the ESR tends to be influenced by a variety of factors of which the level of fibrinogen is important but by no means the only rate determining factor; gammaglobulin levels and haemotocrit also have a strong influence. The measurement of C-RP, ACT or AGP tends to reflect clinical progress of a cancer more closely than the ESR.

3. Oesophageal cancer

There are few reports of tumour markers in oesophageal cancer. Wahren *et al.* [33] observed a CEA >2.5 ng/ml in 35 out of 59 (59%) patients with localised oesophageal cancer; rising to 78% in patients with metastatic cancer. There was also a slight rise of AFP in some patients but this contributed little as a potential marker. In a series of 41 patients with oesophageal cancer investigated by Alexander *et al.* [34], 70% had CEA levels >5 ng/ml; CEA levels >10 ng/ml after therapy were associated with a significantly shortened survival.

4. Carcinoma of the stomach

A high incidence of carcinoma of the stomach is found in Latin America, Japan and some European countries, it is low in much of Africa and intermediate in North America and parts of Europe, where it is tending to decline slowly. Conversely the disease either presents or is discovered generally at a later stage in the Western world than in Japan. This difference is becoming more accentuated as active population screening programmes for stomach cancer have been well established in Japan.

In Western countries laboratory based tests for the diagnosis and prognostic assessment and monitoring of gastric cancer have received far less attention compared to the great effort that has centred on large bowel cancer.

4.1. Aids to diagnosis

The low frequency of elevated levels of classical tumour markers, such as CEA and AFP means that they can play little part in the diagnosis of the disease, and have no role in screening. One promising test is the assay of the level of the tumour-associated sulphated glycoproteins in the gastric juice. One of these foetal sulphoglycoprotein antigens (FSA) described by Häkkinen [36] has warranted its use as a screening test in 214,000 Finnish people and 3% of the rural and 5–7% of the industrial population were positive. Subsequent gastroscopy of 461 led to the detection of 3 histologically proven cancers and one suspected early cancer. Later in 1979, Häkkinen [36] reported that among 34,000 persons tested, 3,000 were FSA positive and 26 were eventually demonstrated to have a gastric cancer; a high incidence of a variety of benign disorders of the stomach, predominantly atrophic gastritis, was present in the FSA positive subjects.

This is an interesting form of non-invasive screening technique but its false positive rate is rather high. On the other hand, Häkkinen considers it could be the basis of a screening system especially in high risk patients. Alterations of the concentration of certain enzymes in gastric juice has been known for a long time to be associated with gastric cancer [37]. The combination of levels of lactic dehydrogenase (LDH) and β-glucuronidase provided a powerful discriminant for gastric cancer in 113 cases of dyspepsia investigated by Rogers *et al.* [38], 41 out of 42 cases of gastric cancer gave positive tests with only 13 out of 113 (11%) false positive results, all in cases with extensive metaplasia. There have been suggestions that a raised level of CEA in the gastric juice is indicative of cancer [39], but is has not become a widely adopted test.

The non-specific elevation of acute phase reactant proteins has been suggested as a possible warning of malignancy in patients complaining of dyspepsia. Grindulis and his colleagues [40] found significant differences in the mean APRP levels in 17 gastric cancers compared to benign lesions in an examination of 107 patients being investigated by gastroscopy but the overlap was too great to be pathognomonic. In our experience of 200 cases of gastric cancer elevation of acute phase proteins, C-RP, ACT and AGP was present in about one half the patients.

A raised β2-microglobulin (β2-m) has been observed by several investigators to occur in about a third of patients with gastric cancer [41, 42]. In a more extensive study of 480 patients, Rashid *et al.* (43) confirmed that a raised β2-m >3mg/l was present in 35% of patients with gastric cancer, 37.8% of patients with pancreatic cancer and in 28% with gastric ulcer. On the other hand there was no elevation in 50 patients with symptoms of dyspepsia and no lesion demonstrated by gastroscopy. In a study of 350 patients, the failure of β2-m levels to provide useful prognostic information in adenocarcinoma has been confirmed by Staab *et al.* (44).

The pre-operative levels of β2-m had no relationship to the patients's survival. The nature of the β2-m response in solid tumours is unknown, but occurs in most common forms of cancer. The most likely explanation is that it relates to the turnover of HLA antigens on the surface of cells that have a high density of these cells, lymphocytes are considered the most likely cell type at present [45]. How the increased β2-m turnover is brought about is unknown; neither is there any obvious connection between this phenomenon and other clinical or immunological disturbances in cancer.

4.2. Assessment of prognosis and monitoring

Once the diagnosis of a cancer is made the values of laboratory tests have different meaning than when the diagnosis remains in doubt. In the context of assessing prognosis the level of the analyte whether in the normal range, moderately or grossly raised can have meaning. The biochemical changes for it is the result from the interplay of factors intrinsic in the tumour, its extent and effect upon the hosts defence mechanism. Staab and his colleagues [46] from Germany have recently described this experience of the pre-operative levels of CEA as a prognostic index in 375 gastric cancers (81 stages I and II, 82 stage III and 212 stage IV). A raised CEA, >4 ng/ml, Roche assay, was present in 123 patients (31%) with a distribution of 18% in stages I and II, 23% in stage III and 37% in stage IV. When the patients within a stage were subdivided according to the pre-operative CEA level no difference in median survival was seen in stages I and II, but significant differences occurred in the CEA sub-groups <4 ng/ml in stage III, and for the CEA ranges 4–10 ng/ml and >10 ng/ml in stage IV.

In Leeds we have asked the question whether the biochemical indices when taken in association with the clinical, X-ray and endoscopic information, can aid in the pre-operative assessment of the patient (47). In the first cohort of 104 patients it appeared that the combination of CEA and the level of the acute phase protein antichymotrypsin, could be useful discriminants. When both analytes were elevated (24 patients) then the median survival was 5 weeks, and when they were both normal (32 patients) median survival was 64 weeks. An intermediary group with one or other of these proteins elevated (48 patients) had an estimated median survival of 15 weeks.

In a second study of 100 additional patients the level of the plasma enzymes phosphohexose isomerase and gammaglutamyl-transferase were brought in as additional analytes. Pre-operatively the site of the tumour in the stomach and the level of C-RP (ACT or AGP could be used alternatively) appeared to provide the best prognostic index before formal staging at surgery. Only two out of 27 (7%) patients with a C-RP >20 mg/l survived longer than 6 months and 16 out of 27 (59%) of them were found to be non-resectable at laparotomy. The post-operative prediction of survival in patients in our second series who had survived 4 or more weeks after surgery was determined by the combination of site and stage alone. Although pre-operative CEA and C-RP levels were related to prognosis, they added no further information once site and stage were taken into account.

4.3. Advanced disease

The pre-treatment blood count can carry important prognostic information in advanced gastric cancer. In a study of 204 patients with metastatic gastric cancer, Bruckner *et al.* (48) observed that prior to chemotherapy the absolute granulocyte counts (<6000/cu mm), lymphocytes (<1500/cu mm) and monocytes (300–900/cu mm) were independent indices of a favourable prognosis; conversely counts outside these limits were a sign of an unfavourable prognosis. If the patient was ambulatory, the median survival of 27.6 weeks improving to 37.6 weeks if two of the haematological indices were in the favourable range. In partially ambulatory patients the median survival was 16.2 weeks, improving to 25.7 weeks if two haematological indices indicated a good prognosis and fell to 11 weeks if they indicated a poor prognosis. Similar prognostic indices have been described for advanced lung cancer which shares with gastric cancer the same fatal outcome [49].

There has been no successful system for monitoring the effects of treatment on metastatic gastric cancer, CEA levels are erratic and their low frequency of positivity makes it unsuitable [50]. In our experience acute phase reactant proteins, in particular α_1-antichymotrypsin and α_1-acid glycoprotein, can provide an indication as to the general evolution of the tumour. In practical terms stable levels of the acute phase proteins within the normal or slightly elevated range correspond to 'stability' of the disease as reflected by the patients' performance status, a progressive rise of APRPs can be expected to occur in most patients with gastric cancer during the last 3–6 months of life. [28]. This 'marker' is more generally applicable than CEA as only about half the patients will eventually show an elevated CEA (Table 1).

Gastric cancer in Caucasians, due to its late presentation, carries a high risk of death. Consequently the most advanced patients are unlikely to survive long enough to be considered for chemotherapy and there will be a difference in the population referred to first line treatment compared to those eventually selected for chemotherapy. The intrinsic variability of the stage and status at first presentation at hospital can produce differences in the composition of various patient populations and this is accentuated when a general hospital population is com-

Table 1. Percentage increased CEA levels in carcinoma of stomach according to stage[a]

Reference	No. of patients	Origin	Percentage raised CEA			
			Stage I	II	III	IV
Tomoda et al. [132]	226	Japan	8.2	25	23	40
Staab et al. [46]	375	Germany		18.5	23	37
De Mello [131]	100	UK		15	35	52
Satake et al. [133]	22 (early)	Japan	0		17	
	70 (advanced)					
Ellis et al. [50]	157 (inoperable)	UK	–	–	–	31

[a] Defined as >4 or 5 ng/ml by Roche assay, or equivalent by other assays.

pared to a special referral institution, as the elderly and most terminal advanced cases rarely reach a referral hospital. This may explain some of the differences in experience of this disease in Europe and North America; and is in marked contrast to studies in Japan which tend to show the full spectrum of the natural history of the disease at first presentation. Clearly, in order to find carcinoma of the stomach earlier in Caucasians we need a change of attitude rather than new technology.

5. Colorectal cancer

5.1. Prognostic assessment

The original Dukes' A, B and C classification, when assessed by careful examination of the specimen resected at surgery, has been found in many series to act as the general guide to prognosis.Since then modifications, such as those proposed by Astler and Coller, [51] have been found to improve the definition of subgroups encompassed with the B group (B1,B2) where B2 is the penetration of the bowel wall and the presence of possible involved lymph nodes. A 'D' category has been added to indicate local or distant metastatic spread beyond the lymph nodes. Others have preferred to use the UICC TNM classification, and various minor modifications of these classifications.

Whatever system is used, it is evident that within the broad categories there are marked differences in overall survival time or tumour free interval after surgery. These differences are still present after taking tumour site, age, sex and histology into account. There are several biochemical factors whose pre-operative levels show a considerable range of values within each of the main clinical and pathological categories: the question is whether this individual variation is a reflection of host and tumour factors that influence prognosis. The two statistical approaches to investigate this question are shown in the Appendix and illustrated by our experience of gastric and colon cancer.

At present the data is fragmented as the analyses run the full range from simple intuitive to sophisticated, nevertheless the salient points are sufficiently self-evident to warrant their collective appraisal. CEA has attracted the most attention: in part this is the result of serendipity since major investment was put into measuring this analyte in the past and now sufficient time has elapsed for the survival patterns of the cohort of patients to have been revealed. In a relatively small group of patients the Roswell Park team have observed that a raised pre-operative CEA carried a worse prognosis for patients with Dukes' B and Dukes' C lesions. Holyoke *et al.* [52] from Roswell Park in Buffalo and Wanebo *et al.* [53] from the Memorial Hospital in New York reported on the significance of pre-operative levels of CEA in 358 patients with colorectal cancer. The recurrence rate was higher in Dukes' B and Dukes' C lesions with CEA >5 ng/ml. There was a linear inverse correlation between the pre-operative levels and the estimated mean time to recurrence in patients with Dukes' B and C lesions ranging from 30 months for a CEA level of 2 ng/ml to 9.8 months for a CEA of 70 ng/ml. In C lesions the median time to recurrence was 13 months if the pre-operative CEA levels were >5 ng/ml and 28 months if <5 ng/ml.

Goslin *et al.* [54] in Boston assessed the pre-operative CEA levels in patients as a method of post-operative stratification after curative resection of colorectal cancer. One hundred and thirty four patients were suitable for study; among the 71 patients with Dukes' B lesions, pre-operative CEA levels were not correlated with risk of recurrence or the time to recurrence. In the Dukes' C lesions, however, an elevated pre-operative CEA was predictive of an enhanced risk of recurrence. Nineteen out of 21 (90%) patients presenting with a CEA > 5ng/ml relapsed in a follow up of 36–72 months whilst only nine out 23 (39%) patients with Dukes' C lesions with a CEA <5 ng/ml had relapsed in the same period.

Two other large studies have been made in Europe. Staab *et al.* [55] in Germany, reported the relationship between CEA and survival in 563 patients observed since 1974 to 1981 and demonstrated that the sub-division of patients according to the surgical criteria of radical resection, palliative resection and non-resectable lesions was a very powerful prognostic parameter. Furthermore, CEA levels of 2–4, 4–10, >10 ng/ml provided an independent prognostic index which was additive to the classical TMN classification or the surgical assessment of prognosis that they have devised. A recent report from Poland on experience of 280 patients showed that CEA correlated with stage and probability of recurrence [56].

However, Blake *et al.* [57] reporting from Pittsburgh were less impressed with the evidence that small elevations of CEA carried much weight as a prognostic factor, though they confirm that levels >10 ng/ml undoubtedly reduced the chance of cure. They were at pains to point out that this was only a statistical probability and should not be interpreted as a certainty for an individual patient.

It is evident from these series seen collectively that pre-operative CEA is a powerful discriminant in the Dukes' C group and the majority of opinion would favour that this is still applicable to Dukes' B lesions. Whether CEA level is the only criterion that has such an effect on prognosis is debatable, other biochemical disturbances that occur in patients with colorectal cancer have not been examined on the same scale.

In our experience with 100 older, pre-operative patients with colorectal cancer we found that the combination of Dukes' stage and pre-operative serum levels of antichymotrypsin, and phosphohexose isomerase, an index of glycolysis, were more effective as indices of survival to 18 months than the combination of Dukes' stage and pre-operative CEA level and that having obtained this information CEA no longer provided any additional information for stratification. This illustrates the importance of not looking solely at tumour associated antigens as prognostic indices as it is possible that *once the diagnosis of the condition is no longer in doubt*, then a variety of non-specific biochemical changes can provide valuable information with regard to prognosis.

5.2. Monitoring patients with colorectal cancer

There is now definite evidence that repeated measurements of the levels of CEA in the blood is probably the most sensitive method for the identification of recurrence or metastatic tumour that has arisen after surgery [58,59,60]. However, whilst all recorded series have several examples of a long lead time between observation of a rising CEA and the clinical identification of recurrence in the absence of exploratory surgery, there are varying proportions of cases in which the clinical identification of recurrence and the elevation of CEA were coincidental and some 15–20% of the patients in which no elevation was present at the time of recurrence.

Many factors influence this type of investigation, in particular the frequency of recall of the patients. The influence of this problem has been discussed by Mach and his colleagues. Evans *et al.* [61] reviewing the literature in 1978 considered that an elevated CEA appears in about one third of sub-clinical recurrent or metastatic large bowel cancers and will provide a lead time of three months or more. The cost effectiveness of this monitoring cannot be ignored and the view has been expressed that the procedure has little value as it makes no difference to the decision-making process that will optimize the well being, effectiveness and duration of the patients' residual life span [62].

The opposite view is expressed by those who believe in second look surgery or the use of adjuvant chemotherapy. The pro's and con's of the different strategies in management is made elsewhere in this book. Here we are concerned with the technicality of laboratory tests for the presence of metastases or recurrence and interpretation of the results (see Chapter 2).

Most authors agree that in any large series of follow-up there will be occasional random elevations of CEA which cannot be explained, the majority of which tend to return to the baseline spontaneously, whilst the majority of the patients who remain tumour free have a CEA that tends to be below 2.5 ng/ml: about 20% of the patients in our series had levels between 2.5–5 ng/ml and several observations had to be made before one could be convinced of the patients' own baseline level. The CEA test is not sensitive to small amounts of tumour such as known involved lymph nodes or tumour present at the resected margin of the specimen or small tumour deposits seen on the surface of the liver. In our experience of minimal residual disease only four out of 43 (9%) patients had unequivocally raised CEA levels two months after surgery where there was known residual tumour [63]. Despite this limited sensitivity sequential CEA measurements have been found helpful in adjuvant chemotherapy for Dukes' B and C colorectal cancers [64].

The insensitivity of the test is the reason why the Mayo Clinic Group [65] are dubious about its use as a routine monitor; this opinion is based on study of 149 patients with Dukes' B2 and C lesions followed up closely; they were seen at least every 15 weeks, until recurrence was documented or they were still tumour free after 1 to 3 years. In 18 patients, there were transient rises of CEA which were not explained by the presence of tumour. In the 34 patients who recurred during the course of the study the authors agree that the CEA is an insensitive indicator of recurrence, 25 out of 34 patients had levels >5 ng/ml but in those series the disease was too advanced to be at a therapeutically advantageous stage; the latter reflecting the inadequacy of the treatment rather than the ineffectiveness of the test.

Holyoke and his colleagues [52] expressed uncertainty with the benefits of second look surgery and resection on the basis of 47 recurrences observed in 161 patients and in only 6 out of 47 (15%) was an abnormality of CEA the sole indication of recurrence. In three patients with a rising CEA, laparotomy failed to confirm the presence of tumour.

Staab *et al.* [66] claimed that an analysis of the rate of increase of CEA can distinguish between localized recurrence and hepatic metastases. In 31 recurrences, localized disease, proven by second look surgery, had a rise of 0.08–0.20 ng CEA/ml in 10 days whereas hepatic metastases had a mean slope of 2.2 ng/ml increase in 10 days. Wood *et al.* [67] have written that the rate of change of the level of CEA is an important factor in selecting patients who are likely to have resectable tumours; their CEA assay had an upper limit of normal of 25 ng/ml, the local recurrences had slopes rising to <75 ng/ml by 12 months; whilst hepatic metastases are fast reaching 100 ng/ml in 6 months. The Memorial Hospital, gastroenterology team [68] reported that among 32 patients with asymptomatic recurrences detected by a rising post-operative CEA, 33 out of 37 laparotomies demonstrated tumour, in 16 cases it was resectable and in 17 non-resectable; once again the lower CEA levels and lower rates of increase occurred in the resectable tumours.

Minton and his colleagues [69], on the other hand, are strong advocates for CEA testing as a way of providing an indication for second look surgery. They advocate the use of normogram to control the variations of the test and take a value that is 2SD above the post-operative low as being a significant increase. Applying these criteria they found that 11 out of 14 (78%) patients with a rising CEA had resectable tumour. Minton's experience seems to be out of line with the estimates of the rate of resectable recurrences which are thought to be more likely in the region of 5–7% [65].

Non-specific indicators can be used for monitoring, such as the measurements of C-reactive protein, and other acute phase proteins, but they are less sensitive for the detection of recurrence than CEA. A progressive increase in their levels can confirm that various treatments are failing to control the evolution of the tumour. In a survey of 55 patients with advanced colorectal cancer attending our chemotherapy clinic, 89% showed an elevated C-RP >10 mg/l three months before death and in 64% the level was >50 mg/l. There is considerable variation from one patient to another in the way in which these non-specific indicators will respond. In the opinion of the Mayo Clinic Group, alkaline phosphatase is one of the most reliable components in standard liver function tests for observing the progress of hepatic metastases [62], and they doubt the value of CEA as an indicator of progression of colorectal cancer. However, this is a somewhat extreme view as monitoring of colorectal cancer was one indication for CEA measurements that was endorsed by the Consensus Meeting on the use of CEA sponsored by the National Cancer Institute [70].

5.3. CEA in screening for colorectal cancer

It is evident that CEA measurements lack the specificity and sensitivity to make it a reliable test for large bowel cancer in asymptomatic subjects or even patients with minimal symptoms. Indeed today a raised CEA in established colon cancer tends to raise a doubt whether the patient will be tumour free 5 years after surgery. It is of interest to look at some of the studies made in the past 10 years as they contain important lessons.

The Community Health survey of the town of Busselton, in Australia, has provided an indication of the usefulness of CEA as a screening system in an asymptomatic population. Considering the 956 unselected persons over the age of 60 years, 44 (4.5%) had a CEA level >5 ng/ml at the beginning of the study. During a 4 year follow up, 6 of these 44 had died of CEA associated cancers, 15 were heavy smokers, 2 had colonic diverticulae, 1 a peptic ulcer. On the other hand, 18 (2%) of 912 CEA negative persons had developed CEA associated cancers during the same time period. The 20 persons who were CEA positive when re-examined after four years, revealed two occult cancers, one of the lung and the other of the colon. It is concluded that the specificity of CEA and the high levels in heavy smokers detract from its usefulness as a population screen [71].

CEA determinations were made in a group of 1800 older aged business executives by the Roswell Park group [52] and two unsuspected cancers were discovered, one in the pancreas, the other in the colon; both were incurable. The group concluded this approach was unreasonably expensive for the yield it provided.

Hence it is unlikely that colonic cancer will be detected by CEA in its pre-invasive phase. Whilst the majority of patients with polyps will have a low or slightly raised CEA <4.0 ng/ml, villous polyps and large adenomatous polyps in older patients or multiple polyps have been reported to be associated with raised CEA levels [72].

The consensus view in 1980 was that CEA was generally unsuitable for cancer screening due to the moderately raised levels that can occur in smokers and a variety of benign conditions of the gastrointestinal tract [70].

6. Pancreatic cancer

Adenocarcinoma of the pancreas presents one of the severest challenges among gastroenterological cancers. The incidence is 4–5% of all cancers, but the prognosis is usually very poor. There is an acute interest in early detection and some progress seems to have been made. Whether this can help to stem the tide is still not known.

6.1. Pancreatic antigens and CEA

In a large investigation of 368 patients suspected as having pancreatic cancer carried out by three major institutions (Mayo Foundation, Memorial Sloan-Kettering and University of Chicago) [20], the final diagnoses showed that 36% of the patients had pancreatic cancer, 11% other cancers, 11% pancreatitis, 30% biliary tract disease and in 12% there was no cause determined for their abdominal pain. A wide battery of tests were used including assays of gastric, parathyroid hormone, calcitonin, glucagon, insulin, C peptide, HCG, RNase, glucose, alkaline phosphatase, POA and CEA. POA was the most useful predictive test in this battery with a correct positive predictive value for pancreatic cancer in 80% and a 73% correct negative predictive value in the other diseases. CEA tended to be less helpful as a discriminant for pancreatic cancer: although it was raised in 85% of patients with carcinoma of the pancreas, it was also raised in 65% of other cancers and 45% of patients with benign disease. On the other hand very high levels of CEA were indicative of advanced tumours but gave no clues as to their site.

Hobbs in 1982 [17] has recently reviewed his experience of POA, in 100 cases of pancreatic cancer, 95% were positive. In a further 128 patients with various other cancers the POA was only rarely positive; but the overlap between the levels of POA in chronic pancreatitis and carcinoma of the pancreas was more liable to be a source of diagnostic error. POA performed very well in the differentiation of obstructive jaundice with only carcinoma of the pancreas giving a positive test.

Zamcheck and Martin [73] in their review of factors influencing circulating CEA levels in pancreatic cancer point out there is a wide range of CEA levels in relation to stage with considerable overlap. Obstruction of the common bile duct, from any cause will tend to enhance the level of CEA, jaundice may influence the clearance of CEA from the circulation by the hepatic parenchyma. The liver is the main site of catabolism of glycosylated proteins of high molecular weight.

Finally, there is general agreement that patients with a raised CEA tend to have a shorter survival time than those in whom this value is normal, but the median survivals differ only by 2 to 3 months. This general opinion of the value of CEA in pancreatic disease was reflected in the British Medical Research Council's report [74] which stated that whilst plasma CEA levels in pancreatic carcinoma tend to be higher than in pancreatitis, their measurement contributed little to the diagnosis or management of pancreatic cancer. This is reiterated in reports of combined CEA and AFP measurements in 66 patients with pancreatic-biliary disease in a Japanese study once more confirming that it is only very high levels of CEA that are diagnostic and then only in widespread tumours [75].

6.2. Ribonuclease (RNase)

Among serum enzyme disturbances in pancreatic cancer those of RNase C levels and alkaline phosphatase have attracted most attention so far. Reddi and Holland [76] using polycytidine (C) as substrate reported that 52 normal subjects had a mean serum RNase C level of 104 ± 24.3 (SD) units/ml. In 30 patients with pancreatic cancer the mean serum level was 383 ± 145 (SD) units/ml, whilst only one in 10 patients with chronic pancreatitis had an elevated value. However, the RNase C assay is non-specific and a low incidence of raised values were observed in several other forms of cancer. Fitzgerald and the Memorial Sloan-Kettering team [77] adopted the RNase C test as designed by Reddi and Holland and took above 250 units/ml as an arbitrary discriminant level for pancreatic cancer. They found raised levels in eight out of 16 patients (50%) with carcinoma of the head of pancreas, and three out of 10 (30%) with other forms of cancer. It is of interest that this group also noted that alkaline phosphatase levels came third in their list of investigations, after computerized transaxial tomography (CTT) and coeliac angiography as the highest percentage correct diagnosis; in their series 82% of patients with pancreatic cancer had a raised level, but there were 33% false positives in a series of 184% patients under investigation.

Others have reported [78, 79, 80] there was too great an overlap of RNase C levels between carcinoma of the pancreas, chronic pancreatitis and other primary malignancies; RNase C levels failed to reflect the clinical changes in cases of pancreatic cancer followed serially during a trial of chemotherapy. Studies of RNase C before and after pancreatectomy have cast doubt that the pancreas is the main source of this enzyme: the liver and granulocytes are thought to be major production sites [81].

6.3. β2-microglobulin

Rashid et al. [82] observed that serum β2-microglobulin levels are raised (>3 mg/l) in 20 out of 37 (54%) patients with malignant obstructive jaundice, but this has no diagnostic value as similar elevations occurred in 12 out of 37 (32%) patients with obstructive jaundice due to gall stones. Serum levels of 'immunosuppressive acid protein', now known to be a fraction of α_1 acid glycoprotein, were elevated in 44 out of 46 (96%) pancreatic cancer patients, 24 out of 26 bile duct cancer patients as well as in all patients with acute pancreatitis and 19 out of 26 (66%) with chronic pancreatitis. The latter reduces its value in differential diagnosis [83].

It would appear that at present POA and alkaline phosphatase [104, 106] are the biochemical tests of choice to obtain information that a patient may have a pancreatic cancer. Relative to the costs of a detailed radiological and endoscopic investigation these tests are cheap; whether they will pick up early cases is more debatable. However, it is clear that the tests cannot be expected to be totally specific: biliary tract cancer is one major differential diagnosis that tends to cross react with POA and will tend to cause abnormalities of the liver function tests which include alkaline phosphatase.

7. Liver cancer

7.1. Liver: metastatic cancer

A profile of biochemical tests, usually consisting of bilirubin, total protein, albumin, globulin, alkaline phosphatase and transaminase levels is a standard investigation in all hospitals. To this may be added gamma glutamyltranspeptidase (γGT) and 5' nucleotidase, and lactic dehydrogenase according to local preference. The general opinion is that of routine enzyme tests, gamma glutamyltransferase (GGT), alkaline phosphatase (AP) and 5' nucleotidase levels are probably the most informative indices of hepatic metastatic cancer in this array [84]. However, when the enzymes such as AP and GGT are used, small deviations above the upper limit of normal are common in primary gastrointestinal tract cancer independent of hepatic involvement and a somewhat elevated working discriminant level may be required.

In large institutions, several additional investigations are available for the detection of hepatic metastases, these include ultrasonic and various imaging techniques and the current question is how can biochemical and imaging techniques be combined in a most cost effective way to make a diagnosis of metastatic cancer in the liver. In general terms there are three contrasting clinical situations: the first is the requirement to identify the presense of relatively small amounts of metastatic tumour, often at the limit of resolution of the various techniques during the preoperative assessment of a patient, or during post-operative surveillance of cancers known to metastasize in the liver. The second is at a far cruder level of resolution in the patient who presents with hepatomegaly in whom metastatic cancer is a probable diagnosis. Finally, there is the search for metastases in patients with tumours in whom the prevalence of metastases tends to be low; in this situation combinations of tests such as γGT and AP are unhelpful [85] and scanning too expensive.

There is considerable body of evidence that the standard liver function tests are insensitive to small tumour burdens and provide little help to the surgeon in his pre-operative assessment. In colon cancer, high levels of CEA are usually indicative of hepatic metastases or the high probability that these metastases will develop. Following the excision of primary colorectal cancer in patients with known hepatic metastases, γGT levels tend to be the first enzyme to rise as the metastases increase in size, followed by alkaline phosphatase, leucine aminopeptidase and 5' nucleotidase. A rise of CEA in these patients is usually the first marker to be disturbed. These events are of a similar pattern in patients receiving chemotherapy as compared to those who are left untreated after surgery [84].

A recent study by Kemeny et al. [86] has compared three imaging techniques and 13 laboratory tests in 80 patients at risk of hepatic metastases but without clinical evidence of hepatic lesions. No test emerged as being ideal, the best combination appeared to be a routine liver function test, one imaging technique and CEA. In Kemeny's study this combination gave a 76% accuracy, but small metastases <2 cm were below the detection limits.

Tartter et al. [87] addressed the problem of what is the most cost effective way of identifying metastases in colorectal cancer. Their experience is based on 327 patients who underwent surgery and had pre-operative CEA or liver scans. Pretreatment alkaline phosphatase measurements were made as a routine; using the cut off limits of 135 IU for AP and 10 ng/ml for CEA, then the combination of these tests had a sensitivity of 86% in 23 out of 26 patients, with hepatic metastases, and a false positivity of 12% in 164 patients. Scanning alone demonstrated metastases in 69% of 35 patients with hepatic metastases. They argued that the combination of AP and CEA measurements could cut the expense by limiting scanning to the patients in whom the tests are abnormal. A similar argument has been proposed by Tempero et al. [88] who believe that liver scans are best reserved for patients whose liver function tests are normal; scans when the biochemistry is grossly abnormal are expensive and unnecessary.

The interesting point that emerges from these two studies is the benefit the surgeon can gain from radioisotopic scanning and ultrasonic examination of the liver in the search for small hepatic metastases. The unnecessary use of high technology to solve questions that can readily be answered with simple techniques is perhaps a mis-use of resource, and an unneccessary burden of cost to the patient, his insurance company or the state.

In patients with hepatomegaly, the differential diagnosis is between neoplastic disease of liver and other causes of liver enlargement. The simple strategy outlined above will suffice; however in our experience the level of serum acid glycoprotein (orosomucoid) is often very helpful, as it tends to be very low in cirrhosis and raised in metastatic cancer. In a recent series 61 out of 72 (84%) of patients with cirrhosis and chronic active hepatitis had an AGP level <1.0 g/l, whilst 57 out of 65 (87%) of patients with hepatic secondaries or malignant obstructive jaundice had a level >1.0 g/l [72]. Among the special enzyme assay tests that might be used to give warning of probable metastatic of primary liver cancer 5' nucleotide diesterase [89] and the isoenzymes of alkaline phosphatase [90,91] both look very promising as indices. As yet they have not been used on a wide scale.

7.2. Screening for hepatoma

The low incidence of hepatoma in Western peoples probably makes population screening by AFP testing cost-ineffective with the possible exception of cirrhotics who are known to be at high risk. In Germany, Lehmann [92] made a survey of 318 cases of cirrhosis and on the basis of raised AFP levels was able to lead to the detection of 15 clinically undiagnosed hepatomas.

Surveys in Dakar, West Africa, yielded 9 cases of hepatoma in 9864 male subjects [93] and in Japan, Koji *et al.* [94] found two undiagnosed hepatomas in 1000 persons living in a hyperendemic area of hepatitis-B virus. However, these results pale into insignificance when set against the Chinese experience in provinces where hepatoma is endemic. The first study from China reported in 1974 on 343,999 people, using a relatively insensitive assay for AFP, discovered 149 AFP positive cases of which 129 (88.4%) were confirmed to have hepatoma [95].

A further massive survey in the Qidong province of China of 1,786,906 persons between 1971–1977 led to the discovery of 1026 cases of hepatoma; using sensitive AFP assay the positivity reached 96.3%. The pick up of stage I disease could be increased to 76% by twice yearly assays in hyperendemic areas. The two-year survival rate for stage I disease was 69% [96]. This is an outstanding example of the use of a biochemical marker to seek cancer in an asymptomatic population at high risk of the disease.

7.3. Hepatocellular carcinoma

There is a marked difference in the relative frequency of hepatocellular cancer in different parts of the world. In North America and Europe primary hepatocellular carcinoma has an incidence generally <1:100,000, far higher levels of incidence occur in parts of Africa where in some areas it is the most common cancer in males. A high incidence of hepatoma is also a feature of Japan and South East Asia.

In general the early diagnosis of primary hepatocellular cancer can be difficult, due to size and functional reserve of the liver. Laboratory tests need to distinguish between the effects of any underlying cirrhosis and hepatocellular carcinoma. The broad experience in European countries and North America shows that if an AFP level of >20 ng/ml is adopted, then 73.86% of patients with hepatocellular cancer will have an elevated value. However, 12.32% of Caucasian patients with liver cirrhosis and 12–31% with chronic hepatitis have a raised AFP which is usually <400 ng/ml [97, 98, 99].

Typical experience of AFP and CEA as tests in the search for primary carcinoma of the liver in an European population is illustrated by a recent report by Bell from Norway [100]. In six years' experience he studied 21 cases of primary hepatic carcinoma, 106 patients with hepatic metastases and 110 alcoholics with liver disease. AFP was strongly elevated in ten out of 14 cases of hepatocellular carcinoma but in none of seven cases of cholangio-carcinoma; CEA was raised in eight out of 14 and five out of seven, respectively. In the 106 patients with liver metastases, a CEA >5 ng/ml was present in 83% and it was >20 ng/ml in 50%. AFP showed a moderate rise in 26% of patients without hepatocellular cancer, and in 31% of the alcoholics the CEA was >5 ng/ml. This experience reflects the lack of specificity of these tests in their lower ranges, AFP is well known to be slightly elevated in several forms of gastrointestinal disease. However, once AFP of CEA are at a high level (>1000 ng/ml and >20 ng/ml, respectively) there is little doubt that the patient has a malignant disease.

Hepatoma in Western countries would appear to run a different clinical course from that seen in high incidence countries. Underlying cirrhosis is not necessarily associated with a worse prognosis in Japan [101] or Uganda [102]. In Uganda, primary hepatoma runs a rapid course with only 20% alive after 2 years in Primack's series. A similar fulminating disease occurs in South African Bantu [103].

In Western Europe the presence of cirrhosis has a deleterious effect on the prognosis of patients with hepatocellular circinoma. The AFP levels tend to be higher in the cirrhotic patients but once the effect of cirrhosis has been taken into account the AFP levels play little part in predicting survival. The range of AFP levels varied greatly in a series of 57 patients with hepatocellular carcinoma from King's College Hospital, London; 11 (27%) had AFP levels 10–1000 ng/ml (slightly raised), 24 (58%) had levels 1000–10,000 and six (15%) >100,000 ng/ml (greatly raised) [83]. This British group considered that CEA contributes little to the diagnosis or surveillance of hepatoma [105], although it might be useful in the few cases with normal AFP levels. This weak CEA response was also seen in black patients in South Africa; in one series 25 out of 72 (39%) cases of hepatoma had a raised CEA, but it was >20 ng/ml in only three [106].

High levels of acute phase reactant proteins have been observed in Japanese [107] and African hepatomas [72]; acid glycoprotein and antichymotrypsin levels are raised above normal, compared to their depressed levels in cirrhosis.

In countries where hepatocellular carcinoma is prevalent the use of a higher cut off level for AFP is common practice, especially as African hepatoma patients tend to have higher levels of AFP than Europeans with the tumour [108]. Using simple radial immunodiffusion techniques and a discriminant level of 10,000 ng/ml, surveys conducted ten years ago showed a positivity of between 53–80% in Japan and several African countries [8]. Radioimmunoassay using a cut off of

>20 ng/ml in Japan showed an overall percent positivity of 89% in 515 patients [8]. However, in three Japanese studies 20.7% of 395 patients with cirrhosis also exhibited a raised AFP. A persistently raised AFP in cirrhosis suggests the development of a hepatoma [109]; levels of >400 ng/ml are particularly suspicious of neoplastic change [8].

The rates of change in AFP levels are a reflection of the differentiation of hepatocellular carcinoma. Matsumoto *et al.* [110] in a study of 96 Japanese patients found poorly differentiated tumours could produce a rise of >10,000 ng/ml in one week, in moderately differentiated tumours the AFP tended to rise at a rate of 1000 ng/ml in 3 to 4 months, and in well differentiated and anaplastic tumours both tend to have levels <200 ng/ml throughout the illness.

8. Future developments

As yet there are no totally reliable biological indicators of early cancer in the gastrointestinal tract, perhaps the most encouraging is POA in pancreatic cancer. Analyses of gastric juice need a high compliance of the population at risk, Häkkinen's [35] studies in Finland can provide the basis of cost-effectiveness calculations. Intensive effort is being made to find and identify new antigens that have cancer-specific properties; the complexities of those already identified are set out in recent reviews [111–112].

8.1. Clinical application

It has been seen that with some exceptions, both tumour specific and non-specific markers are only significantly elevated when the tumour volume is major or has produced some clinical effect. Thus it is unlikely that these markers can have a realistic role in population screening for early gastrointestinal cancer nor can they supplant the need for endoscopic or radiological investigation of the symptomatic patient.

However, it does appear that these markers impart considerable information on the prognosis of tumour bearing patients. Again this may be of limited value where the patient suffers symptoms of a destructive nature, but there are many elderly patients with massive tumours and symptoms only of a debilitating nature who have little to gain in survival time by laparotomy and palliative resection. If the prognosis is seen to be accurately predicted by marker levels, then these patients may be more appropriately treated by supportive measures alone.

It may also be appropriate to run this prognostic data to define subsets of patients who respond positively to certain forms of adjuvant treatment after resection of the primary tumour. Furthermore the levels of various markers may also indicate the appropriate patient for second look surgery. It may so prove that patients with a slow rate of rise in levels of tumour specific markers have confirmed recurrence whereas those with elevated non-specific markers have a widespread metastatic involvement and are thus unlikely to benefit from further exploration. The time has arrived when more practical use is demanded of marker levels and that recognized non-specific markers as an index of host response impart as much practical information as those measuring tumour cell activity.

Non-specific tests obviously present difficulties in interpretation but can add important information for the stratification of patients. This form of stratification may play an important part as we move towards the selection of chemotherapy either in an adjuvant or palliative sense. The drugs available so far for the treatment of gastrointestinal cancer are not especially effective and the force of mortality operating on a normal homogenous group of patients varies widely. We now have the ability to define these subsets more distinctly and the advantage that the biochemical indices are provided by analytes that are stable on storage, and, if necessary, can be sent to a few reference laboratories for measurement.

In the realms of non-specific tests the urinary excretion of the by-products of transfer RNA (tRNA) looks most promising [113]. The basis of this approach is the finding that tRNA methylating enzymes in cancer are hyperactive, compared to their normal counterparts or benign tumours. This leads to the liberation of excess and unusual forms of methylated nucleosides into the circulation and their excretion by the kidney. The separation and quantitation of these products by high performance liquid chromatography has shown that a spectrum of nucleosides are increased in the urine of cancer patients that are normally controlled within narrow limits in health. The evidence is convincing for advanced cancer, the question that is unanswered is whether the system can be simplified to analyse one of two analytes and what will be the minimal tumour load to analysis can detect.

The assay of plasma lipid bound sialic acid, developed by Katopodis and Stock [114] appears to show promise as a simple universal test in cancer as indicated by studies at the Memorial Hospital [115]. The role of this test in the cadre of biochemical investigations needs to be defined, so far it has several features that make it attractive.

Appendix

(by Lesley Struthers, Unit for Cancer Research, University of Leeds).

9. Statistical methodology

Statistical analysis is needed to quantify the effect of a biochemical marker whether it is used as a discriminant factor in the diagnosis of disease or as a prognostic term. The concentration for a given protein, enzyme activity or other type of analyte in body fluids will vary both intrinsically within the control population, and may show a wider variation within a group of patients bearing the same tumour. Preliminary studies of analytes that might be used for a tumour marker are often conducted on small groups of patients representing a variety of tumour types. But at best this type of study could only suggest that a formal study should be made. It is now clear that stage and other powerful biological differences of tumour can make tumour markers superfluous, although a univariate analysis of the data can produce highly significant results. It can be seen from the examples quoted in this review that even large studies involving several hundred patients do not necessarily agree that a marker contains diagnostic or prognostic information. Furthermore, these studies do not usually include any form of randomization. So then results must be treated with caution until they are verified by further studies of a similar magnitude. If the analyte is being examined where there is a comparison of different forms of treatment then it is essential that the biochemical studies should run in parallel with a randomized clinical trial of the treatment.

To make the analysis convenient it is often the practice that the continuous measurements of biochemical markers are divided into groups such as normal, and raised levels (or raised levels can be sub-divided into a series of arbitraty steps). This creates the difficulty of what is the cut off level for a given test (the cut off level being the point of division between those analytes that are normal and those that are raised). In some biochemical markers used in the study of cancer, standard cut off levels have been adopted, for example 2.5 ng/ml and 5 ng/ml for CEA depending on the investigator's confidence in this analyte as a marker. These cut off levels can be calculated by using a set of controls; the controls should be 'normal', healthy persons and a reasonably large number of such persons should be examined. Their age and sex should be appropriate to the clinical setting in which the marker is to be used. If the tumour marker has a normal distribution then a raised value is a measurement above $\bar{x} + 2$ s.d. where $\bar{x}$ is the mean and s.d. the standard deviation. If the distribution is skewed then a log transformation will often give 'normality'. This would give roughly $2\frac{1}{2}\%$ of the 'normal' healthy population with values greater than the cut off value. By using a binary variable instead of the actual value of the biochemical marker, a great deal of information is being thrown away.

Many biochemical measurements can be used as prognostic factors in patients with cancer. However, a biochemical marker will only be of importance if it still can contribute prognostic information once the clinical details are taken into account. Sequential analysis is one way of critically examining whether a marker will fulfil this criterion. A mathematical model is built, starting with the powerful prognostic factors such as tumour stage, tumour differentiation, patient's age, sex etc. Then each potential tumour marker is examined to see whether it can produce any additional effect in the model, the objective being to sub-divide the population with respect to their survival and so the model is gradually built up to eventually include the best combination of prognostic terms or by a similar logic diagnostic terms. A problem that can arise in multivariate analysis is that interaction terms can be important so that all the variables in the final model should have their interaction terms checked. An interaction term between two variables is due to the effect of one variable not having a constant effect with the other on the dependent term. For example, the difference in survival between Dukes' A en B and Dukes' C colorectal cancer, being greater in younger persons than in older patients.

9.1. Discriminant analysis

If patients can be sub-divided into two or more diagnostic groups, then we can test to what extent biochemical markers can help in this grouping by discriminant analysis. The use of a stepwise analysis will mean that only those variables which help to discriminate between the groups will be included in the discriminant function. The variable can include both clinical and biochemical measurements. There are two main types of discriminant analysis: classical discriminant analysis [116], and logistic discriminant analysis [117, 118, 119]. There are advantages and disadvantages with all these types of discriminant analysis and these should be examined before using them. There are a number of statistical packages now available with the facility of using discriminant analysis: BMDP-81, SPSS 9, SAS, and Genstat.

In tumour marker studies that involve two groups, the biochemical measurements are continuous and often have skewed distributions in one group but not the other, which makes logistic discriminant analysis the ideal tool.

9.2. Survival analysis

In a high mortality cancer study, time to death is usually the event of interest but time to other events such as recurrence and remission would use exactly the same methodology. It is often of interest to see whether biochemical measurements taken before treatment are related to survival time. It is also possible to test a biochemical measurement for prognostic effect once clinical factors have been taken into account.

There are a number of statistical methods available for survival analysis and the method used will largely depend on the computing and statistical facilities available. The simplest and most frequently used method is what is now commonly known as the log rank test. Kaplan Meier [120] survival curves are usually used in conjunction with the log rank test to illustrate the differences between survival curves. Both procedures require little statistical assistance, but it is highly recommended that the researcher reads Peto et al. [121] paper before even commencing the study.

The regression model is a more sophisticated statistical method, in which the actual measurements of the biochemical analytes are used rather than discrete measurements. However, this type of analysis usually requires expert advice and access to a large main frame computer. The net advantage is that more information can be obtained that relates to the prediction for an individual patient.

9.3. Kaplan-Meier survival curves

Product limit estimate $P(t)$ of Kaplan & Meier [120]

$$P(t_{(i)}) = \prod_{j=1}^{i} \frac{n_j - 1}{n_j}$$

where the times of death are ordered such that $t_{(1)} \leq t_{(2)} \leq \ldots \leq t_{(i)}$ and n_i is the number of patients still under observation at $t_{(i)}$ including the one that died at $t_{(i)}$.

Log rank test
With two groups A and B

$$X^2 = \frac{(O_A - E_A)^2}{E_A} + \frac{(O_B - E_B)^2}{E_B}$$

where O_A = observations, number of deaths in Group A.
E_A = expected number of deaths in Group A.
O_B = observations, number of deaths in Group B.
E_B = expected number of deaths in Group B.
$E_A = \sum_{i=1}^{k} \frac{\text{No. of deaths on day } i \times \text{No. at risk in Gr. A on day } i}{\text{No. at risk on day } i}$
k = number of distinct survival times.

Using 2 groups X^2 can be compared with Chi-square distribution with 1 df (3.84) at the 5% level. The log rank statistics can be calculated when accounting for another factor. An illustrated example can be found in Peto et al. [120].

In practice X^2 will be calculated in a slightly different way [121, 122].

9.4. Regression models

There are a number of parametric regression models which make assumptions about the hazard function. The hazard function, $h(t)$, is the instantaneous rate of failure at t given the patient has survived to t. The most commonly used models have been the exponential and Weibull, and further discussion about such models and others can be found in Gross and Clarke [124] and Kalbfleisch and Prentice [125].

Cox [126] suggested a regression model in which no assumptions are made about the shape of the hazard and it is related to the marker and clinical measurements by

$$h(t) = h_o(t) \exp(\beta'x)$$
$$\beta'x = \beta_1 x_1 + \beta_2 x_2 + \ldots + \beta_p x_p$$

where $h_o(t)$ remains unknown and $x_1, x_2, \ldots x_p$ are the p variables (biochemical and clinical measurements). A partial log likelihood can be obtained [127] and from it the β's which are allowed to vary are estimated by maximum likelihood and so an estimate of the log-likelihood is obtained to allow for significance testing via the likelihood ratio test. Each biochemical measurement and clinical factor can be tested individually and then the effect of a possible marker can be tested once the prognostic clinical measurements have been accounted for.

A check of the model is essential and this can be performed using the method described by Cox and Snell [128]. If the model is shown to be a reasonable fit of the data, the survivorship function can be estimated [129]. When a survival curve is calculated and a continuous variable is in the model, then an actual value for this variable must be chosen and care should be taken not to choose extreme values. Confidence limits for the survival curves have been calculated by O'Quigley [130].

Acknowledgements

We wish to thank Mrs. M. Birdsall and Mrs. M. Bowen for their help in compiling this review.

References

1. Adinolfi M: Human alphafetoprotein 1956–1978. In: Advances in human genetics, Harris H, Hirschhorn K (eds), New York, Plenum Press, 1979, p 165–228.
2. Ruoslathi E, Seppälä M, Vuopio P, Seksela E, Peltokallis P: Radioimmunoassay of α fetoprotein in primary and secondary cancer of the liver. J Natl Cancer Inst 49: 623–628, 1972.
3. Gitlin D, Boesman M: Sites of serum α fetoprotein synthesis in the human and the rat. J Clin Invest 46: 1010–1016, 1967.
4. Abelev GI, Perova S, Khramkoba PN, Postnikova ZA, Irlin IS: Production of embryonal α-globulin by transplantable hepatomas. Transplantation 1: 174–180, 1963.
5. Tatarinov YS: Detection of embryonic specific α globulin in blood sera of patients with primary

liver tumor. Vopr Med Klim 10: 90–91, 1964.

6. Sell S: Alphafetoprotein. In: Cancer Markers, Sell S (ed), New Jersey, Humana Press, 1980, p 249–293.

7 Sell S: Hepatocellular carcinoma markers. In; Human Cancer Markers, Sell S, Wahren B (eds), New Jersey, Humana Press, 1982, p 133–164.

8. Hirai H: Alpha Fetoprotein. In: Biochemical Markers for Cancer, Chu MT (ed), New York, Marcel Dekker Inc., 1982, p 25–59.

9. Toftager–Larsen K, Petersen PC, Nørgaard-Pedersen B: Carbohydrate microheterogeneity of human alpha fetoprotein. Oncodevelopmental aspects. In: Lectin Biology, Biochemistry, Clinical Biochemistry, Vol 1, Bøg Hansen TC (ed), Berlin, Walter de Gruyter, 1981, p 283–292.

10. Sell S, Stillman D, Gochman N: Serum alpha fetoprotein. Amer J Path 66: 847–853, 1976.

11. Alpert E, Feller ER: Alpha-fetoprotein (AFP) in benign liver disease, evidence that normal liver regeneration does not induce AFP synthesis. Gastroenterology 74: 856–858, 1978.

12. Gold P, Freedman SO: Demonstration of tumor-specific antigens in human colonic carcinomata by immunological tolerance and absorption techniques. J Exp Med 121: 439–462, 1965.

13. Fuks A, Banjo C, Shuster J, Freedman SO, Gold P: Carcinoembryonic antigen (CEA): molecular biology and clinical significance. Biochim Biophys Acta 417: 123–152, 1975.

14. Gold P, Freedman SO, Shuster J: carcinoembryonic antigen: historical perspective. Experimental data In: Immunodiagnosis of Cancer, Part I, Herberman RB, McIntire KR (eds), New York, Marcel Dekker, 1979, p 147–164.

15. Shively JE, Todd CW: Carcinoembryonic antigen A: Chemistry and Biology. In: Cancer Markers, diagnostic and developmental significance, Sell S(ed), New Jersey, Humana Press, 1980, p 295–314.

16. Banwo O, Versey J, Hobbs Jr: New oncofetal antigen for human pancreas. Lancet(i): 643–645, 1974.

17. Hobbs JR: Pancreatic Tumor Markers. In: Human Cancer Markers, Sell S, Wahren B (eds), New Jersey, Humana Press, 1982, p 165–177.

18. Gelder F, Reese C, Mossa AR, Hunter R: Studies on oncofetal antigen, POA. Cancer 42: 1635–1645, 1978.

19. Hunter R, Gelder F, Chu MT, Moosa AR: Markers of Pancreatic Cancer. In: Markers for Diagnosis and Monitoring of Human Cancer, Colnaghi MI, Buraggi GL, Gbione M (eds), New York, Academic Press, 1982, p 135–140.

20. Shimano T, Loor RM, Papsidero LD, Kuriyama M, Vincent RG, Nemoto T, Holyoke ED, Derjian R, Douglas HO, Chu MT: Isolation, characterization and clinical evaluation of pancreas cancer-associated antigen. Cancer 47: 1602–1613, 1981.

21. Potter TP Jr, Jordan T, Jordan JD, Lasater H: Tennessee antigen (Tennagen): Characterization and immunoassay of a tumour associated antigen. In: Prevention and Detection of Cancer, Part 2, Nieburgs HE (ed), New York, Marcel Dekker Inc,1980, p 467.

22. Sampson J, Wong L, Harris OD: The Tennessee antigen in the diagnosis of gastrointestinal malignancy. Aust N Z J Surg 52: 39–41, 1982.

23. Pentycross CR: The Tennessee antigen test, an evaluation in cancer and non cancer patients and in normal subjects. Br J Cancer 45: 223–229, 1982.

24. Gray BN, Walker C, Baynard R, Bennett RC: Tennessee Antigen: The predictive value of pre-operative and post-operative assays in large bowel cancer. Dis Colon and Rectum 25: 539–541, 1982.

25. Björklund B: On the nature and clinical use of tissue polypeptide antigen (TPA). Tumor Diagnostik 1: 9–19, 1980.

26. Andrén-Sandberg A, Isacson S: Tissue polypeptide antigen on colorectal carcinoma. In: Clinical Application of Carcinoembryonic Antigen Assay, Krebs BP, Lalanne CM, Schneider M (eds), Amsterdam, Excerpt Med, 1978, p 139–143.

27. Wagner W, Husemann B, Becker H, Groitc H, Koerfgen HP, Hammerschmidt M: Tissue

polypeptide antigen – a new tumour marker. Aust N Z J Surg 52: 41–43, 1982.

28. Cooper EH, Stone J: Acute phase reactant proteins in cancer. Advances in Cancer Res 30: 1–44, 1979.
29. Pepys MB: C-reactive protein fifty years on. Lancet i: 653–657, 1981.
30. Glenner GG: Amyloid deposits and amyloidosis. New Eng J Med 23: 1283–1292, 1980.
31. Cooper EH, Milford Ward AJ: Acute phase reactant proteins as aids to monitoring disease. Invest Cell Path 2: 293–301, 1979.
32. Arnaud P, Gianazza E: Alpha acid glycoprotein – Structure, genetics and biological significance. In: Marker Proteins in Inflammation, Allen RC, Bienvenu J, Laurent P, Suskind RM (eds), Berlin, de Gruyter, 1982, p 159–169.
33. Wahren BJ, Harmenberg F, Edsmyr F, Jakobsson P, Ingimarsson S: Possible tumour markers in patients with oesophagus cancer. Scand J Gastroent 14: 361–365, 1979.
34. Alexander JC, Chretin PB, Dellon AL, Snyder J: CEA levels in patients with carcinoma of the oesophagus. Cancer 42: 1492–1497, 1978.
35. Häkkinen IPT: A population screening for fetal sulfoglycoprotein antigen in gastric juice. Cancer Res 34: 3069–3072, 1974.
36. Häkkinen IPT: Fetal Sulfoglycoprotein (FSA), In: Compendium of assays for immunodiagnosis of human cancer, Herberman RB (ed), New York, Elsevier, 1979, p 241–246.
37. Faulk WP, Rider JA, Swader JI: Lactate dehydrogenase in gastric juice: Diagnostic adjunct in human stomach cancer. Lancer ii: 1115–1116, 1972.
38. Rogers K, Roberts GM, Williams GT: Gastric juice enzymes: an aid in the diagnosis of gastric cancer?. Lancet i: 1124–1126, 1981.
39. Bunn PA, Cohen MI, Widerlite L, Nugent JL, Mathews MJ, Minna JD: Simultaneous gastric and plasma immunoreactive plasma carcinoembryonic antigen in 108 patients undergoing gastroscopy. Gastroenterology 76: 734–741, 1979.
40. Grindulis KA, Forster PJG, Hubball S, McConkey B: Can acute phase reactants distinguish benign and malignant disease of the upper gut? Clin Oncology 7: 345, 350, 1981.
41. Teasdale C, Mander AM, Fifield R, Keyser JW, Newcombe RC, Hughes LE: Serum β2-microglobulin in controls and cancer patients. Clin Chim Acta 78: 135–143, 1977.
42. Kin K, Sukurabayashi I, Kawai I: β2-microglobulin levels of serum and ascites in malignant disease. Gann 68: 427–434, 1977.
43. Rashid SA, Cooper EH, Axon ATR, Eaves G: Serum β2-microglobulin in malignant and benign diseases of the stomach and pancreas. Biomedicine 33: 112–116, 1980.
44. Staab HJ, Anderer FA, Ablemann LM, Stumpf E, Hiesche K, Fischer R: Circulating β2-microglobulin in malignant disease. Tumor Diagnostik 2: 292–298, 1981.
45. Cooper EH, Plesner T: Beta-2-microglobulin review: its relevance in clinical oncology. Med and Ped Oncology 8: 323–334, 1980.
46. Staab HJ, Anderer FA, Brummendorf T, Hornung A, Fischer R: Prognostic value of preoperative serum CEA level compared to clinical staging – II Stomach cancer. Br J Cancer 45: 718–727, 1982.
47. Rashid SA, O'Quigley J, Axon ATR, Cooper EH: Plasma protein profiles and prognosis in gastric cancer. Br J Cancer 45: 390–394, 1982.
48. Bruckner HW, Lavin PT, Plaxe GE, Storch JA, Livingstone EM: Absolute granulocyte, lymphocyte and monocyte counts: Useful determinant of prognosis with metastatic cancer of the stomach. JAMA 247: 1004–1006, 1982.
49. Chretien PB, Crowder WL, Gertner HR, Sample WF, Catalona WJ: Correlation of preoperative lymphocyte reactivity with clinical course of cancer patients. Surg Gynaecol Obst 136: 380–384, 1973.
50. Ellis DJ, Spiers C, Kingston RD, Brookes VS, Leonard J, Dykes PW: Carcinoembryonic antigen levels in advanced gastric carcinoma. Cancer 42: 623–625, 1978.
51. Astler VB, Coller FA: The prognostic significance of direct extension of carcinoma of the colon

and rectum. Ann Surg 139: 846–852, 1954.

52. Holyoke ED, Evans JT, Mittleman A, Chu MT: Carcinoembryonic antigen as a tumor marker. In: Biochemical markers for cancer, Chu MT (ed), New York, Marcel Dekker, 1982, p 61–80.

53. Wanebo HJ, Rao B, Pinsky CM, Hoffman RG, Stearns M, Schwartz MK, Oettgen HF: Pre-operative carcinoembryonic antigen level as a prognostic indicator in colorectal cancer. N Eng J Med 299: 448–451, 1978.

54. Goslin R, Steele G, MacIntyre J, Mayer R, Sugarbaker PH, Cleghorn K, Wilson R, Zamcheck N: The use of pre-operative plasma CEA levels for the stratification of patients after curative resection of colorectal cancer. Ann Surg 192: 747–751, 1980.

55. Staab HJ, Anderer FA, Brummendorf T, Stumpf E, Fischer R: Prognostic value of pre-operative serum CEA level compared to clinical staging. I. Colorectal carcinoma. Br J Cancer 44: 652–662, 1981.

56. Szymendera JJ, Nowacki MP, Szawlowski AW, Kaminska JA: Predictive value of plasma CEA levels. Pre-operative prognosis and post-operative monitoring of patients with colorectal cancer. Dis Colon and Rectum 25: 46–52, 1982.

57. Blake KE, Dalbow MH, Concannon JP, Hodgson SE, Brodmerkel GJ, Panahandeh AH, Zimmerman K, Headings JJ: Clinical significance of pre-operative plasma carcinoembryoniic antigen (CEA) level in patients with carcinoma of the large bowel. Dis Colon and Rectum 25: 24–32, 1982.

58. Mach JP, Jaeger PH, Bertholet MM, Rusgsegger CH, Loosli RM and Pettard J: Detection of recurrence of large bowel cancer by radioimmune assay of circulating carcinoembryonic antigen (CEA). Lancet 2: 535–540, 1974.

59. Zamcheck N: The present status of CEA in diagnosis, prognosis and evaluation of therapy. Cancer 36: 2460–2470, 1975.

60. Munro Neville A, Cooper EH: Biochemical monitoring of cancer. Ann Clin Biochem 13: 283–305, 1976.

61. Evans JT, Mittleman A, Chu MT, Holyoke ED: Pre and post-operative uses of CEA. Cancer 42: 1419–1421, 1978.

62. Moertel CG, Schutt AJ, Go VLW: Carcinoembryonic antigen test for recurrent colorectal carcinoma. Inadequacy for early detection. JAMA 239: 1065–1066, 1978.

63. Lawton JO, Giles GR, Cooper EH: Evaluation of CEA in patients with known residual disease after resection of colonic cancer. Proc Roy Soc Med 73: 23–28, 1980.

64. Lin CN, McPherson TA, McClelland AR, McCoy L, Kohn M: Value of serial CEA determination in a surgical adjuvant trial of colorectal cancer and gastric carcinoma. J Surg Oncol 14: 275–280, 1980.

65. Beart RW, Metzger PP, O'Connell MJ, Schutt AJ: Post-operative screening of patients with carcinoma of the colon. Dis of Colon and Rectum 24: 585–588, 1981.

66. Staab HJ, Anderer FA, Stumpf E, Fischer R, Slope analysis of post-operative CEA time course and its possible application as aid in diagnosis of disease progression in gastrointestinal cancer. Ann J Surg 136: 322–327, 1978.

67. Wood CB, Ratcliffe JG, Bent RW, Malcolm AJ, Blumgart LH; The clinical significance of the pattern of elevated serum carcinoembryonic antigen (CEA) levels in recurrent colorectal cancer. Br J Surg 67: 46–48, 1980.

68. Attiyeh FF, Stearns MW: Second look laparotomy based on CEA elevations in colorectal cancer. Cancer 47: 2119–2125, 1981.

69. Minton JP, James ILK, Hurtubise PE, Rinker L, Joyce S, Martin EW: The use of serial carcinoembryonic antigen determinations to predict recurrence of carcinoma of the colon and the time for a second look operation. Surg Gynecol Obset 147: 208–210, 1978.

70. National Institute of Health Consensus Development Conference: Carcinoembryonic antigen: its role as a marker in the management of cancer. Ann Intern Med 94: 407–409, 1981.

71. Stevens DP, Mackay IR, Cullen KJ: Carcinoembryonic antigen in a unselected elderly popula-

tion: A four year follow-up. Br J Cancer 32: 147–151, 1975.

72. Doos WG, Wolff WI, Shinga H, De Chabon A, Stenger RJ, Gottlieb LS, Zamcheck N: CEA levels in patients with colorectal polyps. Cancer 36: 1996, 1975.

73. Zamcheck N, Martin EW: Factors controlling circulating CEA levels in pancreatic cancer: some clinical correlations. Cancer 47: 1620–1627, 1981.

74. Medical Research Council – Tumour Products Committee Clinical Subgroup; The diagnostic value of plasma carcinoembryonic antigen (CEA) in pancreatic disease. Br J Cancer 41: 976–979, 1980.

75. Satake K, Cho K, Umeyama K: Alpha-fetoprotein and carcinoembryonic antigen in pancreatobiliary disease with and without jaundice. J Surg Oncol 19: 228–232, 1982.

76. Reddi KK. Holland JF: Elevated serum ribonuclease in patients with pancreatic cancer. Proc Natl Acad Sci USA 73: 2308–2310, 1976.

77. Fitzgerald PJ, Fortner JG, Watson RC, Schwartz MK, Sherlock P, Benua RS, Cubilla AL, Schottenfeld D, Miller D, Winawer SJ, Lightdale J, Leidner SP, Nisselbaum JS, Mendenz-Botet CJ, Poleski MH: Value of diagnostic aids in detecting pancreas cancer. Cancer 41: 868–879, 1978.

78. Corbishley TP, Greenway B, Johnson PJ, Williams R: Serum ribonuclease in the diagnosis of pancreatic carcinoma and in monitoring chemotherapy. Clin Chim Acta 124: 225–233, 1982.

79. Mackie CR, Moosa AR, Go VLW, Noble G, Sizemore G, Cooper MJ, Wood RAB, Hall AW, Waldman T, Gelder F, Rubenstein AW: Prospective evaluation of some candidate tumor markers in the diagnosis of pancreatic cancer. Digestive Diseases 25: 161–172, 1980.

80. Doran G, Allen-Mersh TG, Reynolds KW: Ribonuclease as a tumour marker for pancreatic cancer. J Clin Pathol 33: 1212–1213, 1980.

81. Abramson SB, Rinderknecht H, Renner IG: Ribonuclease C and pancreatic secretory proteins in the peripheral circulation before and after pancreatectomy. Dig Disease Sciences 27: 889–896, 1982.

82. Rashid SA, Axon ATR, Bullen AW, Cooper EH: Serum β2-microglobulin in hepato-biliary diseases. Clin Chim Acta 114: 83–91, 1981.

83. Matsuno S, Kobari M, Matsuda Y, Sato T: Diagnosis of carcinoma of the pancreas by assay of immunosuppressive acid protein. Tohoku J Exp Med 136: 1–10, 1982.

84. Cooper EH, Turner R: Multiparametric approach to biochemical surveillance of large bowel cancer. In: Colorectal Cancer, Prevention, Epidemiology and Screening, Winawer S, Schottenfeld D, Sherlock P (eds), New York, Raven Press, 1980, p 211–218.

85. Baden H, Anderson B, Augustenborg G, Hanel RK: Diagnostic value of gamma-glutamyltranspeptidase and alkaline phosphatase in liver metastases. Surg Gynecol Obstet 133: 769–773, 1971.

86. Kemeny MM, Sugarbaker PH, Smith TJ, Edwards BK, Shawker T, Vermess M, Jones E: A prospective analysis of laboratory tests and imaging studies to detect hepatic lesions. Ann Surg 196: 163–167, 1982.

87. Tartter PI, Slater G, Gelernt I, Aufses AH: Screening for liver metastases from colorectal cancer with carcinoembryonic antigen and alkaline phosphatase. Ann Surg 193: 357–360, 1981.

88. Tempero MA, Petersen RJ, Zetterman RK, Lemon HM, Gurney J: Detection of metastatic liver diseases. Use of liver scans and biochemical liver tests. JAMA 243: 1329–1332, 1982.

89. Tsou KC, Lo KW: 5′ Nucleotide phosphodiesterase and liver cancer. Methods in Cancer Res 19: 273–300, 1982.

90. Voit M, Thyss A, Voit G, Ramaioli A, Cambon P, Schneider M, Lalanne CM: Comparative study of gamma-glutamyltransferase, alkaline phosphatase and its alpha-1-isoenzyme as biological indicators of liver metastases. Clin Chim Acta 115: 349–358, 1981.

91. Yamaguchi K, Futimoto S, Misaki F, Kawai K: Serum alkaline phosphatase (AL-PASE) isoenzyme in gastric and colonic cancer using a simple thin layer electrophoresis polyacrylamide. Gastroenterol Jpn 13: 264–271, 1978.

92. Lehmann FG: Prognostic significance of alpha₁ fetoprotein in liver cirrhosis. Five year prospective study. In: Onco-developmental Gene Expression, Fishman WH, Sell S (eds), New York, Academic Press, 1976, p 407–415.

93. Leblanc L, Tuyns AJ, Masseyeff R: Screening for primary liver cancer. Digestion 8: 8–14, 1973.

94. Koji T, Muneshisa T, Yamaguchi K, Kusumoto Y, Nakamura S: Epidemiological studies of α-fetoprotein and hepatitis B antigen in Tomietown Nagasaki, Japan. Ann NY Acad Sci 259: 239–247, 1975.

95. Co-ordinating Group for the Research of Liver Cancer: Application of serum alpha-fetoprotein assay in mass survey of primary carcinoma of the liver. J Chinese Med 2: 241–245, 1974.

96. Zhu Y: AFP sero-survey and early diagnosis of liver cell cancer in the Qidong field. Zhonghua Zhongliu Zazhi 3: 35–38, 1981.

97. Chayvialle JAP, Ganguli PC: Radioimmunoassay of alpha-fetoprotein in human plasma. Lancet i: 1355–1356, 1973.

98. Ruoslahti E, Pihko H, Seppälä M: Alpha-fetoprotein: Immunological properties. Expression in normal state and in malignant and non-malignant liver disease. Transplant Rev 20: 38–60, 1974.

99. Bloomer JR, Waldmann TA, McIntire R, Klatskin G: Relationship of serum α-fetoprotein to the severity and duration of illness in patients with viral hepatitis. Gastroenterology 68: 342–350, 1975.

100. Bell H: Alpha-fetoprotein and carcinoembryonic antigen in patients with primary liver carcinoma, metastatic liver disease and alcoholic liver disease. Scand J Gastroenterol 17: 898–903, 1982.

101. Okuda K: Clinical aspects of hepatocellular carcinoma – analysis of 134 cases. In: Hepatocellular Carcinoma, Okuda K, Peeters H (eds), New York, Wiley Inc, 1976, p 387.

102. Primack A, Vogel CK, Kyulwazi SK, Ziegler JL, Simon R, Anthony PP: A staging system for hepatocellular carcinoma – prognostic factors in Ugandan patients. Cancer 35: 1357–1364, 1975.

103. Provan JL, Stokes JF, Edwards D: Hepatic artery infusion chemotherapy in hepatoma. Br Med J iii: 346–349,1968.

104. Johnson PJ, Melia WM, Palmer MK, Portman B, Williams R: Relationship between serum alpha-foetoprotein cirrhosis and survival in hepatocellular carcinoma. Br J Cancer 44: 502–505, 1981.

105. Melia WM, Johnson PJ, Carter S, Munro Neville A, Williams R: Plasma carcinoembryonic antigen in the diagnosis and management of patients with hepatocellular carcinoma. Cancer 48: 1004–1008, 1981.

106. Macnab GM, Urbanowicz JM, Kew MC: Carcinoembryonic antigen in hepatocellular cancer. Br J Cancer 38: 51–54, 1978.

107. Matsuzaki S, Iwamura K, Itakura M, Kamiguchi H, Katsunuma T: A clinical evaluation of serum alpha-1-antichymotrypsin levels in liver disease and cancers. Gastroenterol Jpn 16: 582–591, 1981.

108. Greenwood BM, Whittle HC: Immunology of Medicine in the Tropics. London, Arnold, 1981.

109. Kubo Y, Okuda K, Musha H, Nakashima T: Detection of hepatocellular carcinoma during a clinical follow up of chronic liver disease. Gastroenterology 74: 578–582, 1978.

110. Matsumoto Y, Suzuki T, Asada I, Ozawa K, Tobe I, Honjol : Clinical classification of hepatoma in Japan according to serial changes in serum alpha-fetoprotein levels. Japan Cancer 49: 354–360, 1982.

111. Goldenberg DM: Antigens associated with human solid tumours. In: Cancer Markers, Diagnostic and Developmental Significance, Sell S (ed), New Jersey, Humana Press, 1980, p 329–370.

112. Sjögren HO, Wahren B: Gastrointestinal cancer markers. In: Human Cancer Markers, Sell S, Wahren B (eds), New Jersey, Humana Press, 1982, p 105–132.

113. Borek E: Transfer RNA and its by-products as tumor markers. In: Cancer Markers, Diagnostic and Developmental Significance, Sell S (ed), New Jersey, Humana Press, 1980, 445–462.

114. Katapodis N, Stock CL: Improved method to determine lipid bound sialic acid in plasma or

serum. Res Commun Chem Pathol and Pharmacol 30: 171–180,1980.

115. Dnistrian AM, Schwartz MK, Katopodis N, Fracchia AA, Stock CL: Serum lipid bound sialic acid as a marker in breast cancer. Cancer 50: 1815–1819, 1982.

116. Mardia KV, Kent JT, Bibby JM: Discriminant analysis. In: Multivariate Analysis, Birnbaum ZW, Lukacs E (eds), New York, Wiley Inc, 1979, p 300–325.

117. Cox DR: Linear logistic model. In: Analysis of Binary Data, Bartlett MS (ed), London, Methuen, 1970, p 18–19.

118. Anderson JA: Separate sample logistic discrimination. Biometrika 59: 19–35, 1972.

119. Albert A: On the use and computation of likelihood ratios in clinical chemistry. Clin Chem 28: 5, 1113–1119, 1982.

120. Kaplan EL, Meier P: Non-parametric estimation from incomplete observations. J Am Stat Assoc 53: 457–481, 1958.

121. Peto R, Pike MC, Armitage P, Breslow ME, Cox DR, Howard SV, Mantel M, McPherson K, Peto J, Smith PG: Design and analysis of randomized clinical trials requiring prolonged observation of each patient. Part 2. Analysis and examples. Br J Cancer 35: 1–39, 1977.

122. Peto R, Pike MC: Conservation of the approximation (o-e)^2/E in the log rank test for survival data or tumour incidence data. Biometrics 29: 579–584, 1973.

123. Breslow ME: Analysis of survival data under the proportioned hazards model. Int Stat Rev 43: 45–58, 1975.

124. Gross AJ, Clark VA: Some special survival distributions. In: Survival distributions: Reliability Applications in the Biomedical Sciences, Bradley RA, Hunter JS, Kendall DG, Watson GS (eds), New York, Wiley Inc, 1975, p 14–22.

125. Kalbfleisch JD, Prentice RL: Failure time models. In: The statistical analysis of failure time data, Bradley RA, Hunter JS, Kendall PG, Watson GS (eds), New York, Wiley Inc, 1980, p 21–38.

126. Cox DR: Regression models and lifetables (with discussion). J R Stat Soc B 34: 187–220, 1972.

127. Cox DR: Partial likelihood. Biometrika 62: 269–276, 1975.

128. Cox DR, Snell EJ: A general definition of residuals (with discussion). J R Stat Soc B 30: 248–275, 1968.

129. Breslow ME: Covariance analysis of censored survival data. Biometrics 30: 89–99, 1974.

130. O'Quigley J: Regression models and survival prediction. Statistician 31: 107–116, 1981.

131. de Mello J, Struthers L, Turner R, Cooper EH, Giles GR, Yorkshire Gastrointestinal Cancer Research Group: Multivariate analyses as aids to diagnosis and assessment of prognosis in gastrointestinal cancer. Brit J Cancer 48: 341–348, 1983.

132. Tomoda H, Furusawa M, Ohmachi S, Seo Y, Matsukuchi T, Miyazaki M, Kanashima R: Carcinoembryonic antigen in the management of gastric cancer patients. Jpn J Clin Oncol 11: 69–74, 1981.

133. Satake K, Kitamura T, Ishikawa T, Mukai R, Yoshimoto T, Chung YS, Umeyama K: Serum β2-microglobulin and carcinoembryonic antigen in patients with gastric disorders. J Surgical Oncology 17: 225–233, 1981.

2. Newer concepts regarding staging of gastro-intestinal malignancy

J. KIRK MARTIN, JR. and OLIVER H. BEAHRS

1. Introduction

There can be no question concerning the value of staging in cancer treatment. With increasingly complex multimodality treatment, selection of therapy is based on accurate staging. Properly evaluating the extent of disease also allows the physician to discuss precisely the prognosis with the patient [1]. The use of a staging system makes possible valid comparisons between reporting of end results from various centers. Epidemiologic studies are facilitated by proper grouping of patients based on staging. Finally, changing trends in incidence or prevalence of a type of cancer can be quickly demonstrated with appropriate staging.

Staging is not an exact science [2], nor it is always easy to reach agreement on the extent of a lesion at a particular anatomic site. Classification by stage is, however, the best available method to group similar subsets of a disease type to determine appropriate treatment and end results of management.

Staging is based upon the assumption that malignancy develops in a somewhat orderly fashion from a single transformed cell, through a localized tumor, to a tumor with invasion of surrounding structures, lymphatic permeation, and finally to systemic dissemination (Fig. 1). For most malignancies, a statistically significant difference in prognosis can be demonstrated between tumors not yet involving regional lymph nodes and tumors metastatic to regional nodes. Because it is not always *clinically* possible to determine regional lymphatic involvement, differences in staging will exist between pretreatment clinical stating and postsurgical resection staging. It is extremely important to separate cases in groups that are staged chronologically as clinical diagnostic or as postsurgical resection-pathologic for purposes of reporting or comparing data.

J.J. DeCosse and P. Sherlock (eds), Clinical Management of Gastrointestinal Cancer.
© *1984, Martinus Nijhoff Publishers, Boston. ISBN 0-89838-601-2. Printed in The Netherlands.*

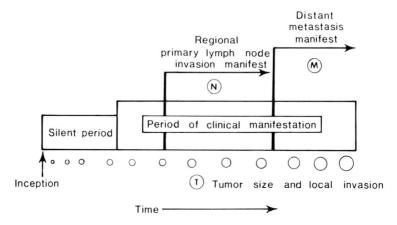

Figure 1. The evolution of a malignancy based on tumor size (*T*), regional lymph node involvement (*N*), and distant metastasis (*M*) is shown. (From *Manual for Staging of Cancer 1978*, p. 1, which was prepared by the American Joint Committee for Cancer Staging and End-Results Reporting.)

2. Staging systems

The most comprehensive and precise classification of cancer stage is the TNM system [3] adopted by the American Joint Committee on Cancer (AJCC) [1]. Three important events in the evolution of a malignant tumor are identified. The extent of the primary tumor (*T*), the status of regional lymph nodes (*N*), and distant metastases (*M*) are recorded. The AJCC classifications are designed, in many instances, to be compatible with the International Union Against Cancer (UICC) system. The TNM system is further described according to the chronology of the period used to establish the stage of the tumor. Five terms are used: cTNM (clinical-diagnostic), sTNM (surgical-evaluative), pTNM (postsurgical resection-pathologic), rTNM (retreatment-clinical diagnostic), and aTNM (autopsy). Definition of the classification is shown in Table 1.

Recommendations regarding staging of cancers have been made for many years. An example is that of Dukes for cancer of the rectum [4,5]. This method, suggested by Lockhart-Mummery and Dukes in 1928, correlated survival of carcinoma of the colon and rectum with progressive stages of intestinal wall and lymph node involvement [6] (Fig. 2). Modifications of the system by Gabriel [7], Kirklin [8], and Astler and Coller [9] all represented refinements in the accuracy of the system. The modification by Astler and Coller probably represents the most widely used form of Dukes' classification today but is still devoid of a category for a tumor that penetrates the bowel wall without regional node involvement. The classification is also limited to pathologically staged tumors and is not applicable to clinical staging.

2.1. Clinical staging

With the advent of increasingly sophisticated diagnostic tests, clinical staging has become more accurate. These methods are especially good at detecting disseminated disease and distant metastases. The use of computerized tomography(CT) and ultrasound will be discussed elsewhere, but suffice it to say that numerous studies have applied and compared the tests and their relative merits in staging [10–13]. The use of CT in assessing pancreatic lesions is particularly valuable [10, 11, 13]. Radioactive scans have also played a part in clinical staging [13, 14]. Fiberoptic endoscopy has been used frequently in diagnosis and staging of gastric cancer [15], and peritoneoscopy may be useful in establishing extent of disease and providing tissue for histologic examination [16, 17]. Coupland and associates [16] found peritoneoscopy to be diagnostic in 86% of 236 patients. The development of fine needle aspiration cytology or core biopsy using CT, ultrasound, or fluorescopic guidance has enabled the radiologist to provide diagnostic tissue

Table 1. Definition of symbols[a]

Three capital letters are used to describe extent of cancer	
T	Primary Tumor
N	Regional Lymph Nodes
M	Distant Metastasis
Type of classification	
c	Clinical-diagnostic
s	Surgical-evaluative
p	Postsurgical resection-pathologic
r	Retreatment
a	Autopsy
This classification is extended by the following designations:	
TUMOR	
TX	Tumor cannot be assessed
T0	No evidence of primary tumor
Tis	Carcinoma in situ
T1, T2, T3, T4	Progressive increase in tumor size and involvement
NODES	
NX	Regional lymph nodes cannot be assessed clinically
N0	Regional lymph nodes not demonstrably abnormal
N1, N2, N3, N4	Increasing degrees of demonstrable abnormality of regional lymph nodes
METASTASIS	
MX	Not assessed
M0	No (known) distant metastasis
M1	Distant metastasis present
	Specify sites of metastasis

[a] This material is taken from p. 4 of the *Manual for Staging of Cancer 1978*, which was prepared by the American Joint Committee for Cancer Staging and End-Results Reporting.

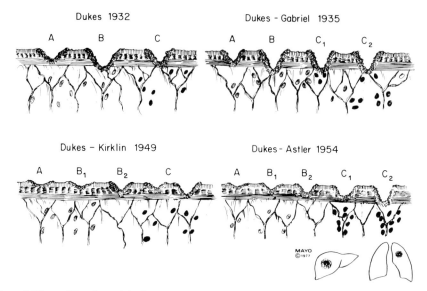

Dukes 1932

Dukes - Gabriel 1935

Dukes - Kirklin 1949

Dukes - Astler 1954

Figure 2. The modifications of the Dukes' staging system are depicted. The most widely used system is currently the Dukes-Astler modification. (From Beart RW, van Heerden JA, Beahrs OH: Evolution in the Pathologic Staging of Carcinoma of the Colon. *Surg Gynecol & Obstet* 146: 257–259, 1978. (By permission of *Surgery, Gynecology & Obstetrics*.).)

from patients suspected of having malignant tumors [18]. Fine needle biopsy has been an important advance in clinical staging and has provided the opportunity for careful operative planning, as well as identification of patients with advanced disease [19]. Adequate samples for cytologic and histologic analyses were obtained in 97% and 89%, respectively, of 150 cases reported by Wittenberg and associates [18].

Despite careful clinical evaluation using multiple diagnostic techniques, some difference will usually be apparent between clinical and surgical staging. The most difficult site to correctly stage is the pancreas; however, liver metastases from colorectal cancers also have proven to be hard to detect [20]. The importance of the problem can be appreciated when early data from our institution's intraoperative radiotherapy experience are examined. Even with the use of all available diagnostic tests, 7 of 21 (33%) patients with pancreatic carcinoma thought to be localized were found to have disseminated disease at operation. The most common finding was hepatic metastases, followed by peritoneal seeding [21]. An update of this experience reconfirms this discrepancy in clinical stage, 16 of 46 patients (35%) felt to have localized pancreatic lesions, in fact, had distant metastases. The use of biochemical testing in detection of liver metastases is discussed by Huguier and Lacaine [22].

2.2. Carcinoembryonic antigen

At the present time, staging reflects the anatomic extent of the tumor. In the future, biological markers will undoubtedly be another parameter in staging of some tumors. An example is the carcinoembryonic antigen. The identification by Gold and Freedman [23] of carcinoembryonic antigen (CEA) in 1965 sparked much investigation into the role of the glycoprotein in the diagnosis of cancer. Two facts have emerged. First, many authors have described the usefulness of the CEA in preoperatively predicting stage of disease [24–34]. Preoperative CEA elevations (greater than 2.5 ng/ml) are present in 81% of colorectal and 90% of pancreatic tumors [37]. Wanebo and associates [33] found CEA levels to correlate with stages of disease. The preoperative levels in patients with resectable Dukes' B and C cancer proved to be an additional cirterion for allocating patients to high or low risk for recurrence. Arnaud [28] noted increasing levels of CEA with advancing stages of disease, and Staab [27] reported results indicating CEA was an independent prognostic parameter. CEA levels above 20 ng/ml are suggestive of liver metastases or disseminated disease [25, 26, 33], and approximately three-fourths of patients with advanced disease will have CEA elevations [33]. Goslin et al.[30] applied preoperative CEA levels to stratify patients with Dukes' C colon cancer. An elevated preoperative CEA should return to normal, usually within one month, following resection of all tumor [28,32,37]. A persistently elevated postoperative CEA is a grave prognostic sign.

Second, CEA has been used to predict recurrent cancer [36–44]. Rising CEA levels will predict recurrent tumor with significant accuracy [36, 39, 41, 43, 44]. Furthermore, the CEA elevations can preceed the clinical appearance of recurrent cancer by months [28, 34, 38]. Unfortunately, this early detection does not always translate into better survival [43]. Martin et al. [44] reported retrospectively that only 6 of 22 patients explored because of rising CEA had resectable tumor. However, in a prospective study, 23 of 38 patients explored for rising CEA had resectable tumor, the increase presumably due to earlier reoperation.

The mean CEA value in patients with resectable recurrences was only 6.5 ng/ml and the time between CEA rise and operation was 1.4 months, whereas in patients with unresectable recurrence the average CEA was 15.6 ng/ml and the interval $4^1/_2$ months.

The rate of rise seems to be of some predictive value, Steele et al. [42] noting that CEA rises greater than 2.1 ng/ml in 30 days were uniformly associated with unresectable recurrences. Attiyeh and Stearns [36] also found lower CEA levels, shorter time intervals to reexploration and slower rates of CEA rise were all directly related to resectability rate.

A promising approach using CEA in the detection of malignancies was reported by Mach and colleagues [45]. Purified ^{131}I-labelled goat antibodies against CEA were injected into 27 carcinoma patients who were subsequently scanned with a scintillation camera. Only the anti-CEA antibodies localized in tumors, and in 11 patients radioactivity was detectable in the tumor at 48 h. Unfortunately, the antibody-derived radioactivity in the tumor was quite small, and they concluded that the method was not yet clinically useful.

Another use of CEA is in suggesting the primary site in patients found to have metastatic disease. Koch and McPherson [46] found a CEA level above 10 ng/ml suggestive of a primary of entodermal origin, breast or ovary. A CEA of below 10 ng/ml was of no use in pointing to a particular primary. Other biochemical markers, such as ceruloplasmin, have not been found to be as useful as CEA. Linder et al. [47] found significantly elevated ceruloplasmin levels in patients with gastrointestinal cancers, and the specificity and sensitivity seemed to be especially high for large bowel cancer. They also found that although levels do not return to normal rapidly following resection, they do return to normal or near-normal levels when the disease is in remission. The authors concluded that despite the fact that ceruloplasmin levels correlated with TNM stage, its use in diagnosis, prognosis, and monitoring was limited.

3. Staging specific malignancies

Staging classifications vary somewhat according to anatomic site. In an effort to review newer concepts of staging, each specific gastrointestinal malignancy will be individually discussed. Where appropriate, alternatives to the TNM system will be mentioned.

3.1. Colorectal cancer staging

Colorectal cancer is the second most common cause of cancer death in both males and females (Fig. 3). The estimated incidence in 1983 is 126,000 cases with over 58,000 deaths [48].

Historically, the Dukes' classification was proposed as a staging system for carcinoma of the colon and rectum [6]. Inadequacies in describing certain colonic tumors have been presented [5], and the TNM classification allows more exact comparison. Survival data for colon and rectal carcinomas have shown sufficient similarity to allow the use of a single classification for both sites [1, 49]. It is important to specify the anatomic location of the malignancy, however, and the traditional terminology is cecum, ascending colon, hepatic flexure, transverse colon, splenic flexure, descending colon, sigmoid colon, and rectum. Anal cancers are usually considered separately owing to their multiple pathological types and potentially different metastatic routes of spread. The rectum is variably defined, but it usually is taken to be the distal 12 cm of bowel above the dentate line. Stage groupings for colorectal cancers are shown in Table 2.

Important pathologic factors assessed in staging colorectal cancers include

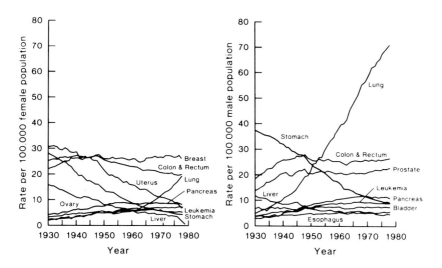

4

Figure 3. Age-adjusted cancer death rates for selected sites, females (left) and males (rights), United States, 1930–1978. Data from the U.S. National Center for Health Statistics and U.S. Bureau of the Census. (From *Ca–A Cancer Journal for Clinicians* 33: 16–17, 1983. Published by the American Cancer Society (By permission).

depth of tumor invasion through the bowel wall, lymphatic involvement, and distant metastases [1, 49, 50, 51]. Stages of disease can be shown graphically to correlate with survival [48, 49, 51]. Data from the American College of Surgeons Commission on Cancer reported five-year survival rates ranging from 76% for patients with localized disease, 43% for patients with regional lymph node metastases, to a mere 5.5% for those with distant metastases [51].

Additional pathologic factors related to prognosis have been examined [52, 53, 54, 55]. The absence of mucinous components in the tumor and the presence of lymphoplasmocytic infiltration in or around the tumor were found to be significant favorable prognostic factors by de Mascarel and associates [54] in France. Dukes' A and B stages were also favorable survival criteria. Patt *et al.* [56] reported a relation to survival for patients with lymphatic sinus histiocytosis and paracortical hyperplasia in colon cancer. Gannon and colleagues [57] noted the presence of tumor associated cytotoxicity is dependent of the stage of disease in patients with colorectal carcinoma. Although lymphatic vascular or perineural involvement did not affect survival when analyzed according to stage in de Mascarel's series, others have found vascular involvement by tumor emboli a poor prognostic sign [53, 58]. Talbot *et al.* [53] examined 703 rectal cancers and identified venous invasion in almost 52%. The authors concluded, '... the corrected 5-year survival rate was significantly worse and liver metastases developed more frequently when venous invasion was present'. Extramural local tumor invasion was reported by Wood and associates [52] to be a poor prognostic factor, and they proposed a modified staging system based, not on lymphatic metastases, but rather on local tumor invasion. Although tumor invasion is clearly an important variable, the TNM classification provides for these data [1]. The use of random liver biopsies in patients with palpably normal livers has been suggested by Rosenbloom and colleagues [55] as a means of more accurate staging, though the yield of unsuspected positive biopsies is unknown.

The incorporation of clinical data with pathologic data to develop more exact staging and prognostic information has been proposed [59, 60, 61]. The calculations involved are somewhat complex, and even if they provide greater specificity than the usual TNM system, their use is likely to be limited. A clinical staging system for rectal cancer has been proposed by Nicholls and associates [62]. The use of clinical staging rather than pathologic staging might, they postulate, enable

Table 2. Stage grouping of cancer of the colon and rectum[a]

Stage 0
　Tis N0 M0
　Carcinoma in situ as demonstrated by histologic examination of tissue (biopsy or other)

Stage I
　Stage 1A
　T1 N0 M0
　T1 NX M0
　Tumor confined to mucosa or submucosa with no demonstrable metastasis to regional lymph nodes and no evidence of distant metastasis
　Stage 1B
　T2 N0 M0
　T2 NX M0
　Tumor involves muscularis but has not extended beyond serosa with no demonstrable metastasis to regional lymph nodes and no evidence of distant metastasis

Stage II
　T3-5 N0 M0
　T3-5 NX M0
　A tumor that has extended beyond the bowel wall or serosa with no demonstrable metastasis to regional lymph nodes and no evidence of distant metastasis

Stage III
　Any T N1 M0
　Any degree of penetration of bowel or rectal wall by tumor with metastasis to regional lymph nodes but no evidence of distant metastasis

Stage IV
　Any T Any N M1
　Any degree of penetration of bowel or rectal wall by tumor with or without metastasis to regional lymph nodes and with evidence of distant metastasis

---

[a] This material is taken from p. 80 of the *Manual for Staging of Cancer 1978,* which was prepared by the American Joint Committee for Cancer Staging and End-Results Reporting.

clinicians to facilitate the choice of patients for local excision or preoperative radiotherapy. In their experience, one major deficiency of clinical staging was the correct prediction of regional lymph node involvement which ranged from only 8% to 55% when compared with pathologic findings. Thus, based on clinical staging, these patients might have been listed and treated as N0 or Dukes' B rather, than N1 or Dukes' C. This could make comparison of treatment options exceedingly difficult. Finally, symptom duration has been related to survival of patients with rectal cancer [63]. McDermott *et al.* [63] found that symptom duration in 1,081 patients with carcinoma of the rectum was not related to sex, age, tumor site or stage, but survival following resection was better for patients with symptoms of greater than 12 months' duration as compared with those having symptoms less than three months. There was also a significant difference between symptoms of more than six months and those of less than six months.

An important consideration in staging colorectal cancer is the detection of synchronous tumors. Welch [64] found the incidence of synchronous large bowel cancer to be 1.7%, and Burns [65] reported the incidence to be 2.7%. Preoperative assessment should include a barium enema or colonoscopy to examine the entire colon, but intraoperative palpation continues to be important.

3.2. Anal cancer staging

The American Joint Committee on Cancer has not established firm guidelines for staging of cancer of the anus. Others argued that, because of the various levels lymph node metastases may be found with anal cancer, the staging classification should be modified from that for the colorectum. Paradis and associates [66] proposed a system incorporating the lymphatic groups commonly affected by metastases. They subdivided Stage III (nodal metastases – N1) into III-A with perirectal lymph node involvement only and III-B with inguinal node involvement. Stage IV then included patients with distant metastases or para-aortic node involvement. The authors also commented on the poor prognosis of patients presenting initially with inguinal metastases.

3.3. Pancreatic cancer staging

Laparotomy and surgical assessment remains the most accurate method of establishing the stage of pancreatic cancer [1,67]. Data pertaining to newer diagnostic methods, including computed tomography, have been previously cited, however, one is still often unable to correctly predict stage of disease preoperatively. Pancreatic cancer is seldom localized.

Of nearly 1,300 patients with cancer of the pancreas treated at our institution over a 25-year period, only 13% were localized [68]. Cancer Patient Survival

Report Number 5 [69], covering 1970–1973, found only 15% localized, 14% with regional metastases and 61% with distant spread at the time of diagnosis. Similarly, the Cancer of the Pancreas Task Force of the American Joint Committee on Cancer found only 12% of tumors to be Stage I and 68% to be Stage IV [70]. There was no statistical difference in survivorship between patients with Stage II and III disease, but the differences between Stages I, II, III, and Stage IV were significantly different at one year ($p<0.05$). Precise staging is particularly important in trying to select and assess newer forms of combined modality therapy such as intraoperative radiation.

3.4. Staging of liver, biliary tract and gallbladder cancer

Staging of primary cancer of the liver, biliary tract and gallbladder was not included in the American Joint Committee on Cancer Manual [1] published in 1978 but is included in the revision published in 1983 [85]. Foreseeing a need to accurately classify these malignancies, Fortner *et al.* [71] published his experience with liver cancer using a three-stage system. Stage I included patients with complete resection, Stage II patients with regional spread or residual disease, and Stage III patients with distant metastases. Survival correlated well with the stages. The value of preoperative angiography in hepatic tumor staging was demonstrated by Adson and Weiland [72]. Over 80% of tumors evaluated surgically were found to be resectable. The use of percutaneous or peritoneoscopic biopsy deserves comment. Their use in histologic confirmation of unresectable lesions is reasonable, but their use in potentially resectable lesions may lead to dissemination of malignant cells [72].

The forthcoming edition of the AJCC staging classification will also stratify patients according to the presence or absence of cirrhosis. The presence of cirrhosis has been reported to be a poor prognostic sign [71].

Bile duct and gallbladder cancers may also be staged using the TNM system. Tompkins and associates [73] examining prognostic factors in bile duct carcinoma found the most significant difference in survival rates appeared to be the location of the lesion. Lesions in the lower third of the bile duct were most often resectable and had a five-year survival rate of 28%, whereas 12% of patients with lesions in the middle third survived five years, and there were no five-year survivors with the lesions of the upper third of the bile duct. Unfortunately, nearly one half (49%) of the cancers were located in the upper third of the bile duct, and only 19% in the lower third.

A staging system for gallbladder cancer was proposed by Nevin and colleagues [74] in 1976, and applied by Wanebo *et al.* [75] in 1982. Whereas Nevin found that survival clearly correlated with stage of disease, Wanebo could demonstrate no prognostically favorable subgroup by microstaging. Like pancreatic cancer, carcinoma of the gallbladder is rarely discovered at a localized stage.

3.5. Gastric cancer staging

The striking decrease in the incidence of gastric cancer during the past several decades has not affected the need to correctly stage this malignancy. The liberal use of upper gastrointestinal endoscopy has permitted the more frequent diagnosis of 'early' gastric cancer. Fielding *et al.* [76] found these favorable tumors, with penetration limited to the submucosa and negative regional lymph nodes, to comprise less than one percent (0.7%) of gastric cancers. Nodal metastases are associated with mucosal lesions in about 9% of cases and with submucosal lesions in 17% [77]. Staging of gastric cancer correlates well with survival, and Cady and associates [78] found location, clinical type (superficial, infiltrative, and polypoid or ulcerative), histologic type (histologic patterns were defined as diffuse, intestinal, mixed, or other), tumor size, and number of lymph node metastases all to be significant.

ReMine [79], reviewing over 2,000 patients with carcinoma of the stomach, found survival to correlate closely with regional node involvement and histologic grade of the tumor. Five-year survival in patients with negative lymph nodes (57.9%) was far better than in patients with positive nodes (14.2%). According to histologic grade, five-year survival ranged from 74% in well-differentiated grade 1 lesions to 21% in undifferentiated grade 4 tumors. Finally, in patients staged according to Dukes' classification, five-year survival was 89.5% for Dukes' A, 55.6% for Dukes' B, and 14.7% for Dukes' C. Size also was found to influence survival.

The TNM system provides for accurate staging of gastric cancer.

3.6. Other gastrointestinal cancer staging

Staging of esophageal cancer has been discussed using the TNM system [2]. Differences in survival are related to tumor depth and nodal metastases. The influence of lymph node involvement was shown nicely by Akiyama *et al.* [80]. In 205 patients with resection of a carcinoma of the esophagus, positive nodes were found in 59%. Five-year survival clearly followed nodal status (54% vs. 15% for negative and positive nodes, respectively). He emphasized that complete nodal dissection, not only of the mediastinum, but also of the abdomen was important for staging. Even with tumors of the upper esophagus, superior gastric node metastases were found in 32% of cases. Conversely, when the tumor is located in the lower esophagus, positive superior mediastinal nodes were found in about 10%.

Carcinoma of the small intestine is unusual, accounting for only about 3% of gastrointestinal malignancies [81, 82]. Preoperative diagnosis is difficult [81, 82, 83], and surgical staging is certainly the most accurate method of assessing extent of disease. Metastases are frequently present at the initial operation. Of 327 patients with small bowel cancer resected at the Mayo Clinic over a 25-year period [83], the ileum was the site in 41% of the neoplams, the jejunum in 36%, the duodenum in 18%, and 5% were not specified. Only five tumors were smaller than 1 cm whereas 48% were larger than 5 cm. Metastases to the liver occurred in 40 cases, of which 62% were carcinoid tumors. Adenocarcinoma made up 39% of tumors histologically, while carcinoid accounted for 21%, lymphomas for 19%, and leiomyosarcomas for 14%. The remaining 7% were miscellaneous types. Norberg and Emas [82] found lymph node metastases to be of no prognostic value in 15 patients. This could have been due to small sample size or advanced stage of the tumors. It would seem to remain an important staging factor.

4. Conclusions

Progress in treating patients with cancer depends on accurate evaluation of results. Meaningful data comparison is possible only with precise, uniform staging of disease. The development of a 'common language' to describe results, as advocated by Miller *et al.* [84] is imperative. Staging of malignancy according to the TNM classification adopted by the American Joint Committee on Cancer would seem to be the logical choice. Data forms for each anatomic site have been developed [1] and their use will aid in the collection of complete data. Their use will also facilitate interinstitutional analysis.

The development of more sophisticated diagnostic tests is improving the ability of the physician to clinically stage cancer, yet the most accurate information is derived from surgical/pathologic staging.

The current recommendations of the American Joint Committee on Cancer for staging of malignant tumors of the alimentary tract, which was published in 1983, are as follows (new ref):

Esophagus

1. TNM clinical diagnostic classification for cervical esophagus only

Primary Tumor (T)
- T0   No demonstrable tumor in the esophagus
- TIS   Carcinoma in situ
- T1   A tumor that involves 5 cm or less of esophageal length, that produces no obstruction, and that has no circumferential involvement and no extraesophageal spread
- T2   A tumor that involves more than 5 cm of esophageal length without extraesophageal spread or a tumor of any size which produces obstruction of that involves the entire circumference but without extraesophageal spread

T3   Any tumor with evidence of extraesophageal spread

Nodal Involvement (N)

Cervival esophagus: The regional lymph nodes in the cervical esophagus are the cervical and supraclavicular nodes.

Thoracic esophagus: Regional lymph nodes for the upper, midthoracic, and lower thoracic esophagus are not ordinarily accessible for clinical evaluation.

NX   Minimum requirements to assess the regional nodes cannot be met
N0   No clinically palpable nodes
N1   Movable, unilateral, palpable nodes
N2   Movable, bilateral, palpable nodes
N3   Fixed nodes

Distant Metastasis (M)

MX   Minimum requirements to assess the presence of distant metastasis cannot be met
M0   No (known) distant metastasis
M1   Distant metastasis present

Stage grouping

Clinical-diagnostic classification for cervical esophagus

Stage I	T1	N0	M0
Stage II	T1	N1, 2	M0
	T2	N0–2	M0
Stage III	T3	Any N	M0
	Any T	N3	M0
Stage IV	Any T	Any N	M1

Postsurgical Resection Pathologic Classification

Stage I	T1	N0	M0
Stage II	T2	N0	M0
Stage III	T3	N0	M0
	Any T	N1–3	M0
Stage IV	Any T	Any N	M1

2. *Definitions for postsurgical resection-pathologic classification*

Primary Tumor (T)

TX   Minimum requirements to assess the primary tumor cannot be met
Tis   Preinvasive carcinoma (carcinoma in situ)

T0	No evidence of tumor found on histological examination of specimen
T1	Tumor with invasion of the mucosa or submucosa but not the muscle coat
T2	Tumor with invasion of the muscle coat
T3	Tumor with invasion beyond the muscle coat *or* with gross invasion of contiguous structures

          T3a Tumor with invasion beyond the muscle coat

          T3b Tumor with gross invasion of contiguous structures

Regional Lymph Nodes (N)

NX	Minimum requirements to assess the regional nodes cannot be met
N0	Regional nodes not involved
N1	Unilateral regional nodes involved
N2	Bilateral regional nodes involved
N3	Extensive multiple regional nodes involved

Distant Metastasis (M)

MX	Minimum requirements to assess the presence of distant metastasis cannot be met
M0	No (known) distant metastasis
M1	Distant metastasis present

          Specify _____.

Stomach

Primary Tumor (T)

TX	Minimum requirements to assess the primary tumor cannot be met
T0	No evidence of primary tumor
Tis	Carcinoma in situ
T1	Tumor limited to mucosa and submucosa regardless of its extent or location
T2	Tumor involves the mucosa, the submucosa (including the muscularis propria), and extends to or into the serosa, but does not penetrate through the serosa
T3	Tumor penetrates through the serosa without invading contiguous structures
T4a	Tumor penetrates through the serosa and involves immediately adjacent tissues such as lesser omentum, perigastric fat, regional ligaments, greater omentum, transverse colon, spleen, esophagus, or duodenum by way of intraluminal extension.
T4b	Tumor penetrates through the serosa and involves the liver, diaphragm, pancreas, abdominal wall, adrenal glands, kidney, retro-

peritoneum, small intestine or esophagus, or duodenum by way of serosa

Nodal Involvement (N)

NX	Minimum requirements to assess the regional nodes cannot be met
N0	No metastases to regional lymph nodes
N1	Involvement of perigastric lymph nodes within 3 cm of the primary tumor along the lesser or greater curvature
N2	Involvement of the regional lymph nodes more than 3 cm from the primary tumor, which are removed or removable at operation, including those located along the left gastric, splenic, celiac, and common hepatic arteries
N3	Involvement of other intra-abdominal lymph nodes which are not removable at operation, such as the para-aortic, hepatoduodenal, retropancreatic, and mesenteric nodes

Distant Metastasis (M)

MX	Minimum requirements to assess the presence of distant metastasis cannot be met
M0	No (known) distant metastasis
M1	Distant metastasis present
	Specify _____ .

Stage Grouping

Stage 0	Tis	N0	M0
Stage I	T1	N0	M0
Stage II	T2 or 3	N0	M0
Stage III	T1–3	N1, 2	M0
	T4a	N0–2	M0
Stage IV	T1–3	N3	M0
	T4b	Any N	M0
	Any T	Any N	M1

Liver

Primary Tumor (T)

TX	Tumor present but cannot be assessed
T0	No evidence of tumor
T1	Small-solitary tumor (<2.0 cm) confined to one lobe
T2	Large tumor (>2.0 cm) confined to one lobe
	a – single tumor nodule
	b – multiple tumor nodules (any size)

T3	Tumor involving both major lobes
	a – single tumor nodule (with direct extension)
	b – multiple tumor nodules
T4	Tumor invading adjacent organs

Nodal Involvement (N)

NX	Nodes cannot be assessed
N0	No histological evidence of metastasis to regional or distant lymph nodes
N1	Histologically confirmed spread to regional lymph nodes in porta hepatis
N2	Histologically confirmed spread to lymph nodes beyond porta hepatis

Distant Metastasis (M)

MX	Not assessed
M0	No known metastasis
M1	Distant metastasis present
	Specify ⎯⎯⎯⎯⎯.

Stage Grouping

Stage IA	T1	N0	M0 without cirrhosis
Stage IB	T1	N0	M0 with cirrhosis
Stage IIA	T2	N0	M0 without cirrhosis
Stage IIB	T2	N0	M0 with cirrhosis
Stage IIIA	T3	N0, N1	M0 without cirrhosis
Stage IIIB	T3	N0, N1	M0 with cirrhosis
Stage IVA	T4	N0–2	M0, M1 without cirrhosis
Stage IVB	T4	N0–2	M0, M1 with cirrhosis

Gallbladder

Primary Tumor (T)

TX	Presence of tumor cannot be assessed
T0	No evidence of tumor
Tis	In situ carcinoma
T1	Invasion limited to the lamina propria or to the muscle layer
T2	Invasion limited to perimuscular connective tissue. No extension beyond serosa or into liver
T3	Involvement of all layers and direct extension beyond serosa or into one adjacent organ or both (must be less than 2 cm into the liver)
T4	Involvement of all layers and direct extension 2 cm or more into liver

or into two or more adjacent organs (includes stomach, duodenum, colon, pancreas, omentum, extrahepatic bile ducts and any involvement of liver)

Nodal Involvement (N)

NX	Minimum requirements cannot be met
N0	No histological evidence of metastasis to regional lymph nodes
N1	Histologically proven metastasis to First Station regional lymph nodes
N2	Histologically proven metastasis to Second Station regional lymph nodes

Distant Metastasis (M).

MX	Not assessed
M0	No (known) distant metastasis
M1	Distant metastasis present
	Specify _____.

Stage Grouping

Stage 0	Tis	N0	M0
Stage I	T1, T2	N0	M0
Stage II	T3, T4	N0	M0
Stage III	T3, T4	N1, N2	M0
Stage IV	T3, T4	N0–2	M1

Extrahepatic bile ducts

Primary Tumor (T)

TX	Presence of tumor cannot be assessed
T0	No evidence of tumor
Tis	In situ carcinoma
T1	Invasion limited to wall
T2	Invasion limited to periductal connective tissues
T3	Involvement of all layers and direct extension into one adjacent major vessel or organ
T4	Involvement of all layers and direct extension beyond secondary ductal bifurcation or into 2 or more adjacent organs including: liver, pancreas, duodenum, stomach, colon, omentum, gallbladder

Nodal Involvement (N)

NX	Minimum requirements cannot be met
N0	No histological evidence of metastasis to regional lymph nodes

N1   Histologically proven metastasis to Second Station regional lymph nodes

Distant Metastasis (M)

MX   Not assessed
M0   No (known) distant metastasis
M1   Distant metastasis

Stage Grouping

Stage 0	Tis	N0	M0
Stage I	T1, T2	N0	M0
Stage II	T3, T4	N0	M0
Stage III	T3, T4	N1, N2	M0
Stage IV	T3, T4	N0–2	M1

Pancreas

Primary Tumor (T)

TX   Minimum requirements to assess the primary tumor cannot be met
T1   No direct extension of the primary tumor beyond the pancreas
T2   Limited direct extension to duodenum, bile ducts, or stomach, still possibly permitting tumor resection
T3   Further direct extension, (incompatible with surgical resection)

Nodal Involvement (N)

NX   Minimum requirements to assess the regional nodes cannot be met
N0   Regional nodes not involved
N1   Regional nodes involved

Distant Metastasis (M)

MX   Minimum requirements to assess the presence of distant metastasis cannot be met
M0   No (known) distant metastasis
M1   Distant metastasis present
            Specify _____.

Stage Grouping

Stage I	T1, T2	N0	M0
Stage II	T3	N0	M0
Stage III	T1–3	N1	M0
Stage IV	T1–3	N0–1	M1

Colon and rectum

Primary Tumor (T)
TX	Minimum requirements to assess the primary tumor cannot be met
T0	No evidence of primary tumor
Tis	Carcinoma in situ
T1	Tumor confined to mucosa or submucosa
T2	Tumor limited to bowel wall but not beyond
T2a	Partial invasion of muscularis propria
T2b	Complete invasion of muscularis propria
T3	Tumor invasion of all layers of bowel wall with or without invasion of adjacent or contiguous tissues
T4	Tumor has spread by direct extension beyond contiguous tissue or the immediately adjacent organs

Nodal Involvement (N)
NX	Minimum requirements to assess the regional nodes cannot be met
N0	Nodes not involved
N1	One to three involved regional nodes adjacent to primary lesions (__)
N2	Regional nodes involved extending to line of resection or ligature of blood vessels (__)
N3	Nodes contain metastasis, location not identified. Specific number examined (__): number involved (__)

Distant Metastasis (M)
MX	Minimum requirements to assess the presence of distant metastasis cannot be met
M0	No (known) distant metastasis
M1	Evidence of distant metastasis
	Specify _____.

Stage Grouping

Stage 0	Tis	N0	M0
Stage I			
IA	T1	N0	M0
IB	T2	N0	M0
Stage II	T3	N0	M0
Stage III	Any T	N1–3	M0
	T4	N0	M0
Stage IV	Any T	Any N	M1

54

References

1. Clinical staging system for carcinoma of the esophagus. CA–A Cancer Journal for Clinicians 25: 50–57, 1975.
2. Manual for Staging of Cancer 1978. Prepared by the American Joint Committee for Cancer Staging and End-Results Reporting, Chicago, Illinois. Administrative sponsor–The American College of Surgeons, Chicago.
3. TNM Classification of malignant tumors. Prepared by The International Union Against Cancer, 2 Rue Du Conseil-General, 1205 Geneva, Switzerland. Second edition.
4. Lockhart-Mummery JP, Dukes C: The precancerous changes in the rectum and colon. Surg Gynecol Obstet 46: 591, 1928.
5. Dukes CE: The classification of cancer of the rectum. J Pathol 35: 323, 1932.
6. Beart RW Jr, van Heerden JA, Beahrs OH: Evolution in the pathologic staging of carcinoma of the colon. Surg Gynecol Obstet 146: 257–259, 1978.
7. Gabriel WB, Dukes C, Bussey HJR: Lymphatic spread on cancer of the rectum. Br J Surg 23: 395, 1935.
8. Kirklin JW, Dockerty MB, Waugh JM: The role of the peritoneal reflection in the prognosis of carcinoma of the rectum and sigmoid colon. Surg Gynecol Obstet 88: 326, 1949.
9. Astler VB, Coller FA: The prognostic significance of direct extension of carcinoma of the colon and rectum. Ann Surg 139: 846, 1954.
10. Hessel SJ, Siegelman, SS, McNeil BJ, Sanders R, Adams DF, Alderson PO, Finberg HJ, Abrams HL: A prospective evaluation of computed tomography and ultrasound of the pancreas. Radiology 143: 129–133, 1982.
11. Haaga JR, Alfidi RJ, Havrilla TR, Tubbs R, Gonzalez L, Meaney TF, Corsi MA: Definitive role of CT scanning of the pancreas: The second year's experience. Radiology 124: 723–730, 1977.
12. Itai Y, Araki I, Tasaka A, Maruyama M: Computed tomographic appearance of resectable pancreatic carcinoma. Radiology 143: 719–726, 1982.
13. Kamin PD, Bernardino ME, Wallace S, Jing B-S: Comparison of ultrasound and computed tomography in the detection of pancreatic malignancy. Cancer 46: 2410–2412, 1980.
14. Knopf DR, Torres WE, Fajman WJ, Sones PJ Jr: Liver lesions: Comparative accuracy of scintigraphy and computed tomography. American Journal of Radiology 138: 623–627, 1982.
15. Winawer SJ, Posner G, Lightdale CJ, Sherlock P, Melamed M, Fortner JG: Endoscopic diagnosis of advanced gastric cancer: Factors influencing yield. Gastroenterology 69: 1183–1187, 1975.
16. Coupland GAE, Townend DM, Martin CJ: Peritoneoscopy–Use in assessment of intra-abdominal malignancy. Surgery 89: 645–649, 1981.
17. Cuschieri A, Hall AW, Clark J: Value of laparoscopy in the diagnosis and management of pancreatic carcinoma. Gut 19: 672–677, 1978.
18. Wittenberg J, Mueller PR, Ferrucci JT Jr, Simeone JF, van Sonnenberg E, Neff CC, Palermo RA, Isler RJ: Percutaneous core biopsy of abdominal tumors using 22 gauge needles: Further observations. American Journal of Radiology 139: 75–80, 1982.
19. Mitty HA, Efremidis SC, Yeh H-C: Impact of fine-needle biopsy on management of patients with carcinoma of the pancreas. American Journal of Radiology 137: 1119–1121, 1981.
20. Metastases in the liver. British Medical Journal 282: 2078–2079, 1981.
21. Gunderson LL, Tepper JE, Biggs PJ et al.: Intraoperative ± External Beam Irradiation. Current Problems in Cancer, Vol. VII, No. 11, May 1983. R.C. Hickey (ed.-in-chief). Yearbook Medical Publishers, Chicago.
22. Huguier M, Lacaine F: Hepatic metastases in gastrointestinal cancer. Arch Surg 116: 399–401, 1981.
23. Gold P, Freedman SO: Demonstration of tumor-specific antigens in human colonic carcinomata by immunological tolerance and absorption techniques. J Exp Med 121: 439–462, 1965.
24. Blake KE, Dalbow MH, Concannon JP, Hodgson SE, Brodmerkel GJ, Panahandeh H, Zimmer-

man K, Headings JJ: Clinic significance of the preoperative plasma carcinoembryonic antigen (CEA) level in patients with carcinoma of the large bowel. Dis Col & Rect 25: 24–31, 1982.

25. Pihl E, McHaughtan J, Ma J, Ward HA, Nairn RC: Immunohistological patterns of carcinoembryonic antigen in colorectal carcinoma. Correlation with staging and blood levels. Pathology 12: 7–13, 1980.

26. Szymendera JJ, Nowacki MP, Szawlowski AW, Kaminska JA: Predictive value of plasma CEA levels: Preoperative prognosis and postoperative monitoring of patients with colorectal carcinoma. Dis Col & Rect 25: 46–52, 1982.

27. Staab HJ, Anderer FA, Brummendorf T, Stumpf E, Fischer R: Prognostic value of preoperative serum CEA level compared to clinical staging. I. Colorectal carcinoma. Br J Cancer 44: 652–662, 1981.

28. Arnaud JP, Koehl C, Adloff M: Carcinoembryonic antigen (CEA) in diagnosis and prognosis of colorectal carcinoma. Dis Col & Rect 23: 141–144, 1980.

29. Wanebo HJ, Rao B, Pinsky CM, Hoffman RG, Stearns M, Schwartz MK, Oettgen HF: Preoperative carcinoembryonic antigen level as a prognostic indicator in colorectal cancer. New England Journal of Medicine 299: 448–451, 1978.

30. Goslin R, Steele G Jr, MacIntyre J, Mayer R, Sugarbaker P, Cleghorn K, Wilson R, Zamcheck N: The use of preoperative plasma CEA levels for the stratification of patients after curative resection of colorectal cancers. Ann Surg 192: 747–751, 1980.

31. Livingstone AS, Hampson LG, Shuster J, Gold P, Hinckey J: Carcinoembryonic antigen in the diagnosis and management of colorectal carcinoma. Archives of Surgery 109: 259–264, 1974.

32. Holyoke D, Reynoso G, Chu TM: Carcinoembryonic (CEA) in patients with carcinoma of the digestive tract. Ann Surg 176: 559–564, 1972.

33. Wanebo HJ, Stearns M, Schwartz MK: Use of CEA as an indicator of early recurrence and as a guide to a selected second-look procedures in patients with colorectal cancer. Ann Surg 188: 481–493, 1978.

34. Lavin PT, Day J, Holyoke D, Mittelman A, Chu TM: A statistical evaluation of baseline and follow-up carcinoembryonic antigen in patients with resectable colorectal carcinoma. Cancer 47: 823–826, 1981.

35. Szymendera JJ, Wilczynska JE, Nowacki MP, Kaminska JA, Szawlowski AW: Serial CEA assays and liver scintigraphy for the detection of hepatic metastases from colorectal carcinoma. Dis Col & Rect 25: 191–197, 1982.

36. Attiyeh FF, Stearns MW Jr: Second-look laparotomy based on CEA elevations in colorectal cancer. Cancer 47: 2119–2125, 1981.

37. Martin EW Jr, Kibbey WE, DiVecchia L, Anderson G, Catalano P, Minton JP: Carcinoembryonic antigen–clinical and historical aspects. Cancer 37: 62–81, 1976.

38. Nicholson JR, Aust JC: Rising carcinoembryonic antigen titers in colorectal carcinoma: An indication for the second-look procedure. Dis Col & Rect 21: 163–164, 1978.

39. Martin ER Jr, James KK, Hurtubise PE, Catalano P, Minton JP: The use of CEA as an early indicator for gastrointestinal tumor recurrence and second-look procedures. Cancer 39: 440–446, 1977.

40. Mavligit G, Gutterman J, Burgess M, Khankhanias N: Adjuvant immunotherapy and chemoimmunotherapy in colorectal cancer of the Dukes' classification. Cancer 36: 2421–2427, 1975.

41. Holyoke ED, Chu TM, Murphy GP: CEA as a monitor of gastrointestinal malignancy. Cancer 35: 830–836, 1975.

42. Steele G, Zamcheck N, Wilson R, Mayer R, Lokich J, Rau P, Maltz J: Results of CEA-initiated second-look surgery for recurrent colorectal cancer. American Journal of Surgery 139: 544–548, 1980.

43. Beart RW Jr, Metzger PP, O'Connell MJ, Schutt AJ: Postoperative screening of patients with carcinoma of the colon. Dis Col & Rect 24: 585–588, 1981.

44. Martin EW Jr, Cooperman M, Carey LC, Minton JP: Sixty second-look procedures indicated primarily by rise in serial carcinoembryonic antigen. J Surg Res 28: 389–394, 1980.

45. Mach J-P, Carrel S, Forni M, Ritschard J, Donath A, Alberto P: Tumor localization of radio-labeled antibodies against carcinoembryonic antigen in patients with carcinoma: A critical evaluation. New England Journal of Medicine 303: 5–10, 1980.
46. Koch M, McPherson TA: Carcinoembryonic antigen levels as an indicator of the primary site in metastatic disease of unknown origin. Cancer 48: 1242–1244, 1981.
47. Linder MC, Moor JR, Wright K: Ceruloplasmin assays in diagnosis and treatment of human lung, breast, and gastrointestinal cancers. JNCI 67: 263–275, 1981.
48. CA-A Cancer Journal for Clinicians. Published by the American Cancer Society. 33: 16–17, 1983.
49. Wood DA, Robbins GF, Zippin C, Lum D, Stearns M: Staging of cancer of the colon and cancer of the rectum. Cancer 43: 961–968, 1979.
50. Hoth DF, Petrucci PE: Natural history and staging of colon cancer. Seminars in Oncology 3: 331–336, 1976.
51. Mettlin C, Natarajan N, Mittelman A, Smart CR, Murphy GP: Management and survival of adenocarcinoma of the rectum in the United States: Results of a national survey by the American College of Surgeons. Oncology 39: 265–273, 1982.
52. Wood GB, Gillis CR, Hole D, Malcolm AJH, Blumgart LH: Local tumour invasion as a prognostic factor in colorectal cancer. Br J Surg 68: 326–328, 1981.
53. Talbot IC, Ritchie S, Leighton MH, Hughes AO, Bussey HJR, Morson BC: The clinical significance of invasion of veins by rectal cancer. Br J Surg 67: 439–442, 1980.
54. de Mascarel A, Coindre JM, de Mascarel I, Trojani M, Maree D, Hoerni B: The prognostic significance of specific histologic features of carcinoma of the colon and rectum. Surg Gynecol Obstet 153: 511–514, 1981.
55. Rosenbloom B, Block JB, Pitch Y: Staging colorectal cancer: Is there a role for liver biopsy? Cancer Treatment Reports 60: 295–296, 1976.
56. Patt DJ, Brynes RK, Vardiman JW, Coppleson LW: Mesocolic lymph node histology in an important prognostic indicator for patients with carcinoma of the sigmoid colon. Cancer 35: 1388. 1975.
57. Gannon PJ, Holyoke ED, Goldrosen MH: Tumor associated lymphocyte cytotoxicity correlated with stage of disease in patients with colon adenocarcinoma. Europ J Cancer 14: 613–617, 1978.
58. Copeland EM, Miller LD, Jones RS: Prognostic factors in carcinoma of the colon and rectum. Am J Surg 116: 875, 1968.
59. Watson FR, Spratt JS, LeDuc RJ: Analysis of variance and covariance for colorectal adenocarcinomas in man as a logical prelude to 'staging'. Journal of Surgical Oncology 8: 155–163, 1976.
60. Feinstein AR, Schimpff CR, Hull EW: A reappraisal of staging and therapy for patients with cancer of the rectum: I. Development of two new systems of staging. Arch Intern Med 135: 1441–1453, 1975.
61. Feinstein AR, Schimpff CR, Hull EW: A reappraisal of staging and therapy for patients with cancer of the rectum: II. Patterns of presentation and outcome of treatment. Arch Intern Med 135: 1454–1462, 1975.
62. Nicholls RJ, Mason AY, Morson BC, Dixon AK, Fry IK: The clinical staging of rectal cancer. Br J Surg 69: 404–409, 1982.
63. McDermott F, Hughes Sir Edward, Pihl E, Milne BJ, Price A: Symptom duration and survival prospects in carcinoma of the rectum. Surg Gynecol Obstet 153: 321–326, 1981.
64. Welch JP: Multiple colorectal tumors: An appraisal of natural history and therapeutic options. American Journal of Surgery 142: 274–280, 1981.
65. Burns FJ: Synchronous and metachronous malignancies of the colon and rectum. Dis Col & Rect 23: 578–579, 1980.
66. Paradis P, Douglass HO Jr, Holyoke ED: The clinical implications of a staging system for carcinoma of the anus. Surg Gynecol & Obstet 141: 411–416, 1975.
67. Holyoke ED: New surgical approaches to pancreatic cancer. Cancer 47: 1719–1723, 1981.
68. Edis AJ, Kiernan PD, Taylor WF: Attempted curative resection of ductal carcinoma of the

pancreas: Review of Mayo Clinic experience, 1951-1975. Mayo Clinic Proceedings 55: 531–536, 1980.

69. Cancer Patient Survival. Report Number 5. Prepared by the End Results Section, Biometry Branch, Division of Cancer Cause and Prevention, National Cancer Institute, Bethesda, Maryland, 1976.

70. Staging of Cancer of the Pancreas. Prepared by the Cancer of the Pancreas Task Force, American Joint Committee on Cancer. Cancer 47: 1631–1637, 1981.

71. Fortner JG, MacLean BJ, Kim DK, Howland WS, Turnbull AD, Goldiner P, Carlon G, Beattie EJ Jr.: The seventies evolution in liver surgery for cancer. Cancer 47: 2162–2166, 1981.

72. Adson MA, Weiland LH: Resection of primary solid hepatic tumors. The American Journal of Surgery 141: 18–21, 1981.

73. Tompkins RK, Thomas D, Wile A, Longmire WP Jr: Prognostic factors in bile duct carcinoma: Analysis of 96 cases. Ann Surg 194: 447–457, 1981.

74. Nevin JE, Moran TJ, Kay S, King R: Carcinoma of the gallbladder. Cancer 37: 141–148, 1976.

75. Wanebo HJ, Castle WN, Fechner RE: Is carcinoma of the gallbladder a curable lesion? Ann Surg 195: 624–631, 1982.

76. Fielding JWL, Ellis DJ, Jones BG, Paterson J, Powell DJ, Waterhouse JAH, Brookes VS: Natural history of 'early' gastric cancer: Results of a 10-year regional survey. British Medical Journal 281: 965–967, 1980.

77. Sogo J, Kobayashi K, Saito J, Fujimaki M, Muto T: The role of lymphadenectomy in curative surgery for gastric cancer. World J Surg 3: 701–708, 1979.

78. Cady B, Ramsden DA, Stein A, Haggitt RC: Gastric Cancer: Contemporary Aspects. The American Journal of Surgery 133: 423–429, 1977.

79. ReMine WH: Carcinoma of the stomach. Chapter 36 IN: ABDOMINAL OPERATIONS, Maingot R (ed), Appleton-Century-Crofts, New York 1980. Seventh edition. Vol 1, pp 521–566.

80. Akiyama H, Tsurumaru M, Kawamura T, Ono Y. Principles of surgical treatment for carcinoma of the esophagus: Analysis of lymph node involvement. Ann Surg 194: 438–446, 1981.

81. Mittal VK, Bodzin JH: Primary malignant tumors of the small bowel. The American Journal of Surgery 140: 396–399, 1980.

82. Norberg K-A, Emas S: Primary tumors of the small intestine. The American Journal of Surgery 142: 569–573, 1981.

83. Pagtalunan RJG, Mayo CW, Dockerty MB: Primary malignant tumors of the small intestine. American Journal of Surgery 108: 13–18, 1964.

84. Miller AB, Hoogstraten B, Staquet M, Winkler A: Reporting results of cancer treatment. Cancer 47: 207–214, 1981.

85. Beanns OH, Myers MH (eds): Manual for staging of Cancer. Prepared by the American Joint Committee on Cancer, Chicago, Illinois. Second edition. J.B. Lippincott Co. Philadelphia PA 1983.

3. Epidemiology of pancreatic cancer

BRIAN MACMAHON

1. Introduction

1.1. An epidemiologic enigma

Cancer of the pancreas is an epidemiologic enigma. Although it accounts for more than 20,000 deaths annually in this country alone no promising hypotheses have been put forward to account for the vagaries of its distribution or to point to etiologic mechanisms. With the exception of a rather weak association of risk with cigarette smoking – itself somewhat mysterious – no external risk factors have been definitively identified. No promising leads have been developed from extensive experimental work in laboratory animals.

1.2. Methodologic problems

Knowledge of the epidemiology of cancer of the pancreas has no doubt been delayed by the difficulty of studying the distribution of the disease in human populations because of the complexity of its diagnosis and the variation by geography, socioeconomic status and other factors in the availability of the necessary resources and expertise. Descriptive statistics have therefore been of variable quality. Because this problem was recognized, there has been, in addition perhaps, a greater reluctance to rely on such sources as death statistics than was really indicated. The rise of cancer registries with their higher quality data gives a better basis for building up the descriptive epidemiology of the disease, but we see, in most areas of the world with reasonable mortality data, generally similar patterns in incidence and mortality data. This *should* be so in an almost uniformly and rapidly fatal disease, but that it *is* so suggests that mortality sources in developed countries are not so bad a source of descriptive data for this disease as they are sometimes thought to be.

A second methodologic problem has to do with the variety of tumors that arise

J.J. DeCosse and P. Sherlock (eds), Clinical Management of Gastrointestinal Cancer.
© *1984, Martinus Nijhoff Publishers, Boston. ISBN 0-89838-601-2. Printed in The Netherlands.*

in pancreatic tissue. It seems likely that adenocarcinomas of the exocrine pancreas have a different etiology than tumors of the islet cells and other less frequent types of malignancy arising in the same organ. Ideally, an epidemiologic review would deal with each histologic type separately. However, demographic data do not distinguish the histologic types of tumor and many *ad hoc* studies have also failed to do so. We must therefore generally assume that the epidemiologic features of 'pancreatic cancer' reflect those of adenocarcinoma of the exocrine gland, the histologic type which accounts for over 90% of all malignant pancreatic tumors. This review will deal only with adenocarcinomas of the exocrine gland, making the assumption just referred to, since, although *something* is known of the common adenocarcinoma, virtually nothing of an epidemiologic nature is known about the rarer tumors.

2. Demographic risk factors

2.1. Age

Cancer of the pancreas is a disease of the elderly and is quite rare under the age of 40. Age-specific mortality rates for white and non-white males for four time periods in the United States are shown in Figure 1. Recent data for white males show a consistent increase in death rates throughout life. Prior to 1964 the rate declined in the very oldest group (85 and over). This decline after reaching a peak is more pronounced in the rates for non-whites, with a peak around age 75 and decline thereafter. Because of its predominance in non-whites and its disappearance in recent data for whites, this decline seems much more likely to be an artefact than real. Possible explanations include errors in census data and less concern to establish the precise cause of death in the very old. Age-specific patterns for females are similar to those illustrated for males.

2.2. Gender

Incidence and mortality data consistently show higher rates of pancreatic cancer for males than for females (Table 1). An excess of males is also seen in large clinical series, and there seems no reason to suspect that it is due to diagnostic bias. The disproportion of males is somewhat lower in clinical series than when incidence or mortality rates are compared but this results from the fact that there are more females than males alive and at risk of developing the disease in the population in the age range at which pancreatic cancer occurs.

There is some variation from place to place in the ratio of male to female incidence rates (Table 1) but it is not striking.

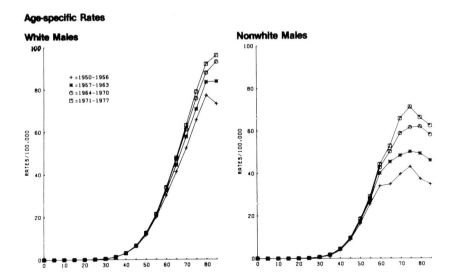

Figure 1. Age-specific mortality rates from pancreatic cancer in U.S. males, 1950–77. From McKay *et al.* [1].

2.3. *Ethnic background*

Table 2 illustrates that, in six US cancer registries, rates of pancreatic cancer are substantially higher for blacks than for whites. Incidence rates for black males and females are approximately double those of the corresponding white gender. There are three curious exceptions. In Los Angeles and Atlanta, while females follow the usual patterns, the rates for white and black males are quite similar. In New Orleans, while males follow the usual pattern, rates for white females are actually higher than those for black females – and also, incidentally, than those for white males.

Figure 2 shows that, in mortality data, the higher mortality rates for non-whites (predominantly blacks) have prevailed since about 1955, but before that the rates for non-whites were lower than those for whites. Using incidence data, Buncher [3] pointed out that the rates of increase between the US National Cancer Surveys of 1947–48 and 1969–71 were substantially greater for blacks than for whites. Because of the diagnostic difficulties already referred to, and the fact that the rate of increase in access to sophisticated medical resources has probably been greater for blacks than whites, we must question both whether there has been an increase in incidence of the disease in either racial group, and the appearance that the increase is greater in blacks than whites. However, it seems reasonable to accept as real the observation that, currently, blacks have substantially higher rates than whites. Indeed, the age-specific patterns shown in Figure 1 suggest that mortality rates in non-whites are rising most rapidly in the older age groups and, as the non-white population adopts the age-specific pattern of the white population, the overall discrepancy in rates will become even greater than it now is.

High rates have been noted in two Polynesian populations for which incidence data are available – the New Zealand Maoris and the Hawaiian and part-Hawaiian population of Hawaii (Table 3). These rates (at least in 1968–72) were among the highest observed anywhere in the world and are two to three times those shown in Table 1. In 1968–72, the high rates affected males particularly, and

Table 1. Truncated[a] age-adjusted annual incidence rates of pancreatic cancer per 100,000 population, from selected cancer registries

Registry	Male	Female
Israel (Jews)	13.8	8.6
Finland	13.3	7.3
US (Whites)[b]	12.3	7.8
Denmark	12.3	7.8
United Kingdom[c]	11.4	6.5
Sweden	11.2	7.1
Norway	10.7	6.8
Japan[d]	10.4	7.0
Canada[e]	10.3	7.1
Slovenia	8.3	4.9
Cali	7.0	4.8

[a] Ages 35–64 only, adjusted in 5 years groups.
[b] Mean of eleven registries (range for males 9.9–17.2) (Puerto Rico and New Mexico not included).
[c] Mean of eleven registries (range for males 8.5–15.0).
[d] Mean of four registries (range for males 8.8–11.9).
[e] Mean of nine provinces (range for males 5.5–14.5).

Data from Waterhouse *et al.* [2].

Table 2. Truncated age–adjusted annual incidence rates of pancreatic cancer per 100,000 population by race, U.S. Registries

Registry	Males		Females	
	White	Black	White	Black
Alameda	11.1	28.8	7.4	14.9
S.F. Bay Area	12.3	25.6	8.4	16.0
Los Angeles	11.3	13.5	4.0	9.2
Atlanta	17.2	18.6	6.6	10.7
New Orleans	11.6	21.8	12.1	8.2
Detroit	11.9	22.0	7.0	13.4

Data from Waterhouse *et al.* [2].

Table 3. Truncated age-adjusted annual incidence rates of pancreatic cancer per 100,000 population in two Polynesian and geographically related populations, 1968–72 and 1973–77[a]

Area	Ethnic group	1968-72		1973-77	
		Male	Female	Male	Female
Hawaii	Hawaiian[b]	31.4	11.4	8.1	11.2
	Caucasian	15.8	12.2	10.3	6.2
	Chinese	11.4	6.4	11.1	11.6
	Filipino	5.7	4.6	8.0	5.4
	Japanese	7.1	6.0	10.6	4.4
New Zealand	Maori	26.6	8.7	18.5	10.9
	White	9.7	4.8	11.3	7.0

[a] Hawaiian and part-Hawaiian.
[b] Data from Waterhouse *et al.* [2, 4].

in these two populations rates for males were approximately three times those for females. However, the data for 1973–77 do not show elevated rates for Hawaiian males, although the high rates in Hawaiian females persist. The small sizes of the population sub-groups in Hawaii make rates over short time spans somewhat unstable. In 1973–77 the high rates in New Zealand Maoris, as well as the large excess over the rate for females, persist but are not so striking as in 1968–72.

2.4. Geography

Because of the diagnostic problems already referred to, apparent geographic differences in frequency of pancreatic cancer are among the most suspect features of the epidemiology of the disease. However, as can be seen in Table 1, while there are apparent differences in incidence rates between areas of the world with well-developed medical resources, the range is not great. The two to three fold range from lowest to highest is considerably less than is found for many other cancers, where ranges of five to ten fold are common and ranges of more than 100 fold occur occasionally, as in cancer of the esophagus.

The geographic variations have led to no etiologic hypotheses, although they have been used to evaluate hypotheses arising from other data – particularly that relating coffee consumption to pancreatic cancer risk.

2.5. Secular trends

As shown in Figure 2, mortality data suggest a slow increase in rates of pancreatic cancer after 1950 – somewhat stronger in males than in females. In whites the

64

Age-adjusted Mortality Rates

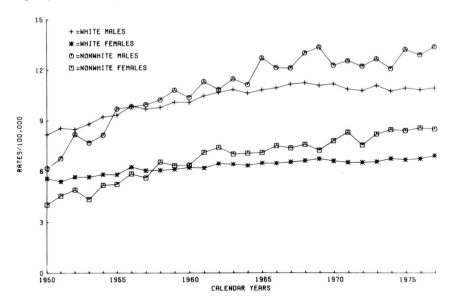

Figure 2. Age-adjusted mortality rates from pancreatic cancer, by race and sex, U.S.A., 1950–77. From McKay *et al.* [1].

rates plateaued in the late 1960s and have been constant since. In non-whites the rates have continued to rise slowly.

Incidence data give a somewhat similar picture. Comparing the Second (1947–1948) and Third (1969–71) US National Cancer Surveys, age adjusted rates rose 22% in white males, 21% in white females, 30% in black males and 126% in black females [5]. Combining data from the Third National Cancer Survey (TNCS) with those for 1973–76 from the Surveillance, Epidemiology and End Results (SEER) program, Pollack and Horm [6] estimated that, for whites, pancreatic cancer incidence declined in males at an annual rate of 0.5% and increased in females at an annual rate of 0.9% over the period 1969–1976. Neither trend is statistically significant and the increase in females is made questionable by problems in comparability of the SEER and TNCS data [7]. Looking only at the 4 years of the SEER program, no evidence of a trend is seen. Recognizing the lack of comparability of the two sets of data for blacks, Pollack and Horm did not examine the incidence trend in this group.

3. Endogenous risk factors

3.1. Diabetes

Although the frequency of clinical diabetes seems to be in excess among patients with pancreatic cancer, a high proportion of patients with the two diseases have developed their diabetes within a short time of the diagnosis of their cancer [8]. It is likely that in most of such patients the diabetic symptoms result from their as yet undiagnosed pancreatic tumor. However, in two studies there is an indication that, even after cases are excluded in which the diabetes developed shortly before the pancreatic cancer, there is an increased risk (approximately two-fold) for pancreatic cancer among diabetic females, but not diabetic males [9, 10]. Why there should be such a relationship in one sex but not the other is puzzling.

3.2. Family history

There has been no systematic study of the risk of pancreatic cancer in the relatives of patients. Unusual clusters – for example, of four siblings all developing the disease [11, 12] – have been reported, but they are rare and in clinical experience family history does not seem to be a prominent feature of this disease.

There appears to be no association of any specific HLA type with the disease [13].

4. Exogenous risk factors

4.1. Tobacco

The most clearly established exogenous risk factor for pancreatic cancer is cigarette smoking. Data from three major follow-up studies are given in Table 4. Heavy cigarette smoking (defined as more than two packs of cigarettes a day in one study [14] and 25 g of tobacco or more in the other [15] is associated with approximately a doubling of the risk of pancreatic cancer. Although absent in one small case-control investigation [17], increased risk associated with cigarette smoking has also been noted in two larger case-control studies [10, 18]. In one study, increased risk was associated with smoking of cigars but not pipes [10], but larger studies indicate no increase in risk for smokers of either pipes or cigars [14, 18].

Relative to the strengths of the associations between cigarette smoking and certain other cancers – notably cancers of the lung, larynx, mouth, bladder and liver – the relationship between cigarette smoking and pancreatic cancer is quite weak. The association is also much weaker than that recently observed between cigarette smoking and risk of chronic pancreatitis [19]. Its interest lies not in any significant opportunity for prevention that it represents but in its potential for leading to understanding of the mechanisms of carcinogenesis in the pancreas and of tobacco carcinogenesis of organs that are not directly exposed to tobacco smoke.

4.2. Alcohol

The relationship between alcohol use and pancreatic cancer has been less extensively studied than has the association with tobacco consumption, but a lack of association has been found in two case-control studies [10, 18], in a proportional mortality analysis of a large series of deaths of alcoholics [20] and in two large follow-up studies of alcoholics [21, 22]. An association with wine drinking was reported in one recent study, but the number of cases was small, the difference between cases and controls was not conventionally significant, and potential confounding factors were not evaluated [17]. Overall, it seems unlikely that alcohol consumption is either a risk factor or has any role in the origin of cancer of the pancreas – a fact that is of interest in light of the clear-cut role of alcohol in the etiology of chronic pancreatitis [19].

4.3. Diet

Some component of diet would seem an obvious candidate for an etiologic role in pancreatic cancer. Unfortunately, for evaluating dietary patterns over the several decades of an individual's life during which the carcinogenic process develops, the available tools are extremely crude. In a large follow-up study in Japan, persons who reported consumption of meat daily or more had approximately 1.5 times the risk of those who ate meat less frequently than daily [23]. The associ-

Table 4. Risk of pancreatic cancer by level of current cigarette consumption relative to an arbitary risk of 1.0 in non smokers, in three follow-up studies.

Study	Non-smokers	Cigarette smokers		
		Light	Moderate	Heavy
Kahn [14]	1.0	1.1	1.4 1.8	2.2 2.7
Doll & Peto [15]	1.0	1.0	1.3	1.9
Hammond [16] – males	1.0		2.4	
– females	1.0		1.8	

ation, though weak, was statistically significant and appeared to be stronger among cigarette smokers. We need not look to the meat or its constituents for an explanation of this observation, for daily consumption of meat must be a marker of many and varied characteristics of the Japanese diet. Indeed, it is possible that high meat consumption is a reflection of high socioeconomic status and adoption of other US customs such as cigarette smoking, and is unrelated to diet. Data for persons of Japanese ancestry in the United States are curious. Rates in Japan are lower than those in US whites (Table 1). Although rates in 'foreign-born' (generally, Japan-born) Japanese parallel those in US whites, rates for persons of Japanese ancestry born in the United States fall back to levels similar to those seen in Japanese in Japan [24].

Moderately low rates of pancreatic cancer have been reported for Mormons [25, 26] and Seventh Day Adventists [27] in the United States – both groups having some dietary customs different from the general population. However, the rates do not seem sufficiently low not to be explained by the fact that both groups proscribe and, in general, practice non-smoking. The exception is an unusually low incidence rate of the disease in Mormon females in rural counties of Utah (3.7 per 100,000) compared to non-Mormon females in the same counties (10.7 per 100,000 [28] which seems too large to explain by differences in cigarette smoking patterns, since only 38% of the non-Mormon females in Utah were current smokers in 1977–79 [29] and this percentage seems likely to be lower in the rural counties.

In sum, comparison of populations with different dietary practices has so far failed to uncover hypotheses postulating etiologic roles for specific components of diet and, in spite of the attractiveness of diet as an area of enquiry in this disease, populations with striking differences in dietary patterns have quite similar rates of pancreatic cancer.

4.4. Coffee

One specific component of diet that has been suggested as worthy of further investigation is coffee. In 1981, in a small case-control study it was reported that, among several other differences, cases had a higher consumption of decaffeinated coffee than controls [17]. Consumption of all forms of coffee was later reported to be similar in cases and controls [30]. A few months after that original publication, in a much larger study, an association with coffee consumption overall and pancreatic cancer risk was reported [18]. The association was statistically highly significant in each sex, and, while no dose-response relationship was evident in males, for both sexes combined, with adjustment for sex, age and cigarette smoking, the dose-response relationship was highly significant. Relative to non-drinkers of coffee, drinkers of one to two cups per day had approximately double the risk of pancreatic cancer, and drinkers of three or more cups per day had approximately three times the risk. Unfortunately, no distinction was made between regular and decaffeinated coffee in this study. Subsequent to this report four small sets of data have been published in the form of letters to the editor. Three are interpreted as failing to confirm the observation [30–32] and one as consistent with it [33]. Each of these data sets is much smaller than that which led to the original observation and further evaluation of this possible relationship is required.

4.5. Occupation

A number of occupations have been indicated by one or another study to be at increased risk for pancreas cancer, but the associations are not strong and none of the isolated observations has been confirmed [3]. Among deaths of members of the American Chemical Society, a proportional mortality study indicated 56 deaths from pancreatic cancer compared to 35 expected [34]. However, no excess of pancreatic cancer was reported in the preliminary report of a study of British chemists [35] or in a cohort study of mortality and cancer incidence among chemists employed by the Du Pont Company [36].

4.6. Ionizing radiation

There has been a suggestion of excess pancreas cancer among British radiologists [37] and among Japanese survivors of the atomic bombs [38]. In both instances the excess is small and of marginal statistical significance. If large doses of ionizing radiation do induce pancreatic cancer they can be responsible for no more than a very small proportion of incident cases.

5. Directions of enquiry

We began this chapter with the statement that cancer of pancreas is an epidemiologic enigma. Not only is the etiology of the disease enigmatic but a review of the literature fails even to identify promising lines of enquiry. Clearly, the association with coffee consumption must be evaluated and, if confirmed, explored as to mechanism. Beyond that, the high rate in the black population of the United States – a rate that promises to become even higher – seems the most promising starting point in a search for hypotheses, although none have yet been offered.

References

1. McKay FW, Hanson MR, Miller RW: Cancer mortality in the United States: 1950–1977. Nat Cancer Inst Monograph 59: 1–467, 1982.
2. Waterhouse J, Muir C, Shanmugaratnam K, Powell J (eds): Cancer incidence in five continents, volume IV. IARC publication No. 42. Lyon: International Agency for Research on Cancer, 1982.
3. Buncher CR: Epidemiology of pancreatic cancer. In: Tumors of the Pancreas. Moossa AA (ed). Baltimore: Wilkins & Wilkins, 1980, p 415–427.
4. Waterhouse J, Muir C, Correa P, Powell J: Cancer incidence in five continents, volume III. IARC publication No. 15. Lyon: International Agency for Research on Cancer, 1976.
5. Seidman H, Silverberg E, Holleb AI: Cancer statistics, 1976 – A comparison of white and black populations. CA 26: 2–13, 1976.
6. Pollack ES, Horm JW: Trends in cancer incidence and mortality in the United States, 1969–76. J Natl Cancer Inst 64: 1091–1103, 1980.
7. Knowlden NF, Burack WR, Burack TS: Cancer: 1. Analysis of recent new case incidence reports. Fund Appl Toxicol 1: 458–468, 1981.
8. Karmody AJ, Kyle J: The association between carcinoma of the pancreas and diabetes mellitus. Br J Surg 56: 362–364, 1969.
9. Kessler II: Cancer mortality among diabetics. J Natl Cancer Inst 44: 673–686, 1970.
10. Wynder EL, Mabuchi K, Maruchi N, Fortner JG: A case-control study of cancer of the pancreas. Cancer 31: 641–648, 1973.
11. Friedman JM, Fialkow PJ: Carcinoma of the pancreas in four brothers. Birth Defects 12: 145–150, 1976.
12. MacDermott RP, Kramer P: Adenocarcinoma of the pancreas in four siblings. Gastroenterology 65: 137–139, 1973.
13. Terasaki PI, Perdue ST, Mickey MR: HLA frequencies in cancer: a second study. In: Genetics of human cancer. Mulvihill JJ, Miller RW, Fraumeni JF Jr (eds). New York: Raven Press, 1977, p 321–328.
14. Kahn HA: The Dorn study of smoking and mortality among US veterans: report on eight and one-half years of observation. Nat Cancer Inst Monograph 19: 1–126, 1966.
15. Doll R, Peto R: Mortality in relation to smoking: 20 years' observations on male British doctors. Brit Med J 2: 1525–1536, 1976.
16. Hammond EC: Smoking in relation to the death rates of one million men and women. Nat Cancer Inst Monograph 19: 127–204, 1966.
17. Lin RS, Kessler II: A multifactorial model for pancreatic cancer in man. Epidemiologic evidence. JAMA 245: 147–152, 1981.
18. MacMahon B, Yen S, Trichopoulos D, Warren J, Nardi G: Coffee and cancer of the pancreas. New Engl J Med 304: 630–633, 1981.
19. Yen S, Hsieh CC, MacMahon B: Consumption of alcohol and tobacco and other risk factors for pancreatitis. Amer J Epidemiol 116: 407–414, 1982.
20. Monson RR, Lyon JL: Proportional mortality among alcoholics. Cancer 36: 1077–1079, 1975.
21. Robinette CD, Hrubec Z, Fraumeni JF Jr.: Chronic alcoholism and subsequent mortality in World War II veterans. Amer J Epidemiol 109: 687–700, 1979.
22. Schmidt W, Popham RE: The role of drinking and smoking in mortality from cancer and other causes in male alcoholics. Cancer 47: 1031–1041, 1981.
23. Hirayama T: A large-scale cohort study on the relationship between diet and selected cancers of digestive organs. In: Gastrointestinal cancer: endogenous factors. Bruce WR, Correa P, Lipkin M, Tannenbaum SR, Wilkins TD (eds). Banbury Report No. 7. Cold Spring Harbor, NY: Cold Spring Harbor Laboratory, 1981.
24. Locke FB, King H: Cancer mortality risk among Japanese in the United States. J Nat Cancer Inst

65: 1149–1156, 1980.

25. Lyon JL, Gardner JW, West DW: Cancer incidence in Mormons and non-Mormons in Utah during 1967–75. J Nat Cancer Inst 65: 1055–1061, 1980.

26. Enstrom JE: Cancer mortality among Mormons in California during 1968–75. J Nat Cancer Inst 65: 1073–1082, 1980.

27. Phillips RL, Garfinkel L, Kuzma JW, Beeson WL, Lotz T, Brin B: Mortality among California Seventh-Day Adventists for selected cancer sites. J Nat Cancer Inst 65: 1097–1107, 1980.

28. Lyon JL, Gardner JW, West DW: Cancer in Utah: risk by religion and place of residence. J Nat Cancer Inst 65: 1063–1071, 1980.

29. West DW, Lyon JL, Gardner JW: Cancer risk factors: an analysis of Utah Mormons and non-Mormons. J Nat Cancer Inst 65: 1083–1095, 1980.

30. Kessler II: Coffee and cancer of the pancreas (Letter to the Editor). New Engl J Med 304: 1605, 1981.

31. Goldstein HR: No association found between coffee and cancer of the pancreas (Letter to the Editor). New Engl J Med 306: 997, 1982.

32. Jick H, Dinan BJ: Coffee and pancreatic cancer (Letter to the Editor) Lancet ii: 92, 1981.

33. Nomura A, Stemmerman GM, Heilbrun LK: Coffee and pancreatic cancer (Letter to the Editor). Lancet ii: 415, 1981.

34. Li FP, Fraumeni JF Jr, Mantel N, Miller RW: Cancer mortality among chemists. J Natl Cancer Inst 43: 1159–1164, 1969.

35. Searle CE, Waterhouse JAH, Henman BA, Bartlett D, McCombie S: Epidemiological study of the mortality of British chemists. Brit J Cancer 38: 192–193, 1978.

36. Hoar SK, Pell S: A retrospective cohort study of mortality and cancer incidence among chemists. J Occ Med 23: 485–501, 1981.

37. Smith PG, Doll R: Mortality from cancer and all causes among British radiologists. Brit J Cancer 54: 187–194, 1981.

38. Beebe GW, Kato H, Land CE: Studies of the mortality of A-bomb survivors. 6. Mortality and radiation dose. Radiat Res 75: 138–201, 1978.

4. Hepatitis B virus and hepatocellular carcinoma

BARUCH S. BLUMBERG and W. THOMAS LONDON

1. Introduction

In this chapter we propose to 1) review the data which supports the hypothesis that persistent infection with the hepatitis B virus (HBV) is required for the development of primary hepatocellular carcinoma (PHC), 2) discuss strategies for primary prevention of PHC, 3) present and discuss a cellular model for PHC in humans which describes the available data on the virus-cancer relation and provide a heuristic model for learning more about the pathogenesis of PHC. An objective of the use of the model and the greater knowledge of pathogenesis would be to develop methods for secondary prevention in persons who are already chronic carriers of HBV.

A goal of cancer research is the prevention of cancers, particularly those that are common in the world, by the discovery of factors that are necessary for their development and reducing or eliminating these factors in a manner which is not, overall, harmful (primary prevention). A second goal is to arrest the progress of the disease if it has already started by removing very small tumors that have not spread (secondary prevention). A third approach, which may be more easily and gentlty accomplished than secondary prevention, is to slow the advance of a potential clinical cancer to a pace that avoids disease perceptible to the individual until very late in his or her possible life span, by which time the host would have died for another reason. This we have called 'prevention by delay.' Developments over the past decade make it very likely that primary prevention for one of the most common cancers in the world, primary cancer of the liver, may be feasible, and current work is directed to an understanding of the other two forms of prevention.

In sub-Saharan Africa, Taiwan, and the populous coastal and southern provinces of mainland China, the incidence of primary hepatocellular carcinoma (PHC) is 25 to 150 cases per 100,000 population. An annual mortality of 100,000 for all of China (population base 850 million) has recently been reported. The incidence of PHC is three to nine times higher in males than females. Hence, the

J.J. DeCosse and P. Sherlock (eds), Clinical Management of Gastrointestinal Cancer.
© 1984, Martinus Nijhoff Publishers, Boston. ISBN 0-89838-601-2. Printed in The Netherlands.

estimated incidence of deaths from PHC in males would be about 17 to 20 per 100,000. Extrapolating these figures to other regions of the world where PHC is a common cancer, we can estimate a worldwide annual incidence of about 1/4 to 1 million cases in men and 50 to 200,000 cases in women. Since PHC is almost always lethal, the incidence and mortality rates per year are about the same [1].

In 1975 [2], we pointed out that advances in our knowledge of the pathology, epidemiology and clinical characteristics of PHC on the one hand, and of the hepatitis B virus on the other made it possible to test the hypothesis that persistent infection with the hepatitis B virus was necessary for the development of (most cases) of PHC. Since that time, a substantial body of evidence which strongly supports this hypothesis has been collected. The quantity and quality of this data are such that it is reasonable to assume that the hypothesis is more likely to be right than wrong and to proceed with the next step; that is, the design of strategies to prevent infection with hepatitis B virus in order to prevent PHC as well as other consequences of HBV infection. Blumberg and Millman, in 1969, introduced a vaccine to protect against hepatitis B infection [3], and this has now been produced in large quantities in the United States and other countries. Based to a large extent on the study of Szmuness and his colleagues in New York, it has been shown within the limits of the studies that the vaccine is safe and effective. It is likely that the vaccine will constitute a major part of public health programs to prevent hepatitis B infection which will be introduced in the near future. The use of such a vaccine which could ultimately prevent PHC could be economically and medically justified because of its effect on other diseases associated with HBV, and its predicted role as a 'cancer vaccine' would be added to this.

In addition to the potential practical importance of this body of scientific information bearing on the HBV-PHC relation, it will be useful in basic studies on how viruses 'cause' cancer. Since (if the accumulated evidence is accepted as convincing) HBV is required for the development of PHC, an understanding of how it does so will provide an explanation of the role of a virus in human carcinogenesis independent of its similarity or difference to existing models derived from other species or experimental observations. This explanation could then form the basis for discovering similar virus relations in other species (which has already happened (see below)) and in humans.

2. Evidence to support the hypothesis that persistent infection with HBV is required for the development of PHC

In this section, the method of 'independent evidence' is used. Although any single item cited may have an alternative explanation, the total body of data taken together is best explained by the stated hypothesis. We have published more detailed discussions of these data, and additional bibliographic references are given in them [1, 4].

2.1.

PHC occurs commonly in regions where chronic carriers of HBV are prevalent and much less frequently in areas where they are not.

2.2.

Case-control studies have shown that 90% or more of patients with PHC who live in areas where HBV is endemic have HBsAg or high titers of antibody against the core antigen in the blood (anti-HBc). These markers can be considered evidence of current or previous persistent HBV infection. In the same areas, controls have markedly lower frequencies of HBsAg and anti-HBc. Even in the United States, where PHC is uncommon, patients with the disease have higher prevalences of HBsAg and anti-HBc than do controls. In other words, in areas of both high and low PHC incidence, serologic evidence of persistent infection with HBV is more common in patients with PHC than in controls (Table 1).

Table 1. Frequency of hepatitis B surface antigen (HBsAg) and antibody against hepatitis B core (anti-HBc) in patients with PHC and controls*

Country	PHC		Controls	
	No. tested	% Positive	No. tested	% Positive
Hepatitis B surface antigen				
Greece	189	55.0	106	4.7
Spain	31	19.3	101	2.0
USA	34	14.7	56	0
Senegal	291	51.9	100	12.0
Mozambique	29	62.1	35	14.3
Uganda	47	47.0	50	6.0
Zambia	19	63.1	40	7.5
South Africa	138	59.5	200	9.0
Taiwan	84	54.8	278	12.2
Singapore	156	35.3	1516	4.1
Japan	260	37.3	4387	2.6
Vietnam	61	80.3	94	24.5
Antibody to hepatitis B core antigen				
Greece	80	70.0	160	31.9
Spain	31	87.0	101	14.8
USA	33	48.5	56	0
Senegal	291	87.3	100	26.0
South Africa	76	86.0	103	31.7
Hong Kong	37	70.3	58	36.2

* Only studies using radioimmunoassay or a test of equivalent sensitivity for HBsAg and in which controls were included are used. These data have not been corrected for age.

Prince [5] has estimated that the relative risk of developing PHC for chronic carriers in the United States and western Europe is about the same as the relative risk for carriers in Asia and Africa. If this is correct, then factors (such as aflatoxins and nitrosamines) which are thought to be related to the development of PHC but which presumably are not as common in the western countries as in the high incidence countries, may not be essential for the development of PHC. They may play a role in increasing the frequency of hepatitis carriers or may accelerate the process of pathogenesis, but there is little direct information about this.

2.3.

Most cases of PHC (approximately 80%) arise in a liver already affected with cirrhosis or chronic active hepatitis or both. If chronic hepatitis and cirrhosis are steps toward the development of liver cancer, then case-control studies of these two diseases should also show higher prevalence of chronic infection with HBV in the cases. Studies in Africa and Korea have confirmed this prediction (Table 2).

2.4.

HBV proteins can usually be demonstrated with histochemical stains or immunologic techniques in the hepatic tissues of patients with PHC. HBsAg and hepatitis B core antigen (HBcAg) are undetectable or present only in small quantities in the tumor cells themselves, but are found in the nonmalignant cells adjacent to the expanding tumor and elsewhere in the liver. These antigens are not found in the livers of uninfected persons nor, in general, in persons with

Table 2. Hepatitis B infection in cases of chronic liver disease and controls in Korea and Mali, West Africa

	N	% HBsAg (+)	% anti-HBc (+)	% anti-HBs (+)
Korea				
Chronic active hepatitis	50	76	94	14
Cirrhosis	35	94	100	6
Controls[a]	104	6	75	54
Mali				
Chronic liver disease[b]	42	46	59	26
Controls	80	5	16	35

[a] Controls are males greater than age 20 in the general population.
[b] Not separated by diagnosis, but most are cases of advanced cirrhosis

antibody to HBsAg in their serum. A particularly pertinent study by Nayak *et al.* [6] in India, which is a relatively low incidence area for PHC, showed that if multiple sections of the liver are examined, HBsAg can be found in some hepatocytes in over 90% of the cases of PHC. Thus, HBV proteins are present in the livers of most patients with PHC from areas endemic for HBV and PHC, and they are also found in the livers of many patients from low incidence areas [6, 7].

2.5.

If persistent HBV infection causes PHC, such infection should precede the occurrence of PHC. To test this hypothesis, it is necessary to identify asymptomatic chronic carriers of HBV and controls who are not carriers and to follow them for several years to see whether PHC develops. A major study of this type is being conducted by Beasley *et al.* in male civil servants between the ages of 40 and 60 years in Taiwan [8]. Approximately 3500 carriers were identified. The controls are an equal number of HBsAg-negative men matched by age and place of origin. Approximately 18,500 additional non-carriers were also identified. The subjects have been followed for four to six years. Eighty-nine cases of PHC have occurred during the follow-up period, and all but three have been in chronic carriers. The one exception arose in a man who had both anti-HBc and anti-HBs, indicating that he had probably been infected in the recent past. Thus far, the relative risk of PHC is more than 200 times greater in carriers than in non-carriers, and 98% (the attributable risk) of the cases have occurred in carriers. This is probably the highest risk known for any of the common cancers.

2.6.

Because PHC usually develops in a liver that is affected by cirrhosis or chronic hepatitis or both, some investigators have argued that any hepatotoxic agent that causes cirrhosis is associated with an increased risk of PHC, and that hepatitis B virus is one such agent. A rigorous test of the hypothesis that chronic infection with hepatitis B virus increases the risk of PHC in addition to producing cirrhosis is to compare the incidence of PHC in patients with cirrhosis who are or are not chronic carriers of HBV. Obata *et al.* have performed such a study in Japan [9]. Seven of 30 HBsAg-positive patients with cirrhosis (23%) but only five of 85 HBsAg-negative patients with cirrhosis (6%) had PHC after about four years. These results are highly consistent with the prediction from the hypothesis.

2.7.

In populations where HBV is endemic (sub-Saharan Africa, Asia, and Oceania), there is good evidence that many of the chronic carriers acquire HBV as a result of infection transmitted from their mothers early in life. That is, the mothers themselves are chronic carriers, and offspring born when the mothers are infectious are likely to become chronic carriers. (Although children of carrier mothers may be exposed *in utero*, at birth, or immediately afterwards, they do not become carriers until after about six weeks to three months.) Within a population, persons infected shortly after birth or during the first year of life will have been chronic carriers of HBV longer than persons of similar age who are infected later in life. Therefore, if the duration of being a chronic carrier is related to the likelihood of having PHC, one could predict that the mothers of patients with PHC would be more likely to be chronic carriers than the mothers of controls of similar age who do not have PHC. Studies in Senegal, West Africa, and in South Korea are consistent with this prediction [10] (Table 3).

2.8.

A further test of the HBV-PHC hypothesis is whether HBV-DNA is present in PHC tissue and whether such DNA is integrated into the tumor cell genome. Summers *et al.*, using livers obtained at autopsy in Senegal, extracted HBV DNA base sequences from 9 of 11 primary liver cancers collected from patients with HBsAg in their serum and from one of four patients who were HBsAg negative but anti-HBs positive [11, 12]. Several cell lines which produce HBsAg have been developed from human primary liver cancer. The first was produced by Alexander in South Africa (PLC/PRF/5) and has been studied in many laboratories

Table 3. Prevalence of HBsAg and anti-HBc in mothers of PHC patients and controls.

	n	HBsAg(+)	anti-HBc(+)
Senegal			
Mothers of PHC cases	28	20 (71.4%)	20 (70.4%)
Mothers of Controls[a]	28	4 (14.3%)	9 (32.1%)
Korea			
Mothers of PHC cases	10	4 (40.0%)	10 (100%)
Controls[b]	34	0	25 (73.5%)

[a] In Senegal controls were mother of individuals matched by sex, age and neighborhood with the PHC cases.

[b] controls in Korea were women randomly selected from a pool of controls such that the mean age and variance were equal to those for the mothers of the PHC cases.

[13]. This cell line produces large quantities of HBsAg 22 nm particles (1.3 mg/ml) but no Dane particles [14]. Marion and Robinson analyzed these cells and demonstrated 4 to 5 ng of HBV DNA per mg of cellular DNA [15]. Gray *et al.* [16] reported that at least six copies of HBV DNA are integrated into the cellular genomic DNA of the liver. Two of the six inserts are incomplete viral genomes, but all six contain the gene for HBsAg. They also isolated RNA transcripts for the HBsAg gene from the Alexander cell line. Brechot *et al.* [17] demonstrated integration of viral DNA in the cellular genomes of three primary liver cancers obtained at autopsy from HBsAg (+) men who lived in Ivory Coast, West Africa. Because only a few bands of integrated DNA were observed in each tumor extract, it is likely that the integration sites were the same within each cell of a given tumor. A third cell line that produces HBsAg has been derived from a human PHC by Aden and Knowles [18]. Recently, Shafritz *et al.* [19], studied percutaneous liver biopsies and post mortem tissue specimens from patients with chronic liver disease associated with persistent HBV infection, and patients with PHC. In 12 patients with hepatocellular carcinoma who had persistent HBV in their serum, integrated HBV DNA was found in host liver cells. It was also found integrated in some patients who had PHC with anti-HBs. In addition, integration was found in the non-tumorous tissue. In carriers of HBV without PHC, integration was seen in two patients who were carriers for more than 8 years, but it was not integrated in individuals who were carriers for less than two years. From this it can be inferred that increasing time of infection increases the probability of integration.

2.9.

In 1971 [20], based on the unusual clinical and epidemiologic characteristics of the hepatitis B virus, we had proposed that it was different from other viruses and that it represented the first of a series of viruses we termed Icrons. (The name is an acronym of the Institute for Cancer Research, ICR, with a neuter Greek ending.) The unique characteristics of the molecular biology of HBV (see below) have supported the notion that HBV is an unusual virus. Recent discoveries of other viruses which conform to the expectations of the Icron model provide additional support for the hypothesis, and these will be briefly described here.

2.9.1. Cancer of the liver and hepatitis virus in Marmota monax

Persistent infection with a virus similar to HBV is associated with a naturally occurring primary carcinoma of the liver in *Marmota monax*, the woodchuck or groundhog [21] (Figure 1). Snyder has trapped Pennsylvania woodchucks in the wild and maintained a colony at the Philadelphia Zoological Garden for the past 20 years. Post-mortem examinations were performed in more than 100 woodchucks, and about 25% of the animals had primary liver cancers. The tumors in

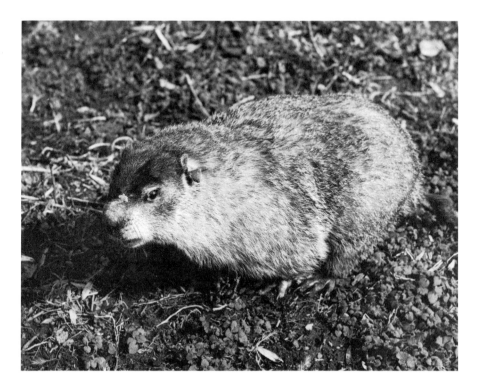

Figure 1. Marmota monax (ground hog, woodchuck).

the animals were usually associated with chronic hepatitis [22]. Snyder brought our attention to his findings and provided us with serum specimens from the infected and diseased animals. Summers, at the Institute for Cancer Research, examined serum samples from these animals for evidence of infection with a virus similar to HBV. He based his investigation on the hypothesis that viruses in the same class as HBV would have a similar nucleic acid structure and similar DNA polymerase. HBV was known to have unique characteristics: it contains a circular, double-stranded DNA genome with a single-stranded region and a DNA polymerase capable of filling in the single-stranded region to make a fully double-stranded, circular DNA. Summers found that about 15% of the woodchuck serum samples had particles containing a DNA polymerase and a DNA genome that were similar in size and structure to those of HBV [23]. Examination of pellets from these serum specimens with an electron microscope showed the three types of particles associated with HBV. Later, Werner *et al.* [24] showed cross-reactivity of the core and surface antigens of the virus in woodchucks (WHV) with the comparable antigens of HBV. A close association between persistent WHV infection and PHC has also been found; DNA from WHV hybridized to the cellular DNA in five woodchuck livers containing PHC but did not hybridize to the DNA in nine livers without tumors. Finally, Summers and his colleagues have demonstrated integration of one or two WHV genomes into tumor-cell DNA in two woodchuck primary liver cancers. Integration appeared to occur at the same unique site in each cell of the tumor. Thus, each tumor was a clone with respect to the integrated viral DNA, a finding similar to that in humans.

Liver cancer in the woodchuck is not what is generally regarded as a laboratory model of a human disease, that is, it was not designed or 'created' by an investigator for research purposes; rather, it is a naturally occurring disease related to a naturally occurring virus, both of which have remarkable features in common with their human counterparts. It provides impressive support for the hypothesis (that persistent infection with hepatitis virus is required for the development of PHC) and also an opportunity to perform observations and studies with an other-than-human species.

2.9.2. Ground squirrel hepatitis virus

The Beechey ground squirrel (*Spermophilus beecheyi*) is a common mammal on the campus of Stanford University in California and a member of the *Squiridea* family, as are the *Marmota*. Marion, Robinson and their colleagues [25] found that the sera of many of these animals had HBsAg reactivity by solid-phase radioimmunoassay. All the sera with reactivity contained virus-like particles with DNA polymerase activity. They designated the virus as ground squirrel hepatitis virus (GSHV), by analogy with HBV, even though initially liver tropism was not shown. (Dead animals were not available for testing.) The particles were similar to the characteristic particles of HBV and WHV with some interesting differences. The elongated particles were more numerous, and their average length was significantly greater than HBV or WHV. There were also more large virion particles, and they were slightly smaller than Dane particles. Essentially all the sera containing viral particles also had endogenous DNA polymerase activity, whereas in humans only sera with both HBsAg and HBeAg have polymerase activity. The DNA is very similar in size and structure with the possible important difference that GSHV DNA has two cleavage sites for the restriction enzyme EcoRI, while HBV DNA and WHV DNA have only a single site.

There is significant cross-reactivity between the surface antigens of HBV and GSHV [25]. Appropriate anti-HBs antiserum can detect essentially all sera which contain GSHV. This implies that there must be closely related configurations of the surface antigen polypeptides. HBsAg has two polypeptide chains of sizes 25,000 and 29,000 daltons. They have nearly identical peptide compositions and similar primary sequences; and, all of the electrophoretic differences can probably be accounted for by the carbohydrate present on the larger but absent from the smaller polypeptide. GSHsAg has two polypeptides of 23,000 and 27,000 daltons, each slightly smaller than the equivalent HBsAg polypeptides; and they also have nearly identical peptide compositions. Gerlich *et al.* [26] suggested that the larger polypeptide of GSHsAg may differ from the smaller by a carbohydrate moiety. They estimated that about 10% less DNA sequence would be required for the 23,000 dalton GSHsAg than for the equivalent 25,000 dalton HBsAg polypeptide. About one third of the peptide spots of the 23,000 (P23) GSHsAg polypeptide are shared in common with the equivalent 25,000 (P25) HBsAg polypeptide, and about one-half of the spots of HBsAg P25 are shared with P23 polypeptide of GSHsAg. Peitelson *et al.* [27] report that the major GSHV core

Table 4. Characteristics of Icrons

	Virus			
	HBV	WHV	GSHV	DHBV
Particles				
Present in large quantities in blood	+	+	+	+
Virion structure double shell	+	+	+	+
Virion diameter, nm	40–45	40–45	47	40
Surface antigen particle, nm	20–25	20–25	18–20	35–60
Elongated surface antigen, length nm	>500	>500	>750	not seen
Core, nm	27	27	~27	27
Tryptophane/tyrosine ratios	high	?	high	?
Dna				
Circular	+	+	+	+
Double and single stranded	+	+	+	+
Dna polymerase	+	+	+	+
Nucleotides (number)	3150	3200	3200	3000
Homology with HBV, %	100	yes	yes	<10%
Ecori sites (number)	1	1	1	1
Antigens				
Surface (hbv, cross-reacting %)	HBsAg	WHsAg (0.1–1)	GSHsAg (large)	DHBsAg
Core (hbv, cross-reacting %)	HBcAg	WHcAg (5–10)	GSHcAg (large)	DHBcAg
e	+	+	?	?
Surface subtypes	Yes	?	?	?
Responses to infection				
Carrier state, % in populations	0.1–20	0–20	0–50	12%
Anti-surface antigen, % in population	anti-HBs 0–50	anti-WHs 25	?	?
Anti-core antigen, % in population	anti-HBc 0–60	anti-WHc	+	?
Anti-e antigen	+	?	+	?
Tropism	liver	liver	?	liver pancreas (?)
Clinical conditions				
Acute hepatitis	+	?	?	?
Chronic hepatitis	+	+	?	+
Cirrhosis	+	?	?	?
Primary hepatic carcinoma	+	+	?	+

polypeptide has 56% homology with its human counterpart as determined by comparing their respective tryptic peptide maps. This greater variability in surface antigen than in core antigens is also a feature of many other enveloped viruses. It generates the interesting concept that for a given genome viruses maintain a greater variability in the surfaces than internally, perhaps as a primary mechanism to restrict host species specificity and to allow for variation of immunological response within the members of the host species.

Cancer of the liver has not been reported in the ground squirrel.

2.9.3. Duck hepatitis B virus (DHBV)

In some regions of the People's Republic of China, where PHC is common in humans, it is also common in domesticated ducks [28]. Scientists in China suggested that the tumors in humans and ducks were caused by a chemical carcinogen in human food and in table scraps fed to domestic ducks. We hypothesized that the ducks were infected with an Icron. In collaboration with Dr. T.-T. Sun of Beijing, sera were obtained from farmyard ducks collected in Chitung County on the north bank of the Yangtze across from Shanghai City. A virus similar in appearance to HBV was seen in the sera of 11 of the 33 ducks [29]. Mason attempted to infect domesticated Pekin ducks (*Anas domesticus*) obtained from commercial breeders in the United States with this presumed virus (Figure 2). In doing so he found that the Pekin ducks were already infected with a virus similar to HBV and to the virus found in their Chinese cousins. (Pekin ducks were imported to America from China in the 19th century.) He and his colleagues found that sera from four of 12 Pekin ducks contained a DNA polymerase that incorporated nucleotide triphosphates into a DNA molecule similar to that found in HBV and WHV. The sera contained virus-like particles of about 40 nm in diameter, similar in appearance to the large virion particles of the other Icrons. Core particles could be separated from the whole virions, and these were similar in appearance and size to the core particles of the other viruses [30].

The DNA in the particles was circular, double and single stranded, and about the same size (3000 bp) as that of the other viruses. Particles which appeared to be analogous to the surface antigen particles of HBV were more heterogeneous in size and shape than the equivalent particles in HBV, WHV, and GSHV. They estimated by liquid hybridization methods that HBV and duck hepatitis B virus (DHBV, as it was called) to have less than 10% DNA homology. Analysis of the tissues of a DHBV infected duck showed most of the viral DNA in the liver. A smaller but significant amount was found in the pancreas. Of 219 ducks of different ages and sex tested, 26 (12%) had DHBV, and it was present about equally in both sexes and in all ages from 1 day to 14 months, suggesting congenital infection. O'Connell *et al.* [31] have found virus in the serum of embryos as early as 5 days of incubation and in the yolk of unincubated eggs. This suggests that in ducks infection of the embryo by the dam may be the major mechanism of virus transmission. Preliminary reports from China indicate that the DHBV is associated with the cancer of the liver found in the ducks.

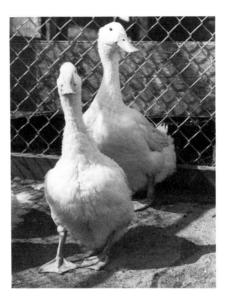

Figure 2. Anas domesticus (Pekin duck).

3. Strategies for primary prevention

Our interpretation of these nine lines of evidence is that, taken together, they strongly support the hypothesis that persistent infection with HBV is required for the development of most cases of PHC, and therefore that the next step is warranted: testing of the hypothesis that decreasing the frequency of HBV infection will in due course decrease the frequency of PHC. The availability of the hepatitis B vaccine produced from HBsAg in human blood [3] and increasing knowledge of the mechanisms of transmission of HBV will make such a study feasible. Since the incidence of cancer is high in HBV carriers, it may be possible to measure the effect of the program within a reasonable time. In any case, independent of its relation to cancer, the control of HBV infection is clearly justified as a public health measure for the prevention of acute and chronic hepatitis and post-necrotic cirrhosis, diseases of major importance in the same regions where PHC is common.

The exact strategies to be used in the forthcoming public health programs will be determined as more experience is gained with the hepatitis B vaccine and the knowledge of the methods of transmission and the natural history of HBV increases. The vaccine appears to be effective in producing antibodies in very young children including newborns. Even though children may be exposed to the virus *in utero* and in early childhood when their mothers (or, less commonly, other family members) are carriers, they do not become persistently infected until about six weeks to two months after birth. In countries of high endemicity a very large percentage of carriers are a consequence of maternal transmission. A program in which vaccine is administered before one to three months might, therefore, in a single generation considerably decrease the frequency of carriers. Infection at an early age is associated with a higher probability of becoming a carrier, while infection in later life is more likely to result in the development of anti-HBs. Hence, even if the vaccination program is not able to completely eliminate infection, if it can be delayed beyond childhood and early growth, it could still have a marked effect on decreasing the frequency of carriers and increasing immunity in the population.

3.1. Intrafamily transmission

In areas of high HBV endemicity, transmission within the family group is extremely important and is likely to lead to the carrier state. We have started a series of family studies, including ethological observations on newborn children and their carrier mothers, to observe behaviors which might increase the probability of infection. The initial family observations have been made in West Africa and in the New Hebrides, areas with a high frequency of hepatitis infection and where traditional living patterns are still followed to a large extent. This may allow us to identify personal sanitation and health practices within the context of the culture which increase the probability of infection. From this, recommendations for simple preventive measures acceptable by the community may be made.

3.2. Insect transmission

There is considerable evidence that mosquitoes and bedbugs can transmit hepatitis. Several species of mosquitoes collected in areas where hepatitis is common in human populations carry the virus. Over 60% of bedbugs captured in beds whose main occupants are hepatitis carriers also carry the virus. The virus may persist in the infected bedbug for up to about five weeks after a single feeding on blood containing hepatitis virus. HBsAg can also be found in the feces of the bedbug up to five weeks after a feeding. The long-term persistence of the virus in an environment, the bed, in which transmission can occur from one person to another, may provide an important mechanism for the maintenance of the infection within families.

Bedbugs and mosquitoes can be controlled by the use of appropriate insecticides and also by traditional and environmental methods not requiring chemicals. Insect-borne infection may be a major mechanism for transmission of virus from a carrier mother (or other family member) to a young child; and, as already said, this is a particularly vulnerable period when carriers may develop. Control of virus-carrying insects, therefore, may have a particularly important impact on the control of chronic liver disease and PHC. There is an additional curious aspect of insect transmission. They may provide a mechanism for transmitting viruses from domestic and wild animals that are close to humans, and since these may contain genetic and other characteristics of their hosts, it may provide a means for the transmission of genetic information between species that are phylogenetically distant but physically proximate.

There are many methods by which hepatitis may be transmitted, which also means that there are many methods by which control can be effected. The use of the vaccine as well as other preventive measures may markedly decrease the high incidence of carriers. If this is so, it can be predicted that, in due course, the incidence of PHC will decrease.

4. A cellular model for primary hepatocellular carcinoma

The relation between HBV and PHC now allows the study of the role of a virus in the pathogenesis of a human tumor. Sufficient information is now available to propose a working model for the virus-cancer relation. A model developed for heuristic purposes should explain all the known data about the phenomenon it is designed to image and have an interesting character that will generate exciting experiments. (Copernicus also added that it should be elegant.) The model starts with the assumption that all (or nearly all) cases of PHC have been infected with HBV; and this was the conclusion arrived at from the hypothesis testing described in the first part of this paper. The observations which have to be accounted for in the model include the following.

1) There is a long incubation period (~20 to 40 years) between the time of infection with HBV and the development of PHC.

2) More males than females develop PHC.

3) HBV is required for the development of diseases in addition to PHC (i.e. acute hepatitis, chronic liver diseases, the carrier state, etc.).

4) In the livers of people with PHC, whole virus, HBsAg and HBcAg appear to occur more commonly and in larger amounts in the cells which have not undergone malignant transformation than in the cells which have.

The model should also explain several other features of HBV infection not directly associated with cancer.

5) The fetus and newborn children (say within the first six weeks) of carrier mothers do not produce HBV even though exposed to virus *in utero*, at the time of birth, and immediately thereafter.

6) Very young children (after about two months and before 10 years) are more likely to become chronic carriers if infected than adults, who are more likely to develop acute hepatitis.

The classical model of viral carcinogenesis indicates that the nucleic acid of the viral agent is integrated into the genome of the host target cell. This genetic

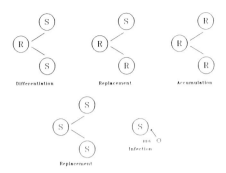

Figure 3. R cells are resistant and S cells susceptible to productive infection with HBV. R cells are less differentiated than S cells. When R cells divide they can produce additional R cells and/or S cells, but S cells can produce only other S cells.

integration results in an alteration of cell characteristics, and malignant transformation occurs. Recent observations have resulted in a modified model in which viral DNA integrates at a site adjacent to a host gene which then directs the process of transformation (promoter insertion). These models explain the process by which a cell becomes a cancer cell, but they do not deal in detail with the emergence of clinical cancer nor with the characteristics listed at the beginning of this section which pertain, in particular, to cancer of the liver.

The model we propose posits the existence of two kinds of liver cells. 1) The S cell, which is susceptible to persistent productive infection (i.e. it produces whole virus, HBsAg particles, etc.) with the expression of viral characteristics within the cell and on its surface. 2) The R cell, which is resistant to persistent productive infection.

This notion had been discussed in our laboratory for several years when in 1980 London introduced the concept that the R cells are immature, less differentiated cells and S cells are fully differentiated, i.e. a characteristic of liver cell maturation is its increased susceptibility to persistent productive infection with HBV. R cells are more likely to divide and when they do so can produce 1) two R cells, 2) one S and one R cell or 3) two S cells. The more differentiated and mature S cells, do not divide often. When they do divide, they produce only other S cells (Figure 3). The fetus and newborns have mostly R cells; at about six weeks to three months there are more S cells and in adulthood nearly all S cells (Figure 4), but some R cells nearly always persist. We will return to the significance of this later.

Productive chronic infection of S cells with HBV leads to slow death of the cells both as a consequence of the response of the host's cellular and serological immune system to the expression of HBV on the surface of the infected cell and the interference with the S cell's metabolism as a consequence of massive viral infection. In the liver, the stimulus for cells to divide is the death of other cells, in

86

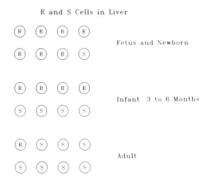

Figure 4. There are few S cells in the undifferentiated fetus and newborn infants, but these increase with time. Adults have mostly S cells.

contrast to, say, the skin where there is constant division and formation of new cells. Hence, in a liver chronically infected with HBV there is continuous cell death and cell regeneration. The death is primarily of S cells, while the R cells, stimulated by the deaths around them, continue to divide producing both R and S cells; the selective balance is tipped in favor of the R cells (Figure 5). Thus, in individuals with persistent HBV infection there would be continuous cell death and continuous cell regeneration. If this process continues long enough, the pathological conditions of chronic active hepatitis and postnecrotic cirrhosis will ensue. Because HBV selectively affects S cells, the S cell population would gradually dwindle, and the R cell population would gradually expand.

If the HBV DNA is integrated into host S cell DNA, and/or if another carcinogenic event occurs in an S cell, it will not be of long lasting consequence because, in due course, the S cells are likely to die. If, however, integration occurs in R cells and/or another carcinogen (i.e. aflatoxin, nitrosamines, etc.) causes transformation (Figure 6), there will be important consequences. The R cells are at a selective advantage relative to the S cells; the numbers of transformed R cells will increase and a clinically perceived cancer will develop if there is uncontrolled division of R cells to form only other R cells.

Since the R cells are continually dividing in response to continuing S cell death, the probability of a transformation event is high. If the death of S cells is slowed or stopped by the control of the HBV infection, then the growth of the cancer may be halted and regression of small cancers may occur if the R cells are no longer at a selective advantage.

This model can explain phenomena not directly related to cancer (items 5 and 6 above). In a fetus or newborn there are very few S cells; hence, if the rare S cells are infected they will die and the infection will quickly terminate since there are few additional susceptible cells (Figure 7). Later in life (after about six weeks) there are a larger number of S cells in which infection may be perpetuated after

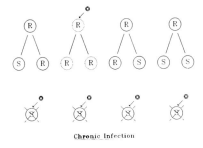

Chronic Infection

Figure 5. Chronic infection of S cells results in death, which may be slow. The R cells are not killed and their numbers increase relative to the S cells. The HBV DNA may integrate into R cells host DNA and transformation may occur (dotted circles). Transformation may also be related to other carcinogens (i.e. aflatoxin, nitrosamines).

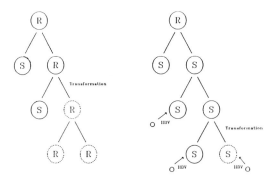

Figure 6. Transformation of R cells can lead to tumors. Normal and transformed S cells will die if infected by HBV.

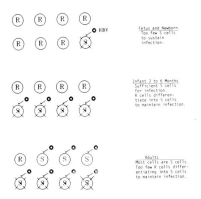

Figure 7. Infection in fetus and newborn infants and adults.

the death of the initially infected cells. There are also sufficient R cells which can divide to provide additional S cells, and a persistent carrier state or chronic hepatitis can ensue. The nature of the liver damage will depend on the extent and nature of the host response to the infected cells. As already noted, the cycles of dying, scarring and regenerating of new cells result in the pathological features of post-hepatic cirrhosis. If an adult is infected with HBV, the S cells will die, but there will not be sufficient R cells to generate new S cells sufficiently rapidly to replace those that were killed. Hence, acute infections are more common in adults.

As long as there are sufficient numbers of R cells from which new liver cells are rejuvenated, liver function will be maintained. In heavy infection, with the death of many S cells, the R cells may be the main supplier of liver function. This may explain the clinical observation that cancer of the liver is often seen in patients with only minimal or moderate liver dysfunction. This results in an apparent anachronism; the R cells, including the transformed R cells, provide liver function until they become so numerous as to destroy the host.

In humans, men are much more likely to develop cirrhosis and PHC than women, even though male and female babies and children are equally exposed to HBV carrier mothers and siblings. Several studies have shown that males are more likely than females to develop persistent infection with HBV [32, 33, 34, 35] and among individuals classified as having persistent infection, females are more likely than males to clear the infection [36]. That is, the male-female difference in risk of cirrhosis and PHC may be accounted for by a greater ability of women to prevent or overcome persistent infection with HBV.

5. Consequences of the model

We are now testing this model and in due course we will know if it is supported or rejected. There are several very interesting consequences of the model which can be acted upon if it is supported. The model is based on cellular development and explains phenomena of maturation, benign infection with hepatitis virus (the carrier state), acute and chronic hepatitis, and cancer. There is no factor that is found uniquely in the cancer cases that cannot be found in conditions without clinical cancer.

The model also suggests an approach to cancer therapy different from that usually used. Most conventional therapies are directed towards the total destruction of cancer cells, even though in the process normal tissues may be damaged or killed which often limits the application of the treatment. The model just described suggests that an effort should be made to enhance the selective advantage of the S cells, i.e. to foster the viability of the noncancerous cells so that they may increase their numbers and prevent the continued growth of tumors.

6. Prevention

The information now available allows us to proceed to test the feasibility of two of the three forms of prevention described in the introduction. The availability of the vaccine and our growing knowledge of transmission and epidemiology of HBV allow the design and execution of strategies for primary prevention by diminishing or eliminating infection, particularly in early childhood.

There are now large populations of southeast Asians in the United States, and many of them are in Philadelphia. We are developing plans to screen volunteers, identify HBV carriers and follow the latter to determine if any develop increases in their alpha fetoproteins (AFP). Chinese investigators, using only AFP testing, have reported that early tumors can be detected in this manner and that their removal increases survival [37]. We will try to determine if this approach is improved by the use of both HBV and AFP screening (also see Chapter 1).

The model, if supported, could lead to an understanding of how prevention by delay might be effected. Methods for delaying integration or for decreasing the deadly infection of S cells might result in a sufficient delay to spare the carriers from cancer during their lifetime, and studies on this problem are now in progress.

Acknowledgements

This paper is adapted from a General Motors Research Foundation publication.

This work was supported by USPHS grants CA-06551, RR-05539, CA-22780 and CA-06927 from the National Institutes of Health and by an appropriation from the Commonwealth of Pennsylvania.

References

1. London WT: Primary hepatocellular carcinoma – etiology, pathogenesis and prevention. Human Pathol 12: 1085–1097, 1981.
2. Blumberg BS, Larouze B, London WT, Werner B, Hesser JE, Millman I, Saimot G, Payet M: The relation of infection with the hepatitis B agent to primary hepatic carcinoma. Am J Pathol 81: 669–682, 1975.
3. Blumberg BS, Millman I: Vaccine against viral hepatitis and process. Serial No. 864,788 filed 10/8/69, Patent 36 36 191 issued 1/18/72, US Patent Office.
4. Blumberg BS, London WT: Hepatitis B virus and primary hepatocellular carcinoma: Relationship of 'Icrons' to cancer. In: Viruses in naturally occurring cancers, Essex M, Todaro G, zur Hausen H (eds). Cold Spring Harbor Conferences on Cell Proliferation, Vol 7, Cold Spring Harbor Laboratory, 1980, p 401–421.
5. Prince AM: Round table discussion: prophylaxis/vaccination. In: Virus and the liver, Bianchi L, Sickinger K, Gerok W, Stalder GA (eds). Lancaster, England: MTP Press, Ltd., 1980, p 399–402.

90

6. Nayak NC, Dhark A, Sachdeva R, Mittal A, Seth HN, Sudarsanam D, Reddy B, Wagholikar UL, Reddy CRRM: Association of human hepatocellular carcinoma and cirrhosis with hepatitis B virus surface and core antigens in the liver. Int J Cancer 20: 643–654, 1977.

7. Omata M, Ashcavi M, Liew C-T, Peters RL: Hepatocellular carcinoma in the USA, etiologic considerations: localization of hepatitis B antigens. Gastroenterology 76: 279–287, 1979.

8. Beasley RP, Lin C-C, Hwang L-Y, Chien C-S: Hepatocellular carcinoma and hepatitis B virus. A prospective study of 22707 men in Taiwan. Lancet 2: 1129–1133, 1981.

9. Obata H, Hayashi N, Motoike Y, Hisamits T, Okuda H, Kubayash S, Nishioka K: A prospective study on the development of hepatocellular carcinoma from liver cirrhosis with persistent hepatitis B virus infection. Int J Cancer 25: 741–747, 1980.

10. Larouze B, London WT, Saimot G, Werner BG, Lustbader ED, Payet M, Blumberg BS: Host responses to hepatitis B infection in patients with primary hepatic carcinoma and their families. A case/control study in Senegal, West Africa. Lancet 2: 534–538, 1976.

11. Summers J, O'Connell A, Maupas P, Goudeau A, Coursaget P, Drucker J: Hepatitis B virus DNA in primary hepatocellular carcinoma tissue. J Med Virol 2: 207–214, 1978.

12. London WT: Observations on hepatoma. In: Viral hepatitis, Vyas GN, Cohen SN, Schmid R (eds). Philadelphia: Franklin Institute Press, 1978, p 455–458.

13. Macnab GM, Alexander JJ, Lecatsas G, Bey EM, Urbanowicz JM: Hepatitis B surface antigen produced by a human hepatoma cell line. Br J Cancer 34: 509–515, 1976.

14. Skelley J, Copeland JA, Howard CR, Zuckerman AJ: Hepatitis B surface antigen produced by a human hepatoma cell line. Nature 282: 617–618, 1979.

15. Marion PL, Robinson WS: Hepatitis B virus and hepatocellular carcinoma. In: Viruses in naturally occurring cancers, Essex M, Todaro G, zur Hausen H (eds). Cold Spring Harbor Conferences on Cell Proliferation, Vol 7, Cold Spring Harbor Laboratory, 1980, p 423–434.

16. Gray P, Edman JC, Valenzuela P, Goodman HM, Rutter WJ: A human hepatoma cell line contains hepatitis B DNA and RNA sequences. J Supramolec Struc 14: Suppl 4: 245, 1980.

17. Brechot C, Pourcel C, Louise A, Rain B, Tiollais P: Presence of integrated hepatitis B virus DNA sequences in cellular DNA of human hepatocellular carcinoma. Nature 286: 533–534, 1980.

18. Knowles BB, Howe CC, Aden DP: Human hepatocellular carcinoma cell lines secrete the major plasma proteins and hepatitis B surface antigen. Science 209: 497–499, 1980.

19. Shafritz DA, Shouval D, Sherman HI, Hadziyannis SJ, Kew MC: Integration of hepatitis B virus DNA into the genome of liver cells in chronic liver disease and hepatocellular carcinoma. New Engl J Med 305: 1067–1073, 1981.

20. Blumberg BS, Millman I, Sutnick AI, London WT: The nature of Australia antigen and its relation to antigen-antibody complex formation. J Exp Med 134: 320–329, 1971.

21. Snyder RL, Ratcliffe HL: Marmota monax: A model for studies of cardiovascular, cerebravascular and neoplastic disease. Acta Zool Path Antv 48: 265–273, 1969.

22. Snyder RL, Summers J: Woodchuck hepatitis virus and hepatocellular carcinoma. In: Viruses in naturally occurring cancers, Essex M, Todaro G, zur Hausen H (eds). Cold Spring Harbor Conferences on Cell Proliferation, Vol 7, Cold Spring Harbor Laboratory, 1980, p 447–458.

23. Summers J, Smolec JM, Snyder R: A virus similar to human hepatitis B virus associated hepatitis and hepatoma in woodchucks. Proc Natl Acad Sci (USA) 75: 4533–4537, 1978.

24. Werner BG, Smolec JM, Snyder R, Summers J: Serological relationship of woodchuck hepatitis virus to human hepatitis B virus. J Virol 32: 314–322, 1979.

25. Marion PL, Oshiro LS, Regnery DC, Scullard GH, Robinson WS: A virus in Beechey ground squirrels that is related to hepatitis B virus of humans. Proc Natl Acad Sci (USA) 77: 2941–2945, 1980.

26. Gerlich WH, Feitelson MA, Marion PL, Robinson WS: Structural relationships between the surface antigens of ground squirrel hepatitis virus and human hepatitis B virus. J Virol 36: 787–795, 1980.

27. Feitelson MA, Marion PL, Robinson WS: Core particles of hepatitis B virus and ground squirrel hepatitis virus. J Virol 687–696, 1982.
28. Kaplan HS, Tsuchitani PJ: In: Cancer in China, New York: Alan R Liss Inc., 1978.
29. Summers J, London WT, Sun T-T, Blumberg BS, in preparation.
30. Mason WS, Seal G, Summers J: Virus of Pekin ducks with structural and biological relatedness to human hepatitis B virus. J. Virol 36: 829–836, 1980.
31. O'Connell A, Urban M, London WT: Naturally occurring infection of Pekin duck embryos by duck hepatitis B virus. Proc Natl Acad Sci (USA), in press, 1983.
32. London WT, Drew JS: Sex differences in response to hepatitis B infection among patients receiving chronic dialysis treatment. Proc Natl Acad Sci (USA) 74: 2561–2563, 1977.
33. Szmuness W, Harley EJ, Ikram H, Stevens CE: Sociodemographic aspects of the epidemiology of hepatitis B. In: Viral hepatitis, Vyas GN, Cohen SN, Schmid R (eds). Philadelphia: Franklin Institute Press, 1978, p 297–319.
34. Blumberg BS, Sutnick AI, London WT, Melartin L: Sex distribution of Australia antigen. Arch Intern Med 130: 227–231, 1972.
35. Blumberg BS: I. History. II. Parental responses to HBV infection and the secondary sex ratio of the offspring. Sex differences in response to hepatitis B virus. Arthritis and Rheumatism 22: 1261–1266, 1979.
36. Goodman M, Wainwright RL, Weir HF, Gall JC: A sex difference in the carrier state of Australia (hepatitis associated) antigen. Pediatrics 48: 907–913, 1971.
37. Tang Z, Yang B, Tang C, Yu Y, Lin Z, Weng H: Evaluation of population screening for hepatocellular carcinoma. Chinese Med J 93: 795–799, 1980.

5. Liver resection for malignant disease

JAMES H. FOSTER

1. Introduction

In the last decade, liver resection for tumor has become an operation which can be done safely by many surgeons. As more experience has accumulated, our understanding of the results which may be achieved has matured and we know better which patients may profit from liver resection for either primary or secondary liver cancer.

It was not always so. During many preceding decades, liver cancer was considered incurable and major liver resection was often a lethal event, even in the major cancer centers. A few pioneers persisted in attempting liver resection for tumor, but because resectable tumors were so rarely found, no single surgeon or group developed much experience. In the more recent past, the lessons of trauma have taught us how to resect liver more safely, and the extensive experience of Asian surgeons with primary liver cancer has led the way to more interest in the United States and Western Europe in liver resection for tumor.

A few centers in this country have done as many as 50 or more resections for tumor in the last ten years, and the experience of many other centers with less volume has also been collected and reviewed. We know more about the natural history of both primary and secondary liver cancers, we are better at distinguishing benign from malignant tumors, and we know better what can be expected from therapies other than resection.

This review will attempt to outline available clinical data which address the questions about whether and when to resect liver for tumor. Based on these data and on a moderate personal clinical experience, the author will conclude with some arbitrary recommendations for patient selection and for the technique of resection.

J.J. DeCosse and P. Sherlock (eds), Clinical Management of Gastrointestinal Cancer.
© *1984, Martinus Nijhoff Publishers, Boston. ISBN 0-89838-601-2. Printed in The Netherlands.*

2. Natural history and the results of non-resectional therapy

An argument for liver resection for cancer must be supported by evidence that resection brings with its attendant dangers some superiority over other therapies and over the natural history of patients with untreated disease. Too often, in our desire to do something for a patient, we forget the first law of therapeutics, which is to do no harm. Anesthesia, operation, chemotherapy, and radiation have all been shown to reduce immunocompetence in the experimental animal. When a patient has established some sort of limited balance with his tumor, we may alter this balance unfavorably or favorably with our treatments.

The mean survival after the diagnosis of primary liver cancer in untreated adult patients is listed in most reviews as 2 to 6 months, with two-year survival being a distinct rarity. This dismal prognosis seems particularly true of the patients from high-incidence areas such as Africa and Southeast Asia where cancer is most often superimposed on non-malignant diffuse liver disease. However, the picture may not be as unhappy in Western countries, especially when primary liver cancer (PLC) occurs in a non-cirrhotic liver. Several long survivors have been reported without treatment and, in one series of 53 patients who eventually died of their disease after a liver resection, the mean survival was 24 months and four patients lived more than 5 years [1].

The histologic variant of PLC recently described by Craig *et al.* [2] and Berman *et al.* [3] and variously called 'fibrolamellar' or 'polygonal cell with fibrous stroma' carries with it a particularly good prognosis – both for cure after resection and for long survival with residual disease with or without resection. Although most PLC's are large when they are discovered, the tumor has a remarkable tendency to grow locally in the liver before metastasizing. In a review of 748 autopsied patients only 52% of the patients who died of PLC had extra-hepatic metastasis at the time of death [1].

Table 1. Natural history of patients with liver metastases from colorectal primary tumors

		Survival after diagnosis of liver metastases		
	Number of patients	Stage	Survival (mos) Mean	1 year survival
Wood *et al.* [5]	15	Solitary	16.7	60%
	11	Localized	10.6	27%
	87	Widespread	3.1	6.%
Pettavel and Morganthaler [6]	12	Minimal	21.5	
	41	Moderate	6.9	
	30	Widespread	1.4	
Blumgart and Allison [7]	15	Solitary		38%
	13	Localized		45%
	76	Widespread		14%

Pediatric patients with PLC who are not cured by resection do poorly. Ninety percent of 76 patients dying with hepatoblastoma and 80% of 82 patients dying with hepatocellular carcinoma were dead within 12 months of diagnosis as reported by Exelby in a series of pediatric patients, and two-year survival with disease was very unusual [4]. Only four of 37 pediatric patients from another series who eventually died of their disease after liver resection survived as long as two years, and they died at 32, 38, 27, and 36 months [1]. Little or no palliation was achieved in either series by radiotherapy or chemotherapy.

As experience with resectional and non-resectional therapy matures, specific data about the survival of patients with cancer metastatic to their liver have become very important in recent years. Retrospective and historic controls are not as acceptable as they were a decade ago; yet we still have no current acceptable data on the survival in prospective trials of untreated control patients. Such data is badly needed. Table 1 lists some of the reported survival data for untreated patients with liver metastases from retrospective reviews. It is very important to note that untreated patients with limited (i.e., potentially resectable) metastases from colorectal carcinoma usually live more than 1 year *without* resection or other therapy. Information about long survival of patients with liver metastases from other metastatic sites is anecdotal. Patients with melanoma and leiomyosarcomas are particularly prone to long survival without therapy, and resection has not yet been shown to improve the prognosis of patients with these uncommon tumors.

3. Diagnostic aids

Human liver tumors are found because they cause symptoms, because of screening programs for populations at high risk, and, to an increasing extent, because modern radiologic techniques such as ultrasonography, radionuclide scanning, and computerized axial tomography are uncovering evidence of mass lesions in the liver of asymptomatic patients.

3.1. History and physical

If symptoms or signs suggest the presence of cancer in the liver, it is often late in the disease. Most patients with resectable disease will be asymptomatic and their lesions will be discovered because a mass is palpated or an astute (or lucky) physician will have ordered a laboratory test. Pain, weight loss, or paraneoplastic syndromes may draw attention to a primary liver cancer. Routine follow-up studies such as alkaline phosphatase, liver scintiscanning, or CEA determinations will uncover a resectable liver metastasis more often than will clinical symptoms.

About 10–15% of primary liver cancers will present with intraperitoneal hemorrhage. If a patient with cirrhosis has bloody ascites, the diagnosis is primary liver cancer until proven otherwise. A careful search should be made in taking the medical history for associated factors such as exposure to aflatoxin, vinyl chloride, thorotrast, arsenic, and alcohol, or for evidence of cirrhosis, alpha-1-antitrypsin deficiency, and those factors associated with hepatitis; e.g., shellfish, drug abuse, contaminated water, blood transfusions, etc. Although birth control pills have been associated with PLC in several case reports, there is yet no verified cause-and-effect relationship. However, oral contraceptive agents have been closely related to the incidence of benign liver cell adenomas. Resectable PLC below age 50, focal nodular hyperplasia, and liver cell adenomas are more common in menstrual age females in the United States of America; [1] hence these lesions should be carefully sought when vague upper abdominal complaints are cause for concern.

3.2. Blood tests

Of the liver function tests commonly performed, the alkaline phosphatase and SGOT are the most often abnormal with liver tumors, although the infrequently performed bromsulphalein retention is more sensitive. None is specific for neoplasia. Erythrocytosis, hypercalcemia, and various endocrine symptoms are occasionally seen with PLC and may be present even if the tumor is small. Alpha-fetoprotein is the most specific blood test for PLC. It is extremely useful in screening populations at high risk and in following both the course of the disease as well as in the differential diagnosis of liver masses. Patients with several benign conditions and extra-hepatic neoplasms may show minor elevations of alpha-fetoprotein, but about 80% of pediatric and adult patients with primary hepatocellular carcinoma will have elevations of alpha-fetoprotein above 30 ng/ml.

Screening populations for alpha-fetoprotein has been very useful in the diagnosis of primary liver cancer in asymptomatic Chinese patients. For example, resection was possible in56% of patients whose diagnosis of PLC was made by alpha-fetoprotein screening but in only 18% of patients with a symptomatic presentation. One-year survival was 64% in screened cases and 15% in the clinically symptomatic. Three-year survival was 62% in the screened patients who were resected [8]. Most of these patients can be presumed to be cured permanently after three disease-free years of close follow-up.

The CEA has limited specificity. It is perhaps most useful in the diagnosis of recurrent colorectal carcinoma. Tartter et al. correlated alkaline phosphatase and CEA determinations with operative findings in patients with primary bowel cancer, and found that if the CEA was greater than 10 ng/dl and the alkaline phosphatase was above 135 international units, there was only a 2% false-negative rate in the detection of liver metastases [9].

3.3. Ultrasonography, scintiscanning, and radiographic aids to diagnosis

Ultrasonography, radionuclide scintiscanning, computerized tomography, and angiography all have an important place in the differential diagnosis of liver masses and in determination of resectability.

The only primary liver cancer that is often cystic is the very rare cystadenocarcinoma, and this can usually be differentiated by ultrasonography from the echo-free simple cyst and the occasionally more complex echinococcal cyst. Cystadenoma and cystadenocarcinoma usually have multiple loculations with thick walls. All of the benign and malignant solid liver tumors fail to pick up technetium 99 sulfur colloid, although focal nodular hyperplasia will occasionally retain enough reticuloendothelial function to be 'warm' on a scintiscan.

The problem with scintiscanning is that it will often miss lesions of 2 cm or less in diameter. Most primary malignant tumors, liver abscesses, and metastatic tumors will pick up Gallium. Computerized axial tomography is more accurate than radionuclide scintiscanning in diagnosing the size and number of liver tumors, but it must depend on differences in tissue density. Contrast enhancement may help or may actually obscure lesions seen before injection of contrast. Metastatic lesions or primary tumors with necrosis and hemorrhage are more likely to be outlined by computerized tomography than are liver cell adenomas and primary hepatocellular carcinomas because, without necrosis, these primary tumors may be of the same density as normal liver.

Selective arteriography is the most invasive, most expensive, and probably the most accurate of the preoperative tests available. It will usually differentiate hemangioma from other tumors. Hepatocellular carcinoma, liver cell adenoma, and focal nodular hyperplasia are usually hypervascular, whereas benign cysts, cholangiocarcinoma, and most metastatic lesions are usually hypovascular. Exceptions to this rule are provided by the vascular metastases from endocrine tumors, melanoma, and leiomyosarcoma. Inferior vena cavography may be useful to determine resectability by demonstrating involvement of the cava or tumor growth from the hepatic veins into the inferior vena cava at the level of the diaphragm. A characteristic pattern of spread for primary hepatocellular carcinoma in both children and adults is growth of the tumor down the portal vein or up into the hepatic veins and eventually into the inferior vena cava.

3.4. Tactics in diagnosis

If the history and physical examination raise the suspicion of liver tumor, the patient should have alkaline phosphatase, SGOT, hepatitis B surface antigen, and alpha-fetoprotein determinations. Ultrasonography and scintiscanning should be done next, with preference of the echogram for a suspected cystic lesion and the scintiscan for a solid lesion. Angiography and computerized tomography are the best tests to diagnose hemangiomas before biopsy. Whether scintiscans or computerized tomograms will prove to be the better way to demonstrate liver metastases remains to be proven, but probably neither is indicated to follow a patient with potential liver metastases unless the alkaline phosphatase or CEA is elevated or there are clinical factors which raise suspicion for liver disease. All patients in whom resection of a significant part of the liver is planned should have preliminary angiography to outline the vascular anatomy.

Before liver resection for carcinoma is undertaken, there are two critical factors which must be assessed. A tissue diagnosis should be made and resectability must be determined. What about needle biopsy? At most sites, this is a useful tool; but it is to be discouraged with liver tumors unless it will provide data which will rule out laparotomy entirely. Needle biopsy is very dangerous with hemangiomas and echinococcal cysts and is relatively dangerous with the hypervascular benign and malignant primary tumors. Needle biopsy of focal nodular hyperplasia may be read by a pathologist as cirrhosis, and a small needle core of tissue from a liver cell adenoma will probably yield a histologic diagnosis of normal liver. Laparoscopy may provide a middle ground by providing evidence about tumor geography and allowing safe needle biopsy under direct vision.

Short of total hepatectomy with transplantation, resectability depends on the lack of evidence of tumor spread beyond the capsule of the liver and on evidence that the tumor does not involve the inferior vena cava or the hilar structures sufficiently to preclude preservation of both inflow and outflow vessels to a sufficient liver remnant. The tests mentioned above may be most helpful; but, more often than not in borderline situations, only full laparotomy with bimanual palpation – usually after the division of some of the suspensory ligaments – will provide evidence sufficient to rule in or rule out resection with certainty. There is no preoperative test which replaces the information which can be perceived by the eyes and through the fingertips of a skilled surgeon. Even smaller tumors deep in the right lobe can usually be found by careful palpation. Specific criteria which preclude resection for various cancers will be mentioned later.

4. Non-resectional therapy

In spite of more than two decades of chemotherapy for both primary and secondary liver cancers, it is still not possible to document an increase in survival of patients so treated. Proponents have touted systemic and then regional applications of chemotherapy with single and multiple drug regimens. Ingenious devices and techniques have been developed to provide continuous arterial perfusion in a home setting, but no well-controlled data have yet appeared which demonstrates superiority of any of these treatments over the natural history of untreated patients with comparable amounts of disease. Comparison of the survival of patients who respond to chemotherapy with those who do not (i.e., 'responders' versus 'non-responders') is as illegitimate as the calculation of a baseball player's batting average by comparing his good days with his bad. A thorough exposition of the data which supports these negative conclusions is beyond the realm of a chapter on liver resection, but the reader is referred to a well-planned prospective trial of systemic versus regional chemotherapy supported by the Central Oncology Group [10] and to a recent monograph on metastatic liver disease [11].

Radiotherapy may provide limited palliation but also has not been shown to increase survival for patients with PLC or with secondary liver cancer. Yttrium spheres and I-131 labeled ferritin have been aimed at liver cancer with some reported success, but survival has not yet been shown to exceed that of untreated patients. Hepatic artery ligation often results in dramatic shrinkage of primary and secondary liver tumors, but return of the arterial supply to the tumor can be documented within a few weeks, and regrowth of the tumor follows along quickly thereafter. The many combinations of ligation, perfusion, and radiation which have been tried are testimony to the unsuccessful results of each therapeutic method alone as well as to the energy and imagination of the investigators, but more than this cannot be claimed at the present time [11].

There are examples where combination therapy has been successful. The embryonal tumors of children provide an excellent example of chemotherapy with resection which has resulted in cure of patients who even have had tumor-spread beyond the capsule of the liver. There are occasional liver tumors which respond to chemotherapy or to hormone manipulation; but, unfortunately, the common varieties of primary liver cancer and metastatic liver disease from the common primary sites such as colon and rectum, lung, stomach, pancreas, kidney, esophagus, and breast rarely respond favorably to the chemotherapeutic agents available today. It is hoped that the pediatric experience may prove to be a model for the future and that resection, chemotherapy, and perhaps radiation can combine to afford many, if not most, patients with primary and secondary liver cancer a chance of cure or significant palliation.

In the meantime, until so-called palliative therapy can be shown to improve the quality or quantity of survival of incurable patients in properly controlled trials, it seems prudent to advise against therapy in asymptomatic patients with unresectable primary or secondary liver cancer. An important exception would be made if those patients could be part of an adequately structured controlled patient trial which would include untreated patients with comparable amounts of disease. The treatment of patients with symptomatic but unresectable liver cancer is more in the realm of art than science. Symptoms usually occur late with liver cancer and, particularly with metastatic disease, survival is usually brief after symptoms occur. Death from liver failure is often reasonably comfortable and follows soon after the onset of jaundice or pain whatever the therapy.

5. The role of resection

How often will a primary or secondary liver cancer be resectable? Are there standard criteria by which to determine resectability? Can resection be done safely? Finally, if a patient survives liver resection for cancer, will significant palliation and/or cure result? Some of these questions can be partially answered on the basis of well-documented recent experience. The questions of resectability, operative morbidity and mortality, and the results achieved by resection of specific tumors are considered separately.

5.1. Resectability

The question of resectability depends on the definition of the word. For our purposes, it means removal of all gross tumor without the assumption of a high operative risk. This chapter excludes total hepatectomy with transplantation or operative maneuvers requiring vessel reconstruction and/or extracorporeal circuits. Our definition usually implies curative intent and thus excludes palliative resection, although one may be indicated occasionally.

Two decades ago, even anatomic lobectomy was fraught with technical dangers and followed by considerable postoperative morbidity and mortality. Metabolic problems were common and hospitalizations were long. Today, with better anesthesia, improved operative techniques, and better post-operative monitoring and support, we can resect up to three-quarters of the mass of the liver without serious metabolic derangement. Our prior troubles were due more to blood loss, hypotension, massive transfusion, sepsis, and late hemorrhage caused by faulty technique than to 'liver failure'. The liver has a remarkable (although still not clearly understood) ability to undergo rapid hypertrophy and hyperplasia when more than 30–40% of its functional volume has been removed. The requirement for metabolic support does not usually exceed ten days even with subtotal resection in uncomplicated cases. Remember, too, that when a surgeon removes 2500 g of tissue for a liver cancer, the uninvolved liver has already hypertrophied before resection, and most of what is removed is tumor and not functional liver. Currently, the resectability of a solitary mass usually depends upon the involvement of the portal structures where they come together at the liver hilum and/or involvement of the out-flow vessels (hepatic veins) near the inferior vena cava.

Does the presence of multiple nodules contribute to unresectability if those nodules do not involve liver hilum or inferior vena cava? Not, perhaps, in the anatomic sense; but, as the reader will see below, widely separate nodules of both primary and secondary cancer usually signify incurable disease. However, satellite nodules around an apparently solitary larger primary or secondary tumor may be related to local portal vein invasion and are not per se signs of incurability.

A resectable tumor can thus be most simply defined as one localized to a single area of the liver which can be safely removed without risk to the in-flow or out-flow tracts of the residual liver. The presence of an underlying cirrhosis in a patient with a liver tumor greatly compromises both the safety of the resection and the curability of the disease, no matter its anatomic location. Liver resection is seldom indicated in the cirrhotic patient except to control hemorrhage in an emergency situation. With modern diagnostic techniques, tumors are being found at an earlier stage. Tumor geography which relates to resectability can often be worked out before laparotomy. In the last decade, this has resulted in fewer unnecessary laparotomies and more resections.

How often will a primary or secondary liver cancer be resectable? In a collected review in 1977 [1] 28% of adult patients with primary liver cancer who came to laparotomy were resected. Table 2 documents more recent experience. Again, about 32% of Asian patients with PLC who were explored were resected. This number increased markedly in those asymptomatic patients whose tumors were found by mass-screening with alpha-fetoprotein. These figures must be tempered by the realization that, at least in Asia, many patients with primary liver cancer never come to laparotomy.

Metastatic cancer in the liver will have spread beyond the possibility of resection by the time it is discovered in most patients. Raven found resectable liver metastases in 5% of patients with primary tumors of the stomach, colon, and

Table 2. Liver Resection for cancer — resectability

Reference	Patients with PLC	Laparotomies	Resections	% Resectable of total patients	of laps
Primary liver cancer					
Foster and Berman (1977) [1]	1378	–	179	12%	–
	–	804	218	–	28%
Balasegaram (1979) [12]	810	535	88	11%	16%
Shanghai (1979 [13]					
AFP Screened cases	134	–	31	23%	–
clinical presentation	1200	–	97	8%	–
Zhaoyou *et al.* (1980) [8]					
AFP screened	66	–	37	56%	–
clinical presentation	220	–	39	8%	–
Mengchao *et al.* (1980) [14]					
AFP screened	16	16	14	88%	88%
clinical presentation	732	356	167	23%	47%
Okuda *et al.* (1980) [15]	4031	1041	361	9%	35%
Lee *et al.* (1982) [16]	935	–	165	18%	–
All malignancies (primary and secondary)					
Fortner *et al.* (1978([17]	–	289	95	–	33%

rectum. Jaffe *et al.* noted 56 solitary nodules in 173 patients for whom they described the geography of the metastatic disease. Bengmark and Hafstrom noted limited, but presumably resectable, disease in 24% of 38 patients with colorectal liver metastases [20]. Wanebo *et al.* found solitary metastasis in the livers of 50 out of 217 patients with evidence of hepatic spread of colorectal cancer [22]. Several other authors have reported similar findings. One can conclude that about 15–30% of patients with colorectal cancer will have disease in their liver at the time of resection of their primary bowel tumor. Perhaps 20–25% of those with liver disease will have a resectable situation in the liver. Thus, four or five of every 100 patients with colorectal cancer may eventually be candidates for liver resection [11].

5.2. Operative mortality and morbidity

One of the major reasons why the place of liver resection for cancer is changing rapidly is that resection has become safer. The risk/benefit ratio has shifted towards patient benefit and away from an operative mortality rate which, in some centers, formerly exceeded 35% after major resection. Table 3 documents the operative mortality after resection which was noted in a national survey several years ago. Some of these resections were done in the late 1960's and early 1970's in hospitals where very few liver resections were being performed. Table 4 updates this experience with more recent reports from Asian and Western countries. The fact that a large majority of Asian patients had diffuse cirrhosis as well as primary cancer accounts for the increased early operative and postoperative mortality. That the operative mortality figure is as low as 14% in the cirrhotic Asian patients is a testimony to the skills of the Asian surgeons, skills which have been refined by

Table 3. Operative mortality[a] — tumor type

Tumor type	Deaths/patients	Deaths (%)
Primary cancer, adults	27/133	20
Primary cancer, children	17/90	19
Metastatic cancer		
colon and rectum primary	8/126	6
other primary	6/51	12
Metastatic carcinoid	3/21	14
En-bloc		
gallbladder Ca	10/35	29
other Ca	6/55	11
Adenoma & FNH	4/99	4
Total	81/610	13

[a] Adapted from Table 11-1, reference 1.

an experience much larger than all but a small handful of Western surgeons.

Table 5 documents a clear relationship between the extent of resection and early mortality, but Starzl's impeccable record with trisegmentectomy (i.e., no death after 20 trisegmentectomies) demonstrates that even the largest resections can be done safely if done expertly [21].

Table 6 attempts to analyze the primary mechanism of operative or postopera-

Table 4. Operative mortality — liver resection for neoplasia

Reference	Patients	No of deaths	Deaths (%)	Note
Asian Reports				
Shanghai 1979 [13]	31	0	–	PLC, preclinical cases (AFP screen)
Shanghai 1979 [13]	370	44	(12)	PLC, clinical presentation
Balasegaram 1979 [12]	88	14	(16)	PLC (51% with cirrhosis)
Balasegaram 1979 [12]	10	2	(20	Metastatic cancer
Okuda 1980 [15]	301	56	(19)	all PLC (79% with cirrhosis)
Mengchao *et al.* 1980 [14]	181	16	(9)	all PLC (126 with cirrhosis)
Lee *et al.* 1982 [16]	165	33	(20)	all PLC (85% with cirrhosis)
	1146	165	(14.4)	
Non Asian Reports				
Starzl *et al.* 1978 [21]	35	0	–	9 metastatic, 26 primary (13 benign)
Fortner *et al.* 1978 [17]	108	10	(9)	4% with regular technique 17% with isolated perfusion
Wanebo *et al.* 1978 [22]	27	2	(7)	all synchronous resection of metastases
Sorenson *et al.* 1979 [23]	31	8	(26)	all lobectomies for PLC
Hanks *et al.* 1980 [24]	21	1	(5)	11 metastases, rest benign and malignant primary
Adson *et al.* 1980 [25] and 1982 [26]	106	2	(2)	all metastatic colon & rectum
Adson *et al.* 1981 [27]	66	3	(4.5)	all primary, 14 benign, 52 malignant
Thompson *et al.* 1981 [28]	12	0		7 metastases, 5 primary, (3 benign)
Logan *et al.* 1982 [29]	19	1	(5)	all metastatic colon and rectum
Aldrete *et al.* 1982 [30]	16	3	(19)	5 metastates, 11 primary (7 benign)
Bengmark *et al.* 1982 [31]	21	3	(14)	all PLC, all deaths in O.R.
Foster J.H. 1982 [32]	57	3	(5)	20 metastases, 37 primary (20 benign)
Total Non-Asian	519	36	(7)	
Overall	1665	201	(12%)	

tive death after liver resection for cancer. In order to construct the table, it was necessary to assign a single cause of death to each patient, although in most cases several factors contributed. However, in spite of this drawback, it is clear that failure to control hemorrhage in the operating room is the leading cause of death in most Western series. Liver failure was the leading cause of death in most Asian series and was usually related to cirrhosis. For example, 15 out of 16 deaths in the experience reported from Shanghai occurred in cirrhotic patients [13]. Late upper gastrointestinal hemorrhage, usually from stress erosions, was another important (and probably preventable) contributor. Death from sepsis was usually related to subphrenic abscess, which in turn was probably related to technical factors such as residual necrotic tissue and dead space.

Three deaths have occurred during 57 resections for tumor by the author. Two occurred early in his experience: one was related to air embolization during a re-resection for fulminant carcinoid syndrome, and the other was a death nine weeks after operation from injury to the major bile duct of the residual lobe. The third death was due to an acute autopsy-proven myocardial infarction on the operating table before any blood loss had occurred in a 77-year-old man with heart disease. It may have been related to decreased venous return after liver torsion to facilitate exposure.

Western surgeons with greater experience have reduced their operative mortality rates to 5% or below. The 9% overall figure reported by Fortner *et al.* can be separated into 17% for patients for whom isolation-perfusion techniques were used, and 4% for patients undergoing 'standard resection'. [17]

We have learned that resection cannot be done with low mortality in the cirrhotic patient and in the elderly patient with cardiac or renal insufficiency. We have also learned to use the CT scan to investigate tumor geography in the area of the inferior vena cava, the area most difficult to assess on the operating table. With better patient selection and with more precise techniques (see below), early mortality should be reduced to a minimum figure well below 5%.

Postoperative complications are still very common after major liver resection. Table 7 documents the incidence of several of the more common ones. Atelectasis

Table 5. Operative mortality — type of resection[a]

Operation	Deaths/patients	Deaths (%)
Extended Right Lobectomy	10/39	26
Right Lobectomy	45/171	26
Left Lobectomy	5/58	9
Left Lateral Segmentectomy	5/70	7
Wedge Excision[b]	17/297	6

[a] Adapted from Table 11-1, Foster JH, Berman MM: *Solid Liver Tumors* [1] plus reference 33.
[b] Includes all resections, however large, which were not included in other categories.

and pleural effusion accompany any major operation in the right upper quadrant, particularly those requiring division of the diaphragm. Subphrenic abscess has become less common as we have learned to avoid mattress sutures, to control bleeding more discretely, and to use drains more effectively and often more sparingly. Liver failure, whether reversible or not, most often occurs in the cirrhotic patient and, thus, should be avoidable by refusing elective resection to such patients.

Metabolic complications such as hypoalbuminemia, coagulopathy, jaundice, etc. are still seen after major liver resection for cancer, but they probably relate more to the effects of operative trauma, anesthesia, hypotension, and multiple transfusions than to the removal of too much liver parenchyma. It is common after a controlled major lobectomy in a non-cirrhotic patient to have *no* significant metabolic complications. Transient abnormalities in laboratory values may be seen for a few days, but they should return to normal by the tenth postoperative day.

Table 6. Liver resection for neoplasia: Causes of operative deaths

References	Deaths/ resections	failure to control hemorrhage	bile duct injury, other technical	liver failure, post-op	Upper gastrointestinal hemorrhage	Sepsis	Cardiopulmonary	Other
Foster and Berman [1]	82/621	26	13	15	4	4	4	5 judgement error 3 air emboli; 2 recurrent Ca.
Fortner *et al.* [17]	10/108	2	2	0	1	0	1	4 coagulophathy + hepatic failure
Sorenson *et al.* [23]	8/31	4	0	3	0	1	0	
Logan *et al.* [29]	1/19	0	0	0	1	0	0	
Adson *et al.* (PLC) [27]	3/66	3	0	0	0	0	0	
Adson *et al.* (met) [25]	2/106	0	0	0	1	0	0	1 late death in 75 year old with complicated course
Balasegaram [12]	14/88	4	0	8	0	2	0	
Lee *et al.* [16]	33°165	9	1	10	3	5	3	2 wound dehiscence
Mengchao *et al.* [14]	16/181	2	0	9	0	1	0	4 coagulophathy
Bengmark *et al.* [31]	3/21	3	0	0	0	0	0	all 3 in O.R.
Foster JH [32]	3/57	0	2	0	0	0	1	

Postoperative low-grade non-spiking fever is commonly seen after major liver resection and often remains unexplained. A careful search for a septic (and drainable) focus should be made; but, more often than not, none will be found. This fever usually subsides in the second postoperative week, and in many patients it appears to be totally unrelated to the use or the cessation of antibiotics. In the current era of improved non-invasive ways to find collections, re-exploration for fever alone after major hepatectomy should probably not be done.

5.3. Survival after liver resection for cancer

If operation can be done safely, and if modern diagnostic tests can effectively exclude spread of tumor beyond the liver, then the only remaining question in regard to liver resection for apparently localized primary and secondary carcinoma is, Will it do any good? Will we ever permanently rid a patient of his cancer by liver resection? Can palliation of the symptomatic patient be achieved by non-curative resection? And, last, the perhaps currently unanswerable but worrisome question, Will unsuccessful operation accelerate tumor growth in those patients who are not cured?

Survival figures are crude yardsticks with which to measure results, but they are perhaps the most objective that we have. They must be compared with the natural history without therapy or with non-resectional therapy. Specific concentration will now be focused on (1) primary liver cancer in adults; (2) primary liver cancer

Table 7. Liver resection for cancer: Post-operative complications

Reference	Number of resections	Subphrenic abscess	Bile leak	Wound infection	Upper GI bleed	Liver failure	Intra-abdominal bleed
Foster and Berman (1977) [1]	621	39	21	–	19	–	13
Fortner *et al.* (1978) [17]	108	22	3	9	2	–	5
Sorenson *et al.* (1979) [23]	31	4	2	2	–	5	6
Balasegaram (1979) [12]	118	4	4	10	–	10	8
Hanks *et al.* (1980) [24]	28	3	0	2	0	0	3
Thompson *et al.* (1981) [28]	12	0	0	2	0	0	2
Lee *et al.* (1982) [16]	165	14	15	–	3	10	12
Totals	1083	86	45				49
		8%	4%				4,5%

in children; (3) metastatic carcinoma; (4) endocrine tumors; and, (5) 'en bloc' resection, i.e., where liver resection is done 'en bloc' to remove a large mass of cancer originating in an adjacent organ and invading the liver by direct contiguity.

5.3.1. Primary liver cancer in adults

Most primary liver cancers (PLC) are not resectable at the time they are diagnosed. Most occur in cirrhotic livers. Many are multifocal or have spread beyond the liver capsule at the time of diagnosis, and others have involved major inflow or outflow structures sufficient to preclude resection. The propensity of primary hepatocellular carcinoma to spread up the hepatic veins and down the portal veins is well documented. Involvement of the hepatic veins is particularly common.

Asian patients with PLC: Without resection, more than 90% of Asian patients will be dead within one year of diagnosis. In reports before 1976, even with resection, only 7% of this most favorable group of patients could be expected to live as long as 5 years [1]. A large majority of Asian patients have diffuse fibrosis and/or cirrhosis, thus increasing their operative risk and their chance of multifocal disease while decreasing their chance for cure with resection. Operative mortality figures have consistently exceeded the rates of five-year survival in this group.

During the last decade, the picture has changed. Asian surgeons have become more wary about resecting patients with cirrhosis [12] and they have had the opportunity to operate upon an increasing number of patients whose tumors have been uncovered by mass screening of populations at high risk with alpha-fetoprotein determinations [8, 13, 14]. The subclinical tumors are smaller, more resectable, and more curable. Table 8 documents the improving overall survival after diagnosis and the marked increase in one-year and five-year survival rates. Thirty-three to 57% of patients will survive 1 year, and five-year survival now exceeds the operative mortality rates. Table 9 contrasts the results of resections for patients whose tumors were found by screening populations with those whose tumor had a clinical presentation. Although the follow-up is short, three-year survival has more than doubled and most recurrences and deaths from PLC occur within 2 years of resection. Most of the patients surviving as long as 3 years are probably cured.

Western patients with PLC: A collected review of reports of the survivors of resection for primary liver cancer noted a five-year survival of 21 of 60 patients (35%) from the literature and 20 of 69 patients (29%) in a nationwide survey of resected cases. That survey noted no long survivors among the ten cirrhotic patients who survived resection, and a 34% five-year survival among the non-cirrhotic patients [1].

More recent reports parallel these results. Adson reported 36% five-year survival and 33% ten-year survival after resection for PLC in 46 patients [27]. Bengmark *et al.* resected 18 patients; of the 16 who survived operation, 12 are dead from 2 to 5 months postoperatively (mean 18 months), and four are alive at 27, 48, 57, and 84 months after hepatectomy [31]. Fortner reported that 100% of the 13 patients who survived 'curative' resection for PLC lived two years, and seven patients were alive more than three years after resection [17]. Iwatsuki *et al.* reported a three-year actuarial survival of 52% in 30 patients after resection for primary hepatic malignancy [34]. Sorenson noted a five-year survival rate of 16% in 23 patients with PLC [23]. Finally, 16 of the 17 patients whom I have resected for PLC survived the operation; 10 patients are dead from 8 to 32 months (mean 15 months), and 6 are still alive without evidence of disease at 5, 6, 18, and 23 months, and at 2 and 3 years [32].

Thus, 'cure' seems possible in about 30 to 40% of patients with localized PLC when it occurs in a non-cirrhotic liver. Current operative mortality is about 12%, or 24 deaths after 115 resections, in recent reports from Western countries [23, 27, 31, 32]. This risk/benefit ratio should improve in the future as operations become safer and the newer diagnostic techniques uncover earlier and smaller lesions.

A word should be said about total hepatectomy and transplantation for primary hepatic malignancy. Calne reported on ten patients who lived at least one year after total hepatectomy and orthotopic liver transplantation for PLC. Two patients were still alive, one at 5 years and the other 15 months after resection with

Table 8. Survival after resection of primary cancer — Asian patients – Recent reports

Survival	Shanghai (1979) [13]	31 screened	112 clinical	Zhaoyou et al. (1980) [8]	66 screened	220 clinical	Mengchao et al. (1980) [14]	16 screened	732 clinical	Okuda et al. (1980) [15]	Hepatocellular Ca only	Lee et al. (1982) [16]	Balasegaram (1979) [12]
All cases of PLC													
– all therapies													
1 year survival		19%			15%						21.5%		
3 year survival		11%			5.5%						5%		
5 year survival											2.4%		
Resected cases													
1 year survival		55%			54%			56%			33.3%	43%	57%
3 year survival		32%						29%			20%	20%	
5 year survival								16%			12%	20%	5%
Unresected cases													
(mean survival)													
1 year survival					8.1%								
3 year survival					0.9%							<1%	
5 year survival					0							0	

evidence of a recurrence. Three other patients had no evidence of carcinoma at the time of their deaths, two more than five years after transplantation [35]. Starzl has reported 21 transplants for clinically evident carcinoma (three in patients less than 15 years of age). Eight patients died post-operatively, of whom seven had no evidence of cancer at autopsy. Of the 13 who survived the transplant, two were alive – one at 10 months, apparently free of disease, and the other at 52 months in spite of the demonstration of miliary metastases in both the abdomen and lung at the time of resection. Two patients who died had no evidence of cancer at autopsy. Starzl also reports the incidental histologic finding of primary malignancy after transplantation in three children for benign disease. One child died postoperatively, but the other two are alive and free of disease at 3 and 11+ years [34]. These results of transplantation are discouraging, but not dismal. One can only encourage these investigators to continue to work out the unique and monumental problems attendant upon transplantation for malignancy.

5.3.2. PLC in children

The primary epithelial cancers of children are hepatoblastoma (which usually occurs in children under two years of age) and hepatocellular carcinoma (which occurs in older children). There is also a rare embryonal sarcoma, most often found in older children. Most pediatric epithelial tumors secrete alpha-fetoprotein and most occur in non-cirrhotic livers. In a 1974 nationwide survey conducted by the Surgical Section of the American Academy of Pediatrics, it was found that

Table 9. Survival after resection of primary liver cancer: Asian patients, screened patients versus clinical presentation

		Shanghai (1979) [13]	Zhaoyou (1980) [8] *et al.*	Menchao (1980) [14] *et al.*
Alpha-fetoprotein screened cases				
number of resected patients		31	66	16
Survival after resection –	1 yr	87%	79%	86%
	3 yr	57%	62%	–
	4 yr		55.5%	
Clinical presentation cases				
number of resected patients		112	220	167
Survival after resection –	1 yr	47%	46%	55%
	3 yr	25%	26%	28%
	4 yr		22.3%	21%

resection was possible in 67% of 129 patients explored for hepatoblastoma and in 36% of 92 patients explored for hepatocellular carcinoma. Operative mortality rates were high, particularly in the younger infant, but survival of resected patients was 76% at one year, 50% at three years, and 34% at 5 years [4].

More recent reports include an extensive Japanese survey and the report of Randolph *et al.* on the experience of the Children's Hospital National Medical Center in Washington, DC. Okuda *et al.* found 72 PLC's in Japanese children 10 years of age and under, of which 64 were hepatoblastomas. Resection was possible in 47 patients with hepatoblastoma, and 61.5% of the resected children survived 5 years [15]. Randolph *et al.* reported on 17 children with primary hepatic malignancy. Twelve had hepatoblastoma, three had hepatocellular carcinoma, and two had embryonal sarcoma. Resection of hepatoblastoma was possible in nine patients and four were still alive, apparently free of disease, at 2, 2, 3, and 4 years after resection. One patient with hepatocellular carcinoma and one with sarcoma were also apparently free of disease after resection and are possibly cured [36].

Because PLC in children is usually found in a non-cirrhotic liver, and because it spreads late, attempts to cure by resection should be aggressive. There are several reports of the imaginative use of combinations of chemotheraphy, radiotherapy, and resection to effect long survival (and presumably cure) in patients with metastatic hepatoblastoma [1]. The author's recent personal experience includes two patients in whom preoperative doxorubicin and cis-platinum therapy for 'unresectable' hepatoblastomas resulted in marked shrinkage, allowing easy resection in one patient. Proximity to the inferior vena cava precluded resection of the small bulk of residual tumor in the other patient. Post-chemotherapy biopsy of both tumors showed little anaplasia, marked necrosis, and even a few islands of mature gastrointestinal epithelium, testifying to the efficacy of these chemotherapeutic agents in controlling this type of embryonal tumor.

This pediatric experience with multimodal therapy may serve as a model for the future therapy of adult patients with PLC when we develop more effective chemotherapeutic agents.

5.3.3. Survival after resection for metastatic liver cancer

The last decade has seen the acceptance of the concept that the resection of liver metastases has a place in the treatment of certain patients with limited disease. As experience has accumulated, the criteria for selection of operative candidates have matured and it is now possible to make specific recommendations. The reported experience of others has been collected [11] and to these data several recent reports can be added to document survival [7, 24, 28, 29, 37]. There is not to date, and perhaps never will be, an adequately controlled prospective study comparing resection with either no therapy, chemotherapy, or radiation therapy for patients with comparable amounts of disease. The results of resection of limited metastases from colorectal primaries and from certain pediatric tumor metastases in terms of long survival and even cure are so much better than those reported after chemotherapy using presently available agents that clinicians are becoming increasingly reluctant to miss an opportunity for 'cure'.

Unfortunately, this claim for the benefits of resection cannot be made for metastases from most other primary sites. Indeed, it appears that long survival after liver resection for tumors such as leiomyosarcomas, melanomas, and endocrine lesions are probably more a function of the tumors' slow growth rate than of the surgeon's ability to remove all residual disease.

Table 10 documents much of the collected survival experience. The largest institutional experience is that of the Mayo Clinic, and it is also the most optimistic. Adson and co-workers have reported 53 wedge resections and 53 major resections for colorectal metastases [25, 26, 38]. In their initial report of 60 resections, the overall five-year survival was 21%, but at least 42% of the patients with solitary lesions lived 5 years (Table 11). Eleven of the 15 patients in that initial report who lived at least 5 years were treated by wedge excision alone. There were no long-term survivors after resection of multiple metastases [38]. In two more recent reports of *major* resection of metastatic colorectal lesions, Adson has noted a five-year survival of 29%, but this figure improved to 46% if only those patients without evidence of extrahepatic metastases are considered. In this latest series, patients with multiple metastases did as well as those with solitary lesions [25, 26].

Logan *et al.* reported the UCLA experience with resection of colorectal

Table 10. Survival after liver resection for metastatic cancer: relation to primary tumor site[a]

Primary tumors	Operative survivors	Survival		Died of recurrence after 5 yr
		2 yr	5 yr	
Colon and rectum	367	136/281 (48%)	61/254 (24%)	14
Wilms tumor	15	8/14	4/10	0
Melanoma	15	2/11	1/11	1
Leiomyosarcoma	12	4/9	1/9	1
Pancreas	8	2/7	1/7	1 (Islet cell)
Uterus and cervix	7	1/5	0/5	–
Stomach	10	1/8	1/8	0
Kidney	7	2/5	1/5	0
Breast	6	0/3	0/2	–
Ovary	3	0/2	0/2	–
Unknown primary	3	0/3	0/3	–
Sarcomas	6	1/3	1/3	1
Others	5	2/4	0/2	–

[a] Adapted from Table 4 *Liver Metastases* Vol 18(3):161–202, Current Problems in Surgery March 1981. *Year Book Med Pub* [11] plus [7],[17], [24], [25], [26], [28], [29], [37].

metastases, having performed 19 resections with one operative death. Six patients were dead from 6 to 25 months after hepatectomy (mean 15 months), but there were 12 patients alive and apparently free of disease, of whom three had lived more than 5 years. Of those patients treated more than 5 years ago, three of nine survive [29]. Muhe *et al.* report a 20% five-year survival of 38 patients after liver resection for metastases from multiple primary sites. There was no long-term survival in patients with tumor originating outside of the splanchnic bed or with multiple metastases, but 26% of the patients with solitary metastases lived 5 years or more [37]. Fortner *et al.* resected 25 patients with colorectal metastases and had two operative deaths. None of the 6 patients undergoing 'palliative' resection lived as long as two years. Three-year actuarial survival was calculated to be 72% for the 17 patients who had 'curative' resection (however, only two patients had survived that long at the time of the report) [17]. Thompson and Little resected colorectal metastases in six patients. Two patients died at 6 and 27 months, but four were alive – three more than 5 years. However, all three long-term survivors had evidence of recurrent carcinoma outside of the liver [28], demonstrating once again that the surgeon must often share credit for long survival with the natural history of the disease.

Wanebo *et al.* recorded a 28% five-year survival after 25 synchronous resections for liver deposits noted at the time of resection of primary colon and rectal tumors [22]. Blumgart and Allison performed six curative and three palliative resections for colorectal secondaries. There were two operative deaths. Only one patient was alive 6 months after resection. Six others died of their disease, the longest at 63 months after liver resection (mean 19 months) [7]. Balasegaram had one five-year survivor after 10 liver resections for metastatic carcinoma in Asian patients [12].

Many of these five-year survival figures are remarkably close to the 30% noted after resection of solitary colorectal metastases found in a nationwide survey several years ago [1]. It is apparent, too, that survival for more than 5 years after liver resection does not always mean 'cure' for patients with colorectal cancer. At least 14 patients have been reported with evidence of disease more than 60 months after liver resection (Table 10). However, a large majority of those who

Table 11. Survival after resection of colorectal metastases: solitary versus multiple lesions[a]

	Solitary	Multiple
Patients at risk for		
5 year survival	165	77
Operative deaths	3	8
5 year survivors	50/165	7/77
	(30%)	(12%)

[a] From Refs. [11], [28], [29].

survive 5 years will be permanently free of disease, and perhaps even those who die late can be considered to have been palliated. Palliative resection where gross disease is left has not been shown to be effective. Adson's experience raises some hope, but that of others suggests that survival will not be effected if tumor is left. Patient morbidity and expense may well be increased by such 'debulking' procedures.

A consensus has been reached by most that the status of the mesenteric lymph nodes taken during colon resection and the interval between bowel and liver resection have little direct correlation with survival after liver resection [1]. Muhe *et al.* found that synchronous resection yielded a 24% five-year survival in 30 patients, while no patient who was resected metachronously lived as long as two years [37]. However, the collective experience from many other reports notes a 21% five-year survival (22 of 106 patients) after synchronous resection and a 22% (22 of 98 patients) after metachronous resection [11], an insignificant difference.

It has become clear that a narrow margin of normal liver suffices as well as a wide one, and that lobectomy is only indicated when tumor size requires it or the safety of resection demands it. Patients with larger lesions do less well, although several patients with huge metastases have become long-term survivors. There is no difference in prognosis after liver resection between patients whose primary tumor originated from the rectum or in any other segment of the large bowel [1].

We are left, then, with reasonably solid data which lead to the conclusion that resection of liver metastases should be recommended when:

(1) the liver metastasis is the only residual disease;

(2) the liver disease is limited in size and location – preferably solitary and small;

(3) the primary tumor was (a) of colonic or rectal origin, (b) a pediatric tumor sensitive to chemotherapy, and (c) a slowly growing, unusual tumor such as leiomyosarcoma, or certain endocrine tumors.

(4) the patient and the surgeon are both well prepared.

5.3.4. *Palliative resection to relieve endocrine symptoms*

Although cure is seldom, if ever, possible by liver resection, significant palliation may be achieved in selected patients with disabling symptoms from metastatic deposits of functioning endocrine tumors. The slow rate of tumor growth and the resulting long natural history of some patients with these rare tumors justifies attempts at symptomatic palliation if gross tumor can be removed. Experience has shown, however, that palliation of endocrine symptoms cannot be expected unless the vast majority (probably 95% or more) of the functioning tumor can be removed.

The malignant carcinoid syndrome provides the classic example of the role of palliative liver resection. In most patients with this disabling symptom complex, the liver metastases will be widespread and resection will not be possible. In a few, disease will be localized and bulky and, thus, eminently suitable for 'debulking'. Pharmacologic therapy is often ineffective in controlling symptoms and in those patients, non-invasive imaging of the liver should indicate whether the disease is suitable for resection.

At least 47 cases have been reported in the literature where metastatic liver deposits have been resected from selected patients with the malignant carcinoid syndrome [1, 7]. In at least five of these patients, two or more resections were performed for control of symptoms. Two of these five patients died on the operating table during a second 'heroic' attempt. Overall, six patients died after 52 resections (12%). Four of 47 patients (8%) died after the initial attempt.

Of the 39 survivors with adequate follow-up information, 38 patients were palliated for from a few weeks to more than ten and one-half years. At least ten of these patients had lived more than 3 years at the time of reporting. The only patient who survived the operation and was not palliated had considerable tumor left in his liver.

There are a few reports of liver resection to palliate other endocrine syndromes. Smrcka et al. relieved hypoglycemia in one patient who became symptom-free for at least four years after liver resection of two metastases from an islet cell tumor [39]. Thompson and Little recently attempted to relieve hypoglycemia from a metastatic islet cell tumor by liver resection. Their patient died with persistent disease one year and eight months after resection with an undocumented amount of palliation [28].

Unfortunately, endocrine liver metastases tend to be multiple and diffuse. Occasionally they are not, and the resectable situation should always be looked for when symptoms become disabling.

An alternative to liver resection for the malignant carcinoid syndrome is provided by hepatic artery interruption. McDermott et al. [40] and, more recently, Bengmark et al [41] have reported palliation after dearterialization and temporary hepatic artery ligation in a few cases. Bengmark, in a literature survey, noted 50% of patients had been palliated for more than three months by hepatic artery interruption. In his personal series, he noted some relief for 13 patients with a malignant carcinoid syndrome lasting for 1 to 42 months (mean symptom-free interval was 3 months). Four of the eight patients who survived at least 1 year were relieved, and two are still symptom-free at 34 and 42 months after temporary interruption of the hepatic artery [41].

5.3.5. Liver resection to satisfy the 'en-bloc' principle

Tumors arising in organs adjacent to the liver such as the stomach, the transverse colon, the gallbladder, the kidney, and the adrenal occasionally invade liver by direct contiguity. Rarely, a lung or esophageal tumor will invade the liver before metastasizing elsewhere. Multi-visceral resection for such locally aggressive cancers has been recommended when obvious disease has not spread beyond the hope of cure. In these cases, all or parts of several organs are resected 'en-bloc' to provide a margin of normal tissues surrounding the cancer.

Will inclusion of a wedge of liver in the resected specimen add risk to the resection, and will it do any good in terms of long-term survival? Appropriate circumstances are found infrequently and most cases are not reported. Table 12 reviews some of the published data.

Gallbladder cancer: Perhaps gallbladder carcinoma remains the most controversial topic in regards to 'en-bloc' resection. The only long-term survivor listed in Table 12 after liver resection for gallbladder cancer had a major lobectomy, but she had a superficial carcinoma that may well have been cured by cholecystectomy alone. It is interesting to note that this patient died $15^{1}/_{2}$ years after liver resection of diffuse cholangiocarcinoma.

Because the gallbladder lies over the junction of the right and left lobes of the liver, a case cannot be made for *either* right or left anatomic lobectomy. Is there a place for wedge excision of the gallbladder bed, perhaps combined with dissection of the lymph nodes along the common bile duct and behind the head of the pancreas? Data sufficient to answer that question definitively are not yet in, but the reported experience is not very encouraging. Table 13 summarizes data collected from 14 reports since 1970 [42]. Many of the included patients may have had limited disease, yet only two patients of the 85 with adequate follow-up are alive without disease more than 5 years after liver resection.

Adson makes the best case for extended resection including wedge excision of the gallbladder bed, but his numbers are small and more time will be needed to learn the lessons of this experience [43]. For the present, liver resection is probably indicated only for those patients who have gallbladder cancers which are not clinically evident and are found incidentally at operation. The disease should be sharply limited, yet proven by frozen section to extend through the muscularis. If such a cancer is reported by a pathologist two days after cholecystectomy for benign disease, perhaps a case can be made for re-exploration in a few months for a 'second look'. Such an interval might allow the incurable aggressive carcinoma to declare itself while not precluding limited delayed excision by wedge liver resection of persistent, indolent, local disease. There is yet no

Table 12. 'En-bloc' liver resection for adjacent cancers[a]

Primary tumor	Patients	Operative deaths	5-yr survivors[2]
Gall-bladder	57	10	1/41
Stomach	54	3	6/44
Colon	23	2	3/14
Kidney	9	1	0/3
Adrenal	3	1	0/2
Lung	1	0	0/1

[a] Adapted from Chapter 10, *Solid Liver tumors,* Foster JH, Berman MM: W.B. Saunders, 1977 [1].
[b] Excludes operative deaths.

Table 13. Liver resection for gall-bladder cancer (14 reports since 1970)[a]

	Operation	
	Wedge excision	Major 'lobectomy'
Patients	62	24
Operative deaths	10	9
Dead with disease in less than $3^{1}/_{2}$ yr	41	13
Alive, free of disease at less than 5 yr	4	1
Alive with disease at less than 1 year	3	0
Lost to follow-up	1	0
5-year survivors	3[b]	1[b]

[a] Adapted from Table 6, Foster JH, Chapter on Carcinoma of the Gallbladder *Surgery of the Gall Bladder and Bile Ducts.* Ed. Way LW, Dunphy JE. W.B. Saunders, Philadelphia 1984 [42].

[b] 1 patient after wedge excision and 1 patient after lobectomy died *with* disease after 5 yr.

evidence which supports 'en-bloc' liver resection for patients with superficial papillary 'pathologist cancers' which involve only the mucosa of the gallbladder.

Gastric cancer: Bulky gastric carcinomas may invade the left lateral segment of the liver. Wedge excision of part of that segment can be readily accomplished using mattress sutures, blunt suction technique, or even the crush-clamp technique advocated by Lin [44]. That only six of 44 patients so treated survived 5 years is discouraging (see Table 12), but adding the liver resection should not increase morbidity significantly and will result in an occasional cure in patients with locally aggressive gastric tumor. If tumor has involved the quadrate or caudate lobes, the risk of resection will probably outweigh any possible benefit to the patient.

Colon carcinoma: When the liver is involved by direct invasion of a tumor of the right transverse colon, it is usually only the lower anterior edge of the liver which is involved. This, too, can be readily and safely resected and may lead to an occasional 'cure'.

6. Technique of liver resection for cancer

The finer details of operative technique which allow safe liver resection for cancer are more thoroughly and more appropriately discussed and illustrated elsewhere [1, 45–48]. In the next few paragraphs, I will try to summarize and editorialize, in somewhat dogmatic fashion, to leave the reader with a clear view of my own current prejudices. Those prejudices have changed and continue to change with more experience.

6.1. Pre-operative requirements

Hemostatic mechanisms must be intact to allow safe major liver resection. Hyperbilirubinemia and hypoalbuminemia are ominous findings which usually signal incurability, if not unresectability. The chest must be free of disease. Computerized axial tomography is certainly more effective than standard chest X-ray and probably more effective than regular tomography in excluding pulmonary metastases.

Angiography is recommended for all patients except those with small and peripheral tumors. Selective arteriography may uncover disease unsuspected by other tests and will alert the surgeon to the frequent variations in the arterial anatomy of the human liver. Inferior venacavography should be performed when caval involvement is suspected or is suggested by CT scan, particularly for patients with bulky hepatocellular carcinomas.

6.2. Operative evaluation

A decision for resection should not be made unless (1) there is no disease outside the liver; (2) a margin of normal liver can be taken around the tumor without risking either the inflow or outflow vessels and ducts of the remaining liver; and, (3) when the residual liver looks healthy, i.e., non-cirrhotic and without metastases.

Exceptions occur to every rule. Direct invasion of a limited area of diaphragm does not preclude resection of an otherwise resectable primary or secondary liver cancer – involved diaphragm should be taken 'en-bloc'. Certain endocrine metastases may be enucleated without a margin of normal liver if they lie close to vital structures, and resection of primary liver cancer may occasionally be indicated in the patient with cirrhosis to control continuing spontaneous hemorrhage.

A step-wise approch to operative evaluation is recommended. A limited abdominal incision will allow inspection. If no contraindication is found, the incision can be enlarged to allow thorough palpation and inspection of the liver, the regional node-bearing areas, and the rest of the belly. If all is well, the incision can be further lengthened to allow bimanual palpation of the liver. If involvement of the inferior vena cava is suspected, division of the falciform ligament back to the inferior vena cava superiorly and careful palpation through the foramen of Winslow inferiorly will help to resolve this issue.

Thoracic extension of an abdominal incision is not often needed for adults and almost never required for children or for patients with tumors in their left lobe. Although more difficult for the surgeon and more uncomfortable for the patient, I still prefer extension into the right thorax over median sternotomy for large right lobe tumors because it allows careful palpation of the right lung and hilum for metastatic disease, it provides better exposure for diagnostic evaluation and operative control of the difficult hepatic vein/inferior vena cava junction, and because wide radial incision of the right diaphragm allows displacement of a huge tumor into the chest, thus allowing safe access to the liver hilum and to the minor hepatic veins entering the caudate lobe.

6.3. How much liver to resect

Peripheral tumors, even if large, can usually be resected by wedge excision since non-anatomic division of peripheral parenchyma will not risk vessels and ducts to the remaining liver. Wedge excision of significant parts of the more central liver near the gallbladder bed or quadrate lobe may result in necrosis or sequestration of more peripheral liver and chronic biliary fistula. Much is made of the segmental anatomy of the liver [44], and, indeed, the surgeon should know his intrahepatic anatomy. However, segmental excision, which theoretically preserves more liver, may actually increase the operative risk to the patient and provide little benefit. Non-cirrhotic patients tolerate uncomplicated anatomic lobectomy so well that attempts to save one of the major segments of the right lobe are not warranted.

For practical purposes, there are only four types of liver resection to be recommended: (1) wedge excision of peripheral lesions; (2) right or left anatomic lobectomy for larger lesions or lesions near the dome of either lobe; (3) left lateral segmentectomy; and, (4) extension of either right or left lobectomy by taking one or more adjacent segments of the opposite lobe. Starzl calls extended resection 'trisegmentectomy' [46]. Central resections of either the quadrate or caudate lobes are large wedge excisions.

The clearly-demonstrated, but not-so-well understood, ability of the human liver to regenerate by hypertrophy and hyperplasia allows resection of up to 75–80% of the liver without important lasting metabolic defects. Remember, too, that when a huge tumor fills the right lobe, the left lobe will already show compensatory hypertrophy before operation, and most of what will be removed will be tumor and not functional liver.

6.4. Control of inflow and outflow vessels and ducts

Hilar dissection before anatomic resection is usually straightforward. Most problems are caused by failure to appreciate arterial anomalies or the *immediate* bifurcation or trifurcation of the right portal vein and bile ducts. The arteries are best identified during initial dissection by pushing pulsating structures up towards the surgeon with a finger in the Foramen of Winslow. All hilar dissection, including clearing of the quadrate lobe for extended right lobectomy, can and should be done outside of the liver capsule.

Arguments persist about hepatic vein control before or after, transection of liver substance. Those with more experience do it later in most patients. An occasional patient will have an easily accessible right or left middle hepatic vein/ inferior vena cava confluence which can be controlled outside of the liver parenchyma, but most patients will not. It is much safer to leave control of most major hepatic veins until they can be approached anteriorly through transected parenchyma.

6.5. Parenchymal transection

There are many ways to cut through the liver. For most surgeons and most patients, however, techniques which are simple, reasonably rapid, and which do not require fancy tools or techniques are to be preferred. I decry transection with either the hot or cold knife and I have no experience with the laser. Mattress sutures produce cuffs of necrosis and risk vessels and ducts in residual liver. They may still be useful for certain peripheral wedge excisions. Large and specially designed clamps are used by many and are recommended to reduce blood loss. Often they are difficult to apply centrally. Their very effectiveness in temporarily halting bleeding and bile leakage may lull the surgeon into less-than-complete ligation with subsequent bleeding or fistula formation.

Once the capsule is transected, liver parenchyma should be divided bluntly with ligation of all ducts and vessels as they are encountered. Finger fracture is faster but less discrete than blunt suction. The principles are well-established; leave no dead tissue, occlude every macroscopic transected duct and vessel, and do no harm to the residual liver. Remember that there is little collateral inflow or outflow potential for the veins and ducts of the liver. If you tie off the right hepatic duct, you must remove all of the right lobe to avoid bile fistula.

My own preference is to use a narrow suction tip to bluntly tease apart parenchyma while controlling the tumor with my non-dominant hand. A practiced assistant clips or ties all encountered vessels *before* they are cut. Formal capsule incision precedes this step and guides the surgeon as he works his way down through liver tissue. Team work and speed reduce blood loss. Metal clips are used for all but the largest vessels [1].

6.6. Preparation for closure

Minor venous oozing will usually stop after a few minutes of compression. Persistent arterial bleeding should be sutured discretely. Clamps will tear and compound the problem. Approximation of the capsule may assist hemostasis but usually is not required. Raw surfaces do not require resurfacing. Unless duct injury has occurred, normal-size bile ducts should not be decompressed. Peritoneal drainage after elective controlled resection is probably overdone in most instances. A few days of gentle suction through one or two drains will suffice for most patients. Get the drains out early if they are not productive.

7. Conclusions

When primary liver cancer occurs in a non-cirrhotic liver, it should be considered as a curable disease until proven otherwise. Only resection will cure, although chemotherapy and radiotherapy may be required adjuvants for certain pediatric tumors. Preoperative testing using newer imaging techniques is useful in determining resectability, but the surgeons' eyes and hands remain the most sensitive instruments presently available to assist in making final decisions in borderline cases. Metastatic disease should also be resected in highly selected instances, mostly with colorectal tumors. Patients with smaller and apparently solitary lesions do better, but the status of the mesenteric nodes, the margin of normal liver tissue resected, and the interval between the bowel and liver resections do not appear to influence the results after liver resection for metastatic disease.

What should be recommended for a patient in whose liver the surgeon has found an apparently solitary, but pre-operatively unsuspected metastasis, at the time of colon resection? If the lesion is peripheral and safely resectable through the existing incision, excision biopsy is recommended. If circumstances are not ideal, the surgeon should carefully evaluate the rest of the liver with particular attention to the relationship of disease to the inflow and outflow vessels, and he should biopsy the suspected lesion. All liver nodules in gastrointestinal cancer patients are not metastases, particularly in women. A baseline postoperative scan and CEA determination should be done and then the patient should be watched carefully for a few months (e.g. 3–4 months). If the disease is not rapidly progressive, if thorough re-evaluation reveals no other disease, and if both the patient and the surgeon are properly prepared, the metastatic focus should be resected.

Patients with disabling symptoms from localized liver metastasis from endocrine tumors may be palliated by liver resection. Other patients with invasive, but localized, gastrointestinal cancers may occasionally be candidates for wedge excision of adjacent liver to satisfy the 'en-bloc' principle.

Liver resection for cancer can be done safely in the 1980's and will yield highly satisfactory results if limited to patients with 'curable' disease. Palliative liver resection, or debulking operations, cannot be recommended (except to relieve endocrine symptoms) until more evidence is obtained that they will benefit the patient.

References

1. Foster JH, Berman MM: Solid liver tumors, Vol 22 in series, Major Problems in Clinical Surgery. Philadelphia: WB Saunders, 1977.
2. Craig JR, Peters RL, Edmondson HA *et al.*: Fibrolamellar carcinoma of the liver: a tumor of adolescents and young adults with distinctive clinico-pathologic features. Cancer 46: 372–379, 1980.
3. Berman MM, Libbey NP, Foster JH: Hepatocellular carcinoma. Polygonal cell type with fibrous stroma: an atypical variant with a favorable prognosis. Cancer 46: 0142–0149, 1980.
4. Exelby PR, Filler RM, Grosfeld JL: Liver tumors in children in the particular reference to hepatoblastomas and hepatocellular carcinoma: American Academy of Pediatrics, Surgical Section Survey – 1974. J Pediatr Surg 10: 329, 1975.
5. Wood GB, Gillis CR, Blumgart LH: A retrospective study of the natural history of patients with liver metastases from colorectal cancer. Clin Oncol 2: 285, 1976.
6. Pettavel J, Morgenthaler F: Protracted arterial chemotherapy of liver tumors: an experience of 107 cases over a 12-year period. Prog Clin Cancer 7: 217, 1978.
7. Blumgart LH, Allison DJ: Resection and embolization in the management of secondary hepatic tumors. World J Surg 6: 32–45, 1982.
8. Zhaoyou T, Binghui Y, Chenlong T *et al.*: Evaluation of population screening for hepatocellular carcinoma. Chin Med J 93: 795–799, 1980.
9. Tartter PI, Slater G, Gelernt I *et al.*: Screening for liver metastases from colon cancer with CEA and alkaline phosphatase. Gastroenterology 78: 1275, 1980.
10. Grage TB, Shingleton WW, Ar J, *et al.*: Results of prospective randomized study of hepatic artery infusion with 5-fluorouracil vs. intravenous 5-fluorouracil in patients with hepatic metastases from colorectal cancer: a central oncology group study (COG 7032). Front Gastrointest Res 5: 116, 1979.
11. Foster JH, Lundy J: Liver metastases. Curr Probl Surg 18: 161–202, 1982.
12. Balasegaram M: Hepatic resection for malignant tumors. Surg Rounds, 14–44, Sept 1979.
13. Shanghai Coordinating Group: Diagnosis and treatment of primary hepatocellular carcinoma in early stage. Chin Med J 92: 801–806, 1979.
14. Mengchao W, Han C, Xiaohua Z, *et al.*: Primary hepatic carcinoma resection over 18 years. Chin Med J 93: 723–728, 1980.
15. Okuda K, Liver Cancer Study Group of Japan: Primary liver cancers in Japan. Cancer 45: 2663–2669, 1980.
16. Lee NW, Wong J, Ong GB: The surgical management of primary carcinoma of the liver. World J Surg 6: 66–75, 1982.
17. Fortner JG, Dong KK, Maclean BJ, *et al.*: Major hepatic resection for neoplasia. Ann Surg 188: 363–371, 1978.
18. Raven RW: Hepatectomy. Copenhagen: Imprimerie Medicale et Scientifique, 16: 1099, 1955.
19. Jaffe BM, *et al.*: Factors influencing survival in patients with untreated hepatic metastases. Surg Gynecol Obstet 127: 1, 1968.
20. Bengmark S, Hafstrom L: The natural history of primary and secondary malignant tumors of the liver: I. The prognosis for patients with hepatic metastases from colonic and rectal carcinoma by laparotomy. Cancer 23: 198, 1969.
21. Starzl TE, Koep LJ: Surgical approaches for primary and metastatic liver neoplasms, including total hepatectomy with orthotopic liver transplantation. Prog Clin Cancer 7: 181–193, 1978.
22. Wanebo HJ, Semoglou C, Attiyeh F, *et al.*: Surgical management of patients with primary operable colorectal cancer and synchronous liver metastases. Amer J Surg 135: 81, 1978.
23. Sorenson TA, Aronsen KF, Aune S, *et al.*: Results of hepatic lobectomy for primary epithelial cancer in 31 adults. Amer J Surg 138: 407–410, 1979.
24. Hanks JB, Meyers WC, Filston HC, *et al.*: Surgical resection for benign and malignant liver

disease. Ann Surg 191: 584–92, 1980.

25. Adson MA, Van Heerden JA: Major hepatic resections for metastatic colorectal cancer. Ann Surg 191: 576–583, 1980.
26. Adson MA: Invited commentary on Muhe E, Gall FP and Angermann B: Resection of Liver Metastases. World J Surg 6: 210–215, 1982.
27. Adson MA, Weiland LH: Resection of primary solid hepatic tumors. Amer J Surg 141: 18–21, 1981.
28. Thompson JF, Little JM: Liver resection for neoplasm. Aust NZ J Surg 51: 274–279, 1981.
29. Logan SE, Meier SJ, Ramming KP, et al.: Hepatic resection of metastatic colorectal carcinoma. Arch Surg 117: 25–28, 1982.
30. Aldrete JS, Asdemir D, Laws HL: Major hepatic resections: Analysis of 51 cases. Am Surg 48: 118–122, 1982.
31. Bengmark S, Hafstrom L, Jeppsson B: Primary carcinoma of the liver: improvement in sight? World J Surg 6: 54–60, 1982.
32. Foster JH: Personal and previously unpublished experience.
33. Attiyeh FF, Wanebo HJ, Stearns MW: Hepatic resection for metastasis from colorectal cancer. Dis Colon Rectum 21: 160–162, 1978.
34. Iwatsuki S, Klintman JBG, Starzl TE: Total hepatectomy and liver replacement (orthotopic liver transplantation) for primary hepatic malignancy. World J Surg 6: 81–85, 1982.
35. Calne RY: Liver transplantation for liver cancer. World J Surg 6: 76–80, 1982.
36. Randolph JG, Altman RP, Arensman RM, et al.: Liver resection in children with hepatic neoplasms. Ann Surg 187: 599–605, 1978.
37. Muhe E, Gall FP, Angermann B: Resection of liver metastases. World J Surg 6: 210–215, 1982.
38. Wilson SM, Adson MA: Surgical treatment of hepatic metastases from colorectal cancers. Arch Surg 111: 330, 1976.
39. Smrcka J, et al.: Arteriographic demonstration and successful removal of metastatic islet cell tumors in liver. Diabetes 16: 598, 1967.
40. McDermott Jr WV, Paris AL, Clouse ME, et al.: Dearterialization of the liver for metastatic cancer. Ann Surg 187: 38, 1978.
41. Bengmark S, Ericsson M, Lunderquist A, et al.: Temporary liver dearterialization in patients with metastatic carcinoid disease. World J Surg 6: 46–53, 1982.
42. Foster JH: Carcinoma of the gallbladder. In: Surgery of the gallbladder and bile ducts, Way LW and Dunphy JE (eds). Philadelphia: WB Saunders, 1984.
43. Adson MA: Carcinoma of the gallbladder. Surg Clin North Am 53: 1202–1216, 1973.
44. Lin TY: A simplified technique for hepatic resection. Ann Surg 180: 285, 1974.
45. Bismuth H: Surgical anatomy and anatomical surgery of the liver. World J Surg 6: 3–9, 1982.
46. Bismuth H, Houssin D, Castaing D: Major and minor segmentectomies 'reglees' in liver surgery. World J Surg 6: 10–24, 1982.
47. Starzl TE, Koep LJ, Weil III R, et al.: Right trisegmentectomy for hepatic neoplasms. Surg Gynecol Obstet 150: 208–214, 1980.
48. Starzl TE, Iwatsuki S, Shaw BW, et al.: Left hepatic trisegmentectomy. Surg Gynecol Obstet 155: 21–27, 1982.

6. Current concepts in the treatment of esophageal cancer

DAVID KELSEN

1. Introduction

Malignant tumors of the esophagus are highly virulent neoplasms. In the United States, there has been no improvement in five year survival statistics over the past two decades, in spite of technical advances in both surgery and radiation therapy; only 5–10% of all newly diagnosed patients will be long-term survivors. Although relatively uncommon in the United States, the disease is endemic in other parts of the world. The vast majority of esophageal tumors are epidermoid carcinomas. In a study from Memorial Hospital involving 1,918 patients, Turnbull and his colleagues found that 95% had epidermoid cancer, with most of the other cases involving adenocarcinomas [1]. While most other series have noted a similar histologic pattern, occasionally up to 15% of patients were found to have adenocarcinomas [2]. Whether these studies have included large numbers of gastroesophageal cancers, or whether this represents an unusually large number of patients with adenocarcinoma arising in Barrett's esophagus, is unclear. In either case, conventional treatment has been unsatisfactory, and intensive investigations in the epidemiology, early diagnosis, staging and treatment of patients with esophageal cancer are ongoing.

2. Epidemiology

The incidence of esophageal cancer varies markedly. In some areas, epidermoid carcinoma of the esophagus is among the most common of tumors, whereas in others, it is exceedingly rare. Incidence rates for men between the ages of 35–64 years are shown in Table 1, taken from the excellent review by Haas and Schotenfeld [3]. In some countries only mortality rates are reported. Because it is highly lethal, the vast majority of patients with esophageal cancer can be expected to die of their disease; Doll has established a ratio of 1.19 times the mortality as indicative of its overall incidence [4]. As can be seen, there is a seven

J.J. DeCosse and P. Sherlock (eds), Clinical Management of Gastrointestinal Cancer.
© *1984, Martinus Nijhoff Publishers, Boston. ISBN 0-89838-601-2. Printed in The Netherlands.*

to 40 fold difference in incidence between high and low risk areas. Caucasian males in the United States and Canada have low rates of 2.2–5.8 cases per 100,000, whereas in China and Iran, the equivalent incidence is 109–206 [4]. The Transkei in South Africa and parts of the Soviet Union also have a high incidence rate. Areas of moderately high incidence include France (25.5), the United States for non whites (20.5), and Puerto Rico (35.2). In the Brittany Coast area of

Table 1. Truncated incidence rates in males for esophageal cancer, selected countries

Population	Rate
Africa	
Mozambique, Lourenco Marques	11.8
Nigeria, Ibadan	2.6
South Africa (colored)	28.0
South Africa (white)	6.1
South Africa Durban (African)	98.9
South Africa Durban (Indian)	14.7
South Africa, Johannesburg (Africa)	21.8
Uganda, Kyadondo	5.5
America	
Canada	2.2
United States (white)	5.8
United States (non-white)	20.5
Puerto Rico	35.2
Chile	18.9
Venezuela	4.8
Asia	
Singapore (Chinese)	24.6
Japan	20.7
Israel	4.2
Iran, Gonbad	206.4
USSR (Turkmenistan)	110.5
USSR (Uzbekistan)	48.5
USSR (Georgia)	7.9
Northern China	109.0
Europe	
Austria	4.9
Belgium	6.2
Denmark	3.9
France	25.5
Germany (Federal Republic)	4.8
Italy	6.5
Portugal	11.5
Switzerland	15.1
Sweden	3.4

Incidence rates are given as average annual rates per 100,000 persons aged 35-64 years. From Haas and Schottenfeld (with permission).

France, the rate of 56.1/100,000 is twice that of the rest of the country, with a particularly high male:female ratio of 56:1. Although in most areas males predominate, Iran is an exception with slightly more women having the tumor.

Whether the incidence of esophageal cancer is increasing or whether there have been improvements in case reporting is unclear. In part, this is because documentation in underdeveloped countries has been relatively sparse. However, there is suggestive evidence that, in at least one high risk area, the disease is actually increasing. Prior to the 1920's, esophageal cancer was rarely seen in the Transkei area of South Africa. Burrell reported that a survey performed in the mid 1960's indicated that the disease was first noted approximately 25 years before the survey, with older inhabitants 'emphatic that it was unheard of in their young days'[5]. Esophageal cancer, known to the Bantu as a 'defilment of the gullet' is now endemic in this area. On the other hand, the disease was apparently well known in China even in antiquity. In Linxian Province, 'hard of swallowing disease' has been noted for at least 2000 years; a temple to honor the throat god was extant until 1927 [6].

The epidemiologic studies that have been performed have thus tried to determine the environmental and genetic factors that have led to the large differences in incidence of this disease.

Animal data involving esophageal neoplasms has come primarily from China and Africa. Chinese studies involving carcinomas of the pharynx and esophagus in chickens date back to the early 1970's [6]. The incidence rate among chickens in Linxian Province was seven times that of other provinces, and paralleled the rate of esophageal cancer among humans. Interestingly, over 50% of diseased fowl were kept by families who either had a member with esophageal cancer or were neighbors of such a family. Ninety-seven percent of the tumors in chickens were epidermoid carcinomas. Equally fascinating was a study of the incidence of esophageal cancer in the chickens of families that had migrated to a low risk area, but who still had a high incidence of esophageal tumors (82.0 cases/100,000 versus 21.53 cases/100,000 for the native group). In parallel with the human data, chickens belonging to the immigrants had a higher incidence of esophageal tumors. Since neither the water supply nor the soil tilled appeared to be contributing factors, the method of food preparation was implicated.

In Africa, large animals such as cattle, sheep, and hogs have been noted to have an increased incidence of carcinoma of the esophagus or rumen [7]. In Kenya, Plowright noted that as many as 2.5% of cattle grazing in one area, the Nasampolai Valley, had developed epidermoid carcinoma of the rumen [7]. In the Cape Province of South Africa, 8% of sheep in one farming area developed esophageal cancer during a ten year period observation [8]. The disease appeared to be related to two factors: use of a new anti-parasite solution and grazing in plateau grasslands. Only animals having both factors present developed esophageal tumors.

Among humans, a number of agents have been suspected to be carcinogenic. In the United States and in European countries, alcohol and tobacco abuse are the two most commonly associated habits. In France, death rates for esophageal cancer and for alcohol abuse have been significantly correlated. In the United States, heavy drinkers were more likely to develop this disease. In Africa, the use of maize as a staple food and its use in making home-brewed beers has been implicated in high risk areas. Some studies suggest a synergism between alcohol and tobacco exposures. However, alcohol or tobacco abuse is clearly not the only cause of esophageal cancer, as the high incidence seen in Iran is in a population which neither smokes nor uses liquor.

Less commonly seen conditions that also cause an increased incidence of esophageal cancer include lye ingestion, achalasia, Plummer-Vinson syndrome, the rare dermatologic abnormality of tylosis palmaris et plantaris, and, perhaps, reflux esophagitis. For patients with lye-induced strictures and achalasia, the increased incidence of the disease is high enough to suggest the need for close follow-up, especially as these patients may chronically have dysphagia, so that the most commonly seen presenting symptom of cancer may be ignored. Late diagnosis probably explains the extraordinarily poor prognosis for esophageal cancer when seen in the setting of achalasia. In one series, less than 15% of patients had resectable disease [9].

3. Diagnosis and staging

Mass screening programs have been most successful in areas of high incidence, such as China. The techniques used in China are relatively simple and can be performed by paramedical personnel. The mainstay of screening is 'Lawang' ('pulling in a net'), which involves use of an inflatable balloon which is covered by a nylon mesh. The tube is swallowed by the patient, balloon inflated, and the tube withdrawn by the technician. Smears are then made for cytological evaluation. If the cytologic specimens are positive, or highly suspicious, barium contrast and endoscopic procedures, with or without toluidine blue staining, are performed.

Using this procedure the yield of early cases is high: in 1974, 14,000 patients over age 30 were screened at Yaocun Commune; 75% of tumors detected were early lesions. Many of these were not detectable by X-ray or by endoscopy. Patients found during the screening programs were more likely to have a T_1 lesion, or even carcinoma *in situ,* as compared to patients who underwent investigation because of symptoms, and their improved prognosis appears to be related to the earlier stage of the disease. In one Chinese series involving 237 patients whose tumor had been discovered during screening procedures and who had stage I tumors, the five year survival rate was 85.9%; 56.6% were ten year survivors [10]. On the other hand, the five year survival rate for patients with more advanced disease (stages III or IV) was 30.3%. Because of the high incidence of esophageal cancer, patient acceptance of these and other surveillance techniques are good. Whether such methods can be used in specific high risk populations in western countries (such as those with prior head and neck cancer) is unclear; but with the relatively low incidence of this tumor in the United States, mass screening of the general population may not be cost effective.

Unlike the Chinese experience, few patients in the United States have the incidental discovery of an esophageal cancer while still asymptomatic. Almost invariably, dysphagia or odynophagia have been present for 1 to 6 months, and frequently even longer before a diagnosis is made. In addition to patient delay in seeking medical attention, it is not at all infrequent to have a physician dismiss the patient's complaints as non-specific, prescribing, for example, antacids. The first barium esophagram may be performed only after persistant dysphagia for weeks to months.

Once an esophageal tumor is suspected, and barium contrast studies confirm an abnormality, the initial diagnostic study that is usually performed is an upper gastrointestinal endoscopy and biopsy to confirm the diagnosis and determine cell type. The barium swallow itself will also be an important part of the staging procedure.

In addition to a careful physical examination, barium esophagram and esophagoscopy, the following studies are usually obtained: a 12 channel screening profile, including serum alkaline phosphatase, lactic dehydrogenase, and SGOT as measures of liver function; bone and liver scans are performed if the alkaline phosphatase is elevated. In all patients whose primary tumor is at the level of the carina or higher (i.e. <25 cm from the incisor teeth), bronchoscopy is mandatory in order to rule out asymptomatic invasion of the tracheo-bronchial tree. This finding automatically places the patient in the extensive disease group, indicates inoperability, and means that the patient is at high risk to develop the disasterous complication of a tracheoesophageal fistula.

During the last decade, several additional techniques to allow more accurate staging of newly diagnosed patients have been studied. These procedures are of interest because of the high percentage of patients who undergo exploration but who are found to have unresectable disease, or unsuspected hepatic or other visceral metastases, and because of the substantial operative morbidity and mortality in this frequently debilitated population. Thus, pre-operative knowledge of the presence of unresectable tumor is of considerable importance. In addition, as multimodality regimens involving pre-operative radiation or chemotherapy become more effective it is essential that objective evaluations of response, as well as pre-treatment staging, be as accurate as possible. The finding of metastatic disease outside the local-regional field is especially important if preoperative radiation therapy is planned, as tumor outside the radiation portal will presumably progress during the 4 to 6 weeks before surgery.

Among the techniques used to evaluate periesophageal structures and regional lymph nodes are azygography, mediastinoscopy, and computerized tomography (CT).

Azygography involves the injection of a water soluble contrast material into a rib (usually the tenth rib). If the hemiazygous vein is visualized, this almost invariably means obstruction of the azygous, either by direct extension or by nodal enlargement. Narrowing of the azygous has the same implication. Segarra and Carious used this approach to evaluate 26 patients before surgery [11]. Seventeen had normal azygograms; of these 13 patients had resectable disease. Of the nine patients with abnormal azygograms, the tumor was unresectable in all eight in whom the block was at the level of primary tumor (indicating direct tumor extension). In the one patient with involvement of the azygous at a distance from the primary, only nodal metastases were present and the esophagus could be removed.

Mediastinoscopy has also been used, in association with staging laparotomy, to evaluation regional and distant nodal disease. Murray and his associates studied 30 patients who appeared to have disease limited to the esophagus after a standard work-up [12]. Sixty percent had primary tumors of the upper two-thirds of the esophagus. All patients had pre-operative radiation before mediastinoscopy or laparotomy. Five of 30 patients had a positive mediastinoscopy; in four, the lymph nodes were fixed. None of these patients were explored. Of the 25 patients with negative mediastinoscopies, nine of 17 who had resections had positive lymph nodes. Celiac metastases were found in 16 of 26 patients who had a laparotomy, of whom eight went on to undergo resection of the primary tumor. Murray concludes that resection was palliative in this setting.

Guernsey and his colleagues had evaluated the use of staging laparotomy alone in 40 patients with tumors in the thoracic esophagus [13]. All appeared to have resectable disease after a standard evaluation. Sixteen were found to have unsuspected metastases to abdominal lymph nodes. The incidence of positive celiac nodes was highest in the mid and lower esophageal lesions. In 12 patients, nodal metastases were grossly evident at surgery. All 16 patients died within 11 months.

The advent of computerized tomography (CT) has added a non-invasive technique for evaluation of mediastinal and abdominal structures which may prove of value not only for staging patients prior to any therapy but for evaluating response to pre-operative radiation or chemotherapy. Several groups have now compiled a substantial experience in CT scanning for malignant tumors of the esophagus. Daffner studied 35 patients with known esophageal carcinoma who were being evaluated for potential resection [14]. Twenty-nine patients had obliteration of paraesophageal fat planes at varying parts of the esphagus; 28 had mediastinal invasion at the time of surgery. Six patients had normal CT scanning of the thorax; four had no tumor in the mediastinum at surgery. Thirty-three patients also had scans of the abdomen; among the 19 patients in whom the CT was positive, 16 were confirmed at surgery to have abdominal metastases. Among the 14 patients who had negative abdominal scans, 11 were found to be free of tumor at exploration. CT scanning may make invasive procedures such as azyography, mediastinoscopy, and staging laparotomy obsolete.

Following diagnosis and staging procedures, patients seen at Memorial Hospital are divided into two groups: those in whom the tumor is clinically limited to the local-regional (LR) area are considered candidates for potential curative therapy. These patients have clinical stage I or II tumors using the AJC TNM classification (Table 2) [15]. We do not currently use invasive staging procedures, and are beginning to investigate CT scanning pre-operatively. For the present, abnormal CT scans suggesting paraesophageal invasion or abdominal nodal metastases do not exclude patients from surgery. Approximately 50 to 60% of our patients have LR disease. The remaining 40 to 50% either present with metastases to distant sites or have had a local recurrence following definitive surgery and/or radiation therapy. They are considered to have extensive disease, and are treated with palliative intent.

Table 2. TMN classification

Primary Tumor (T) (for all three segments of the esophagus)

T0	No demonstrable tumor in the esophagus
TIS	Carcinoma in situ
T1	A tumor <5 cm in esophageal length with no obstruction, no circumferential involvement and no estraesophageal spread
T2	A tumor >5 cm in esophageal length with no extra-esophageal spread or a tumor of any size which obstructs or has circumferential involvement and with no extraesophageal spread
T3	Any tumor with esophageal spread

Nodal involvement (N)

Cervical esophagus: the regional lymph nodes in cervical esophagus are the cervical and supraclavicular nodes

N0	No clinically palpable nodes
N1	Movable, unilateral, palpable nodes
N2	Movable, bilateral, palpable nodes
N3	Fixed nodes

Thoracic esophagus:

NX	(clinical evaluation) Regional lymph for the upper, midthoracic, and lower thoracic esophagus that are ordinarily not accessible for clinical evaluation
N0	(surgical evaluation) No positive nodes
N1	(surgical evaluation) Positive nodes

Distant Metastasis (M)

MX	Not assessed
M0	No (known) distant metastasis*
M1	Distant metastasis present

4. Treatment

Surgery for the potentially curable patient

Despite generally poor results, surgery remains the standard treatment for the patient with potentially curable local-regional esophageal cancer. The lack of other proven methods has, until recently, led most physicians to accept attempted resection despite its having the highest operative mortality seen with any routine surgical procedure. In addition to allowing a small but definite cure rate, resection and anastomosis usually means permanent relief from dysphagia.

Two major techniques are used to restore alimentary tract continuity: esophagectomy with colon interposition, and esophagectomy with esophagogastrostomy.

The major rationale for the use of colon interposition resides in the ability to perform an extrathoracic, usually cervical proximal anastomosis, thus decreasing the severity of complications following an anastomotic leak. A leak in the neck is less serious than one in the chest. None the less, a review of several series using the colon for reconstruction indicates that this technique is formidable, with a substantial morbidity and mortality.

Wilkins and Burke reviewed their results using colon bypass in 40 patients, of whom 37 had malignancy and 3 had benign strictures [16]. There were a total of six operative deaths (18%), and a 5.2% anastomatic leak rate. It should be noted that the colon bypass preceded planned esophagectomy in most patients, but was also used to bypass an unresectable tumor in 13. Huguier and his collegues used the colon as an esophageal replacement in 46 patients [17]. There were 11 postoperative deaths; 29% of patients had an anastomatic leak in the neck.

Postlewait and collegues treated 29 patients with esophageal cancer using colon interposition [18]. There were eight operative deaths, and three patients had nonfatal leaks. They reviewed a total of 285 additional cases from the literature and found an overall 24.5% mortality. El-Domeiri reviewed 88 patients treated, at Memorial Hospital, with colon interposition [19]. Most of these patients received radiation therapy before placement of the colon bypass. As was the case in other studies, a fistula at the cervical anastomosis was common, occurring in 41.3%. Operative mortality was 22.6%. Of the 53 patients who survived the operative procedure and had adequate follow-up, only 51% were able to resume a normal diet. Thirty-two percent were not able to use the colon bypass at all, and continued to use a gastrostomy tube.

In all of these series, the major cause of death was ischemic necrosis of the interposed colon. Pulmonary dysfunction was infrequent. Nine patients in Huguier's series died of nonhemorrhagic shock, whose etology was apparently unclear. Because anastomatic leak in the neck was so common, strictures occurred in 12% of patients. Dilation of an anastomatic stricture following colon bypass may be difficult, and surgical revision is usually needed. Most colon procedures require several steps. Attempts at single-stage operations, although certainly feasible, appear to have a higher operative mortality than do staged procedures.

In summary, colon interposition has the advantage of allowing a cervical anastomosis, thus avoiding the dangers of an intrathoracic anastomatic leak. However, it usually requires several stages to completion, has a substantial operative mortality, and a fairly high stricture rate. Considering the extremely short survival of these patients, a treatment plan that includes several major operative procedures spread over a number of months is probably undesirable.

4.1.1. Esophagectomy with esophagogastrostomy

Esophagectomy followed by an esophagogastrostomy is the second major form of reconstruction of the alimentary tract. Its major advantage is that it is a single stage procedure, which is technically relatively easy to perform. Until recently, the major disadvantage has been the high rate of intrathoracic anastomatic leaks, with the associated risks of mediastinitis and death. However, the introduction of mechanical stapling devices has resulted in a decreased incidence of leakage and simplified performance of the anastomosis. As a result, esophagogastrostomy has become more popular. Steichen and Ravitch reviewed the use of stapling devices in esophageal surgery [20]. Several different instruments are currently available, including the EEA (End to End Anastomosis), GIA and TA-55. Basically these devices allow rapid and safe performance of the anastomosis, employing double rows of metal staples. Details of the technique can be found in Steichen's review.

The most common complication we have seen is a fairly high incidence of anastomotic strictures (approximately 25%) which, however, are usually handled easily by dilation. In addition to technical advances seen using the stapling devices, improved nutritional support services and better post-operative care appear to have decreased the operative mortality seen following esophago-gastrectomy. The Lewis approach, involving a vertical upper abdominal incision and right anterolateral thoracotomy, is now widely used. A combined thoracoab-dominal, left sided incision is still favored by some for lower third or gastro-esophageal junction tumors. With either approach, more recent studies suggest that the operative mortality, in experienced hands, should be less than 10%.

In a nonrandomized study, Wilson and co-workers compared esophagogastros-tomy, with radiation therapy for midthird esophageal lesions [21]. There were 20 patients in each group. In the surgery arm, there was one operative death (5%), and four major post-operative complications. Ellis reviewed his experiences at the Lahey Clinic [22]. Of 82 patients undergoing exploration, 72 had resectable disease. The operative mortality was 2.8%. Approximately 25% had post-opera-tive complications. Similarly, Piccone and his collegues used the Lewis procedure to resect middle-third esophageal carcinomas in 55 patients [23]. The operative mortality was 3.6%. Carey, Plested and Hughes explored 39 patients with middle and lower third lesions [24]. There were no post-operative deaths among 37 who had resectable disease, although 16 patients had minor or major post-operative complications. It thus apears that using current techniques, the operative morbidity and mortality for esophagogastrectomy is acceptable. However, the overall, long term results have remained poor.

Earlam and Cunha-Menlo have extensively reviewed the results of series where surgery was a major part of the treatment plan [25]. Although they did not separate those programs using surgery alone from those including pre or post-operative radiation, and although many series included substantial numbers of patients with adenocarcinoma, the statistics for the 20 year period 1960–1979 are quite helpful in giving an over-all picture of the disease during that time. Data were included from 122 series involving 83, 783 patients. The mean operability rate was 58%; 39% of patients had resectable disease. Operative mortality was 25% (a mean of 13 deaths out every of 58 operable patients). The one-year survival was 31% for patients with operable disease and 45% for those with resectable disease; at 24 months, survival fell to 14% for operable patients and 20% for those with resectable tumors.

This review, which encompasses results from throughout the world, provides a good idea of the dismal prognosis for this tumor. By extracting from their report those series published since 1972 and adding those published since 1980, an idea of surgical results in the last decade, including the period when the stapling devide and nutritional support began to gain widespread acceptance, can be obtained. These more recent studies are shown in Table 3. Again, the treatment plan for these patients may have included other modalities besides surgery (usually radiation). The operability rate is probably unrealistically high, as some larger series, such as that of Giuli and Gignoux, include only operable patients. The results of these studies indicate that the operability rate was 82.8%, and resections were possible among 52.7%. The operative mortality was 22%; at one year, 22.8% patients were alive; but by 5 years, only 3.6% had survived.

4.1.2. Surgical palliation

The main aim of surgical palliation of advanced esophageal cancer is to restore nutritional function by relieving or bypassing the mechanical obstruction caused by the tumor.

The easiest and probably most unsatisfactory solution to the problem is the placement of a feeding gastrostomy. Although this is technically simple to perform even in severely debilitated patients, gastrostomy does not restore the ability to swallow; patients with high-grade blockage are still unable to handle their own secretions. The technique generally means an inhospital stay of 5 to 10 days, and does have an associated mortality of 5 to 10%. If possible most investigators would rather avoid using a feeding gastrostomy.

Dilatation of the tumor-obstructed segment has been used successfully to allow ingestion of at least a soft diet. The major disadvantage of this procedure is the need for repeated applications; in addition, dilation may not be feasible if the

Table 3. Surgery in esophageal cancer 1972-1982

Author	Number of patients	% op	% res	% res mort	Survival (%)		Ref.
					1 yr	5 yr	
Amer Joint Committee	917				24	5	26
Angorn	924	13	11				27
Applequist	701	54	24	23		4	28
Belsey	198	85	76	26	20	2	29
Boyd	56	100	100	9	43		30
Buck	118	26	19	35			31
Carey	37	100	11				24
Cedarquist	966	15	7	45	8	2	32
Chinese	1228	100	94	1			33
Drucker	45	100	100	4			34
Ellis	82	100	88	2.8			22
Gary-Bobo	755	30	22	12	23	5	35
Giuli	2400	100	100	30	14		36
Hambraeus	50		100	26	38		37
Hankins	234	21	18	54	27	1	38
Hunt	387				10		39
Jackson	292	75	74	19	18	5	40
Just-Vera	4342					1	41
Kelsen	110	90	61	12		5	42
Leverment	452	84	69	34	51		43
Lortat-Jacob	4000	44	26	53	17	3	44
Lowe	600	31			6	1	45
Marks	415	33	24		7	5	46
McKeown	403	97	92	11			47
Milne	600	96	84	27			48
Mohansingh	969	78	62	15	10		49
Nakayama	6282	66	40	5		1	50
Parker	609	28	19	41		2	51
Pelletier	75	76	48		9	4	52
Picconi	89	93	91	10			53
Rambo	486		32		22	6	54
Ross	182	45	26				55
Rossetti	482	41				4	56
Roussel	1402	31	22				57
Sanfelippo	432	61	41				58
Segol	8	100	100	13	75	13	59
Seitz	164	35					60
Skinner	110		53	43	21	3	61
Smith	41	63			29	5	62
Stoller	127	43			11	1	63
Stone	86	79	60	12		7	64
Takita	153	26				1	65
Van Houtte	136		12	13	19	5	66
Wahlers	205				21	1	67
Webb	52	100	44	30	25	2	68

patient has a long segment that is obstructed. When used by skilled operators, complications of perforation and fever were rare (10% of patients but <2% of dilations [69].

Intraluminal tubes have been widely used over the past 20–30 years in patients with unresectable disease (either with or without metastases) or in those with localized recurrences following a resection or definitive radiation therapy. Most tubes require a gastrostomy to allow placement. They are generally either pulled through the lesion from below, or pushed through from above. The advantages of an intraluminal tube over dilatation include a single procedure rather than multiple applications, and potential use in longer lesions. However, in addition to the need for gastrostomy, intraluminal tubes can not be used for upper lesions (cervical or high thoracic). The narrow inner lumen of most tubes usually limits the patient to a soft diet, but relief of dysphagia to at least this extent is seen in 60–90% [70–73]. An operative mortality of 10–20% has been reported by most investigators; hospitalization averages 8 to 10 days. Late complications include tube migration, chronic reflux of gastric contents if the tube traverses the lower esophageal sphincter (which increases the risks of aspiration pneumonia) and, rarely, perforation and hemorrhage if the tube penetrates the esophageal wall. In a review of over 2500 cases using standard intraluminal tubes, usually placed via a gastrostomy, the non-fatal complication rate was 28% [73]. More recently, Boyce and his colleagues have used an intraluminal tube that does not require gastrostomy for placement [74]. As is the case for standard tubes, the per-oral technique cannot be used for high lesions (cervical or upper thoracic). Complications when using this technique appear to be substantially less common than those seen with an operatively-placed tube.

Many surgeons feel that even in the presence of advanced disease, a palliative resection or a bypass procedure is preferable to gastrostomy, dilatation, or an intraluminal tube. The rationale for the use of a major surgical procedure in the face of incurable disease is that one has, in general, definitively treated the patient's major symptom, dysphagia. Solids are usually handled easily and patients can enjoy a normal diet until death from intercurrent disease. This type of approach is usually used in the 40 to 60% of patients who have operable (local-regional) tumor but who are found, at the time of surgery, to have clearly incurable disease.

The definition of a palliative resection varies, but in general means that either gross tumor was left behind, that microscopically positive margins were present, or that metastatic tumor was resected (e.g. celiac lymph nodes) as part of the procedure. Since the five year survival rate for esophageal is so poor, many surgeons approach all patients with even operable tumors with the understanding that the treatment planned is for palliation, and if an occasional patient is cured, that is an extra dividend [29].

A number of different procedures have been used for palliative resections. Except for bypass techniques, they are identical to those discussed above for surgery of the potentially curable patient.

Bypass procedures using the stomach to anastomose above the level of the obstruction have been fairly widely used and appear to have an operative morbidity and mortality similar to that of patients undergoing resection. In one series of 55 patients, a 7.5% operative mortality was seen. Of the 51 who survived surgery, only three did not have an improvement in swallowing function [30]. The complication rate was 33% and mean survival was only 5 months. Similar results were seen in a group of 119 patients with middle-third lesions who had a palliative resection. The median survival was again 5 months, and the operative mortality 28% [29].

The major disadvantage as far as any surgical intervention is concerned is the significant operative morbidity and mortality (10–30%) attendent. Patients in whom palliative procedures are performed have as can be seen from the series discussed above, a median life expectancy of 5 to 6 months. For this reason, radiation therapy is used by many physicians in patients with locally advanced disease.

4.2. Radiation therapy

Radiation therapy for esophageal carcinoma can be given with curative (radical) intent, or for purposes of palliation only. Pearson has defined the indications for curative radiation therapy to include:
  (1) a diagnosis of epidermoid or undifferentiated cancer;
  (2) no evidence of distant metastases;
  (3) the primary lesion is less than 9 cm in length;
  (4) the tracheo-bronchial tree, thyroid, stomach, and vertebrae have not been invaded by the tumor;
  (5) reasonably good general medical condition.
The recommended dose of curative radiation, in Pearson's experience, is 4800–5300 rads to a volume of 15 af096.5 cm delivered in 20 equal fractions [75]. At Memorial Hospital, doses of 5500 rads are given using a multiple port technique, the first 4,000 rads via standard anterior-posterior parallel opposed portals, and the final 1500 rads given via tangential fields (thus decreasing the risk of spinal cord toxicity).

Survival is usually the end point of most trials; few studies involving the use of radiation in the treatment of esophageal cancer, either with radical therapy for potentially curable disease, or using palliative doses, have attempted to quantitate the effectiveness of radiation in inducing objective tumor regression. Recent studies from Memorial Hospital, involving investigational chemotherapeutic regimens, have indicated that serial radiographic studies can be used to quantitate the responses in the primary site. Pre and post treatment barium esophagrams were required in these chemotherapy studies. In most cases, the radiographic assessment of response was compared to pathological evaluation following surgical resection, or endoscopic confirmation in non-operable patients [42].

A complete response (CR) required both a normal barium esophagram as well as endoscopic confirmation of regression, including negative cytology or pathologic review of the resected specimen and *all* tissues sampled at surgery indicating that no viable tumor remained. A partial response (PR) thus means either a more than 50% decrease in the tumor mass as seen by repeat barium esophagram, or that the esophagram was now normal, but viable tumor (microscopically or macroscopically), was found at endoscopy or surgery. A minor regression, which is not used in calculating response rates but which may give substantial symptomatic relief, means that definite improvement in the barium esophagram is seen, but this involves less than 50% tumor decrease. Radiographic examples of tumor regression as seen by barium esophagram have been reported [42, 76]. Only occasional radiation therapy studies have made similar assessments. In one trial, by Kolaric and his colleagues, four of 12 patients receiving radical radiation therapy (5,000–7,000 rads) had partial regressions lasting for a median of 6 months [77]. Most other studies have used survival as an endpoint, and, again, discuss this only in relation to patients treated for cure. However, a few reports have described improvement in dysphagia, which at least gives some idea of tumor regression.

Van Andel and his colleagues used radiation therapy alone in 67 patients with advanced disease who were treated with palliative intent [78]. Three to five thousand rads were delivered to the tumor over a 2 to 4 week period. One-half had 'reasonable to good' relief of dysphagia. Survival was poor, with only three patients living for more than one year. Wara *et al.* used a higher dosage of 5,000–6,000 rads in a group of 129 patients [79]. One-fifth were unable to complete the treatment plan usually because of progressive disease. Of the 80% who finished radiation, two-thirds, 54% of the entire group, had relief of dysphagia for at least 8 weeks, but in only 11% was swallowing improved for more than 6 months. Placement of a celestin tube was required in 30 patients. The Eastern Cooperative Oncology Group has recently completed a study comparing radiation therapy alone with the use of radiation and bleomycin [80]. The dosage of radiation was 5,000–6,000 rads. Among those receiving radiation only, in whom an assessment of improvement in dysphagia was made, 18 of 37 (49%) had improved swallowing.

Thus, objective response data, combined with symptomatic improvement, suggest that approximately 50% of patients receiving 3000 to 6000 rads will have enough tumor shrinkage to substantially relieve their dysphagia. This improvement will last for 2 to 6 months. The other 50% will have little or no improvement.

Radiation toxicities and complications, when given with curative intent, can be substantial. They include esophagitis, tracheo-esophageal or esophageal-aortic fistula, mediastinitis, pneumonitis, and myelosupression. In the study by Earle *et al.*, mild myelosupression (white blood cell nadir counts between 2,000 and 4,000) occurred in nine of 37 (24%) patients; two patients (6%) had severe leukopenia (less than 2,000 white cells/mm^3) [82]. Tracheo-esophageal fistulas were seen in three of 37 (9%) patients in Earle's study, and one of 12 in Kolaric's study. Elkon *et al.* treated 50 patients with curative intent [81]. Three patients had significant radiation toxicity: one developed transverse myelitis, one perforated his esophagus and died of mediastinitis, and one had severe pulmonary fibrosis.

Radiation esophagitis usually begins during the second week of therapy, and becomes most severe during the fourth week of a 4 week schedule. Earlam and Cunha-Menlo have pointed out the difficulty in assessing the true complication rate of radical radiation therapy since many patients will develop progressive disease during treatment [82]. In these cases, the total dose of radiation is lowered, the treatment volume is reduced, or therapy is stopped entirely and the patient is listed as having had palliative radiation. In one study, 20% of patients had early termination of radiation [79].

There are no direct comparisons between surgery and radiation therapy as far as survival is concerned. Since most patients with potentially operable disease do indeed undergo exploration, radiation series are probably heavily weighted with poor risk patients. Table 4 from Earlam and Cunha-Menlo summarizes survival data from a number of radiation studies using supervoltage techniques [82, 83–129]. As can be seen, survival results are poor: at 12 months, only 18% of patients were still alive. Two year and five year survival rates were similar (8% and 6%), suggesting that the two year mark might be a reasonable one for prediction of 'long-term' survival. These data suggest that radiation may not be significantly worse than surgery as far as long-term survival is concerned. However, as discussed above, palliation of dysphagia is probably not as good.

When patients with esophageal carcinoma relapse following radiation, tumor recurrence can be either local or distant. Elkon reviewed the sites of recurrence in 30 patients who had received curative dosages [81]. Since they were not, in general, explored surgically, patients were clinically staged retrospectively by the length of the lesion and the presence of metastases. The overall local recurrence rate in the radiated field was 44%; an additional 26% had marginal recurrences (at the edge of the port). Patients with longer lesions (stage II or III) had a higher rate of local recurrence than did those with stage I (<5 cm long) tumors (64% vs 25%). However, the number of patients in each subgroup was small. Pearson had noted a similar local recurrence rate ≈50% of patients treated with radical radiotherapy had regrowth of tumor in the radiated field. Distant disease was at least as common as local failure, with a number of patients relapsing at both sites.

The failure of either radiation or surgery to cure substantial numbers of patients is not surprising in view of the findings of several autopsy series. In the most recent of these, Anderson and Ladd reviewed the autopsy records of 79 patients dying of esophageal cancer [130]. As this was a Veterans Administration Hospital study, all patients were males. 94% had residual active tumor at au-

Table 4. Results of radiation therapy 1954-1979

First author	Year	No. patients	Palliative RT (%)	Survival (%) 1 yr	5 yr	Ref.
Appelquist	1972	188	31		3	85
Buschke	1954	60	22	33	4	86
Cederquist	1978	700	45		4	87
Cossu	1967	154		16	2	88
Ebarhardt	1970	41			5	89
Eichorn	1966	872			4	90
Gary-Bobo	1978	530		14	2	91
Gunderson	1976	169			19	92
Gynning	1965	355	22	25	6	93
Hankins	1972	181	34		1	94
Heinze	1973	110		14	2	95
Holsti	1969	132		31		96
Humphrey	1968	188		18	1	97
Krishnamurthi	1965	100	22	12	4	98
Kuttig	1966	27			7	99
Lawler	1969	68	93		1	100
Lawrence	1976	169			19	101
LeBorgne	1963	294			3	102
Lederman	1966	196		19	1	103
Leon	1971	196			1	104
Levit	1970	25		12		105
Lewinsky	1975	85			0	106
Lowe	1972	224		11	3	107
Marcial	1966	197	23	28	4	108
Marks	1976	82	60		2	109
Martinez	1964	362		8	1	110
Meynard	1965	110		16	1	111
Millburn	1968	64	61		9	112
Miller	1962	33	76			113
Moor	1968	17	100			114
Moseley	1968	26	100		4	115
Mustard	1956	125		18	1	116
Nakayama	1967	100			6	117
Pearson	1978	288	83		20	118
Pelletier	1972	21		10		119
Pierquin	1966	115			3	120
Robertson	1967	39			8	121
Ross	1974	40			13	122
Skinner	1976	21		18		123
Stoller	1977	53		8		124
Takita	1977	57			2	125
Vanhoutte	1977	120	28	22	2	126
Verhaeghe	1971	300	30	21		127
Voutilainen	1975	140		28	7	128
Wahlers	1975	205	39	21	2	129
Walker	1964	35			6	130
Wara	1976	129		18	1	131
Watson	1963	19	54		21	132

topsy. Nine percent of patients were found to have only local tumor; the remaining 85% had disseminated disease, with 82% having residual local tumor as well. The most common sites of metastases were lymph nodes, lung, and liver; the latter two sites were involved in approximately 50% of patients. With a median survival of 4 months, the extensive nature of tumor found at post-mortum examination cannot be ascribed to a prolonged interval between diagnosis and death. Similarly, Attah and Hadju reviewed 113 autopsies performed at Cleveland Metropolitan General Hospital [131]. 73% had metastatic disease. Again, lymph nodes, lung, and liver were the most common sites. Bosch *et al.* found that 32% of their patients had no local disease at autopsy, but more than one half of these had died in the immediate post operative period. Overall, 51% had lymph node or visceral metastases at autopsy [132].

These and other autopsy series have established that in the majority of patients, esophageal cancer is disseminated at the time of diagnosis. Localized treatment planning alone is thus doomed to failure. Clearly, development of effective systemic therapy would allow treatment of both the primary tumor and metastatic disease.

4.3. Chemotherapy

4.3.1. Single agents

Because the vast majority of patients with esophageal cancer have or will develop systemic disease, effective chemotherapy should, at least theoretically, play a major role in their management. However, surprisingly few antineoplastic agents have undergone sufficient testing in this disease. If one accepts the need for at least 19 adequate patient trials for any given agent to determine if it is active (if 19 patients are adequately studied, and not one response is seen, it can be assumed with 95% confidence, that the drug in question will have therapeutic activity in less than 15% of patients), then only 10 drugs have had at least minimal phase II studies in epidermoid carcinoma of the esophagus (Table 5). For the medical oncologist, adenocarcinoma of the esophagus is a different disease, usually treated with the same agents used in gastric cancer.

Bleomycin, an antitumor antibiotic, is the most widely used single agent. Data compiled from a number of different studies, involving various schedules and routes of administration, indicate that major objective tumor regression (complete or partial remissions − CR + PR) were seen in 17% of patients [133–135]. The median duration of response was usually quite brief (1.5 to 2.5 months), and rarely of significant clinical benefit. Bleomycin's major toxicities include mucositis, fever, chills and pulmonary fibrosis (usually seen after cumulative doses exceeding 200 units). Myelosupression is uncommon.

Methotrexate, an inhibitor of folic acid reductase, was studied by the Eastern Cooperative Oncology Group (ECOG) [136]. In a small group of 26 patients three responses were seen. Major toxicities of methotrexate include my-elosupression and mucositis. During the same trial, 5-Flurouracil, a pyramidine analogue, was given to 23 patients; four (17%) responded. The median duration of response for both drugs was approximately 2 months.

Adriamycin, another antitumor antibiotic, has undergone two separate studies: one by Kolaric *et al.*, in patients with locally advanced disease, and one by ECOG in patients with systemic disease [136, 137]. In the first study, six of 18 patients had partial responses, and Kolaric concluded that the drug was active. However, in a more recent study by ECOG, only one of 20 patients had a brief regression. Adriamycin probably has only modest activity in this disease. Its major toxicities are nausea and vomiting, alopecia, myelosupression, and a congestive cardiomyopathy seen after total cumulative doses exceeding 450–550 mg/m^2.

Mitomycin C is the third antitumor antibiotic which has been studied in esophageal cancer. In its initial trials, from India and Japan, modest activity was seen, with four of 27 (15%) patients having partial responses [138]. In a more recent study by the ECOG, a higher response rate was noted (8/24) but, at the dosage and scheduled used, toxicity was prohibitive with severe myelosupression being seen in 31% of patients [136]. Overall, mitomycin has moderate activity in esophageal cancer. CCNU, a nitrosourea which functions as an alkylating agent, has undergone a small Phase II trial and also had modest activity.

Methyl-glyoxal bis (gualylhydrazone) (MGBG) is an inhibitor of polyamine synthesis that was first studied by Falkson in the early 1970's. Using a daily dosage schedule, he found that this agent was active but toxicity, including mucositis, was severe [139]. Interest in MGBG was renewed after Knight *et al.* demonstrated that toxicity using a weekly schedule was markedly decreased [140]. A trial of MGBG using the weekly schedule has recently been completed at Memorial

Table 5. Chemotherapy of esophageal carcinoma. Single agent activity

Drug	Patients studied	Patients responding (%)
		(Complete/Partial)
Bleomycin	64	11 (17)
Methotrexate	26	3 (12)
5-Flurouracil	23	4 (17)
Adriamycin	39	7 (18)
Cisplatin	61	11 (18)
Vindesine	35	5 (15)
Mitomycin C	48	12 (25)
CCNU	19	3 (16)
Methyl-GAG	45	9 (20)
VP-16	20	0 (0)

Hospital [141]. Most of the patients in this study had received prior chemotherapy with either cisplatin-bleomycin or cisplatin-vindesine-bleomycin (see below). In most chemotherapy trials, prior treatment with other agents decreases the chances of response. None the less, activity was seen using MGBG, confirming Falkson's observations, and toxicity was substantially less. Interestingly, all responding patients had received prior chemotherapy suggesting that, in at least some patients, MGBG was not cross-resistant with cisplatin, bleomycin, and vindesine.

Vindesine is an investigational vinca alkaloid which has undergone extensive testing over the last 4 to 5 years. In esophageal cancer, 35 patients have been treated using a weekly or semi-weekly schedule. The majority of those patients were studied at Memorial Hospital, and a number of them had received prior therapy with cisplatin-bleomycin [142]. Modest activity in the 15% range has been noted, with a median duration of response of 5 months. Vindesine's major toxicities are myelosupression and a peripheral neuropathy.

Since the initial report of the activity of cisplatin-bleomycin, three phase II trials of cisplatin as a single agent have been completed [136, 143–144]. Dosages used have ranged from 50 mg/m^2 on days 1 and 8 to 120mg/m^2 every 3 weeks. Among the 61 patients treated, 11 have had a partial regression. Nausea and vomiting, renal damage, involving the proximal tubule, were the major toxicities. Myelosupression was usually mild.

Finally, VP-16-123 (etoposide) an epipodophyllotoxin derivative, had shown some activity against esophageal cancer in preliminary phase I (dose finding) trials. However, a recently completed study from Memorial Hospital has failed to confirm this, with no responses being seen among the 20 evaluable patients [145], Again, many of these patients had received prior chemotherapy.

In summary, of the ten drugs having undergone at least minimally adequate testing, eight have had modest to moderate activity (15–20%). The median duration of these remissions are usually quite brief.

4.3.2. Combination chemotherapy

During the last 5–6 years, a number of trials involving multi-agent combinations have been performed. The rationale for such trials lies primarily in the effectiveness of combination chemotherapy in the treatment of other malignancies, such as the leukemias and lymphomas, and breast, ovarian, and testicular cancers. Multi-agent combinations in esophageal cancer had been hampered by the paucity of single agent data, discussed above. The results of these studies are summarized in Table 6. This data includes only those studies in which chemotherapy was used alone; trials of concurrent chemotherapy and radiation, in which the activity of the chemotherapeutic agents themselves cannot be ascertained are discussed below.

Cisplatin and a bleomycin infusion were initially used at Memorial Hospital in 1976 because the combination appeared to be highly active in advanced epidermoid carcinoma of the head and neck. They were initially given to patients with advanced disease and then, after responses had been seen in this group of patients, cisplatin and bleomycin were given pre-operatively or before radiation therapy. Evaluation of response in patients with metastatic disease involved the standard criteria of complete remission (100% disappearance of all known disease for a minimum of one month), partial response ($\geq$50% but <100% decrease in the sum of the two longest perpendicular diameters of all measurable disease) and minor response (>25% but <50% decrease). Measurable disease in this population included lymph node, subcutaneous, or pulmonary metastases, or tumors that were measurable by computerized tomography. For those patients in whom the primary lesion was one of or was the only measure of response, the criteria of response involving serial barium esophograms, endoscopy, and pathological review of the resected specimen, were as outlined above.

Overall, 61 patients were evaluable for response [145]. Major objective regressions were seen in 15%. For patients with metastatic disease, the median duration of response was 6 months. Duration of remission for patients receiving combined modality therapy including chemotherapy, surgery and/or radiation cannot be ascribed to cisplatin-bleomycin alone, and are discussed in detail in the section on combined modality therapy. The major toxicities of cisplatin-bleomycin included nausea and vomiting, which was almost universal, nephrotoxicity (peak serum creatinine $\geq$2.5 mg%) seen in 20% of patients, and pulmonary fibrosis, which was seen in 2%. There were two drug related deaths (4%). Myelosupression was minimal.

Because vindesine had shown activity in its phase II trial, including responses in patients who had previously been treated with cisplatin-bleomycin, and because of its different toxicities and mechanisms of action, it was added to cisplatin-bleomycin (Figure 1). In this trial, which was completed in 1981, 68 evaluable patients were treated [148]. Twenty-four had extensive disease, and 44 localized tumor. The overall major objective response rate was 53%. In patients with local-regional disease, treated before surgery or radiation, the response rate was higher

Table 6. Esophageal cancer combination chemotherapy

Drug combination	Patients studied	Response (%) (CR/PR)	Median duration (months)
DDP BLEO	61	15	6.0
DDP/DVA/BLEO	62	50	7.5
BLEO/ADRIA	16	19	4.0
DDP/MTX/BLEO	22	27	3.5
DDP/Mito/BLEO	17	54	–

DDP = Cisplatin, DVA = Vindesine, BLEO = Bleomycin, ADRIA = Adriamycin, MTX = Methotrexate, Mito = Mitomycin.

ESOPHAGEAL II
Combined Modality Therapy

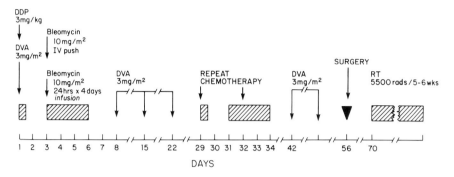

Figure 1. Combined modaluty therapy of local-regional esophageal cancer using cisplatin, bleomycin and vindesine. (Reprinted with permission from the *Annals of Thoracic Surgery.*)

than that seen in the group with extensive disease (63% vs 33%). The generally poorer performance status of the patients with metastases may be the explanation for the lower response rate seen in this group. In general, both for esophageal cancer and other solid tumors, patients with a poor performance status (a measure of their general medical condition) are less likely to respond to chemotherapy and are more likely to have substantial toxicity.

Although there were no complete remissions, by our criteria, among the 34 responding patients, eight had complete radiographic resolution of the primary tumor. Endoscopic or pathological review, however, indicated residual macroscopic or microscopic tumor in either the primary tumor or lymph nodes, and they are thus considered as partial responders. Two patients who had bronchoscopically-proven invasion of the trachea, without an overt fistula, had complete healing, including negative cytology, on rebronchoscopy.

The median duration of response for patients with extensive disease, treated primarily with chemotherapy alone, was 7 months. The toxicities of the cisplatin-bleomycin-vindesine regimen, although substantial, were usually well tolerated. Nausea and vomiting following administration of cisplatin was ameliorated by use of the new antiemetic metochlopramide. Nephrotoxicity was again seen in 20% of patients. Alopecia was common, as was a peripheral neuropathy from Vindesine and/or Cisplatin. Although only one patient developed a clinically apparent pulmonary fibrosis, asymptomatic changes in the vital capacity were noted in 8%. The dose limiting toxicity, however, was myelosupression. The median white blood cell nadir was 1700/mm³; eight patients had an episode of fever during the nadir period. There were two drug related deaths (3%), one from sepsis and one from nephrotoxicity.

In addition to these two trials from Memorial Hospital, several other multi-agent combinations have recently been reported. Kolaric and his collegues combined bleomycin and adriamycin after their initial studies had indicated adriamycin's activity [149]. These trials, in which a concurrent randomized arm received the same agents plus radiation therapy to the primary lesion, involved patients with local-regional disease. The results of the bleomycin-adriamycin combination were disappointing: although their initial trial with adriamycin had demonstrated 33% activity, in the follow-up study with the two agents, only 19% of patients responded. Results of their studies with chemotherapy and radiation are discussed below.

Ladd and collegues treated a group of 17 patients with cisplatin, bleomycin and mitomycin C or mitomycin, bleomycin and vincristine [150]. The response rate of 54% was encouraging, but, at the dosage and scheduling use, toxicity was prohibitive, with 22% having drug related deaths.

Vogel and collegues treated a small group of 11 patients with a combination of cisplatin, methotrexate and bleomycin [151]. Five patients had major responses; the median duration of response was 6 months. Using a similar combination, Fiorentino treated an additional 11 patients; two had partial remissions [152]. Overall, cisplatin methotrexate and bleomycin in this dosage schedule had 27% activity.

Thus, multi-agent chemotherapeutic programs are now undergoing more widespread trial. Most combinations involve the use of cisplatin in a variety of dosages. The highest response rate seen to date (in a fairly large group of 68 patients), was obtained using cisplatin, vindesine and bleomycin. This response rate is 2–2.5 times greater than that seen with either cisplatin, bleomycin or vindesine when used alone or with the cisplatin-bleomycin combination. Thus, it now appears that epidermoid carcinoma of the esophagus should no longer be considered to be totally resistant to chemotherapy. However, even with newer combinations, many patients do not respond to initial therapy, and remission durations are relatively brief. New drug investigations should continue to have a high priority.

4.4. Combined modality therapy

4.4.1. Surgery and radiation therapy
The dismal outcome for patients with local-regional tumor treated with either surgery or radiation therapy alone has led a number of investigators to combine these two modalities. Preoperative radiation has been widely used in an attempt to increase the resection rate by causing local tumor regression and thereby improving survival. Results of these studies are summarized in Table 7 [152–158]. Although almost all of these studies are nonrandomized, several of them involve large numbers of patients. Selection criteria appears to have varied substantially, as some series, such as Akakura's have resection and operability rates of almost 100%, whereas in others, such as Parker's, only one-third to one-half of patients

entering the study had surgery. Operative mortality ranged from 6.2% to 31% except for the two Japanese series five year survival rates were disappointing, being well under 10%. Guernsey's trial, in which the radiation therapy dosage averaged 6,000 rads, indicated that toxicity could be severe: 4 deaths (10%) could be attributed to complications of radiation.

Recently, Lannois and his colleagues reported their results of a controlled, randomized trial of pre-operative radiation versus surgery alone [159]. The dosage of radiation was 4000 rads delivered over 8–22 days. Surgery involved an esophagectomy and esophagogastrostomy. There was no significant different in either resection rate or long term survival between the two arms of the study: 76% of patients receiving pre-operative radiation had resectable disease, compared with 70% of the surgery only group. At five years, 9.5% of preoperative radiation patients were alive, whereas for surgery only, 11.5% were five-year survivors. The average survival was 4.5 months after pre-op RT, and 8.2 months after surgery. Pre-operative radiation did not, however, increase operative mortality. This randomized study suggests that pre-operative radiation is of no value in improving long-term survival; the earlier, uncontrolled American trials support this finding. In addition, since resection rates were not improved either, pre-operative radiation did not appear to allow improved palliation.

4.4.2. Chemotherapy, surgery, and radiation therapy

Combined modality programs involving chemotherapy, surgery and radiation have undergone less intensive study than have radiation and surgery probably because, until quite recently, there have been no chemotherapeutic programs of proven effectiveness in esophageal cancer. Initial trials with single agent chemotherapy plus surgery involved only small groups of patients. More recently, as described above, combination chemotherapy has undergone its initial evaluation. Pre-operative chemotherapy with cisplatin and a bleomycin infusion was begun,

Table 7. Pre-operative radiation in esophageal carcinoma

Author	Pre-op dose (Rad)	No. pts	% To surgery	% resct.	% Rx mort.	AVG. survival	% Total treated alive 5 yrs
1) Akakura	5–6,000	117	100%	82%	20.5%	unstated	25%*
2) Parker	4,500	138	34	87	31.0	unclear	2
3) Guernsey	5–6,600	40	58	87	31.0	unclear	2.5
4) Marks	4,500	332	41	73	18.0	unclear	6
5) Nakayama	2,000	191	unstated	73	6.2	unclear	30+
6) Kelsen	2,000	19	87	54	12.0	9 mos.	5
	4,500	57	87	54	12.0	9 mos.	5
7) Lannois	4,000	67	93	76	2.3	4.5 mos.	9.5
	control	57	85	70	2.1	8.2 mos.	11.5

at Memorial Hospital, in 1976. The rationale for pre-operative chemotherapy resided in treating both the primary tumor and potential systemic metastases.

After activity had been noted in patients with advanced, metastatic disease, a trial of pre-operative cisplatin and bleomycin was begun. In this study completed in 1979, 34 patients with local-regional disease received a single course of chemotherapy before surgery [158]. Response to chemotherapy was evaluated by barium esophagram, performed on day 18; surgery (involving an esophagectomy and esophagogastrostomy) was performed on day 21. Following Surgery, a second course of chemotherapy and radiation therapy (3200 rads delivered over a 4 week period) was given. All patients underwent exploration; 76% had resectable disease. The response to chemotherapy had been similar to that seen in patients with metastatic disease (17% complete and partial regressions). Operative mortality was 11%. Compared to our experience with pre-operative radiation therapy, cisplatin and bleomycin yielded a higher resection rate with no increase in operative mortality (76% vs 54% resection rate, 11% vs 12% operative mortality). Since resected patients in general have improved palliation in that their dysphagia is usually permanently relieved, pre-operative cisplatin-bleomycin appeared to be at least as good as, if not superior to, pre-operative radiation in this study. However, long-term survival was not increased. The median duration of survival following cisplatin-bleomycin was 9 months with 10% of patients living for >3 years. It was concluded that this lack of improvement in survival was a result of the only modest anti-neoplastic activity of the two drug combination.

Following the identification of Vindesine as another active agent, which appeared, in at least some patients with advanced disease, to lack cross resistance with cisplatin-bleomycin, it was added to the initial combination. During the period 1979–1981, a second group of 34 patients with local-regional tumor was treated with the three-drug combination of cisplatin, vindesine and bleomycin (DVB) [148]. Only two courses of chemotherapy were given, as our earlier experience with cisplatin-bleomycin had indicated that this elderly population would not tolerate maintenance chemotherapy. Initially, one cycle of DVB was given before and one after surgery. When it became apparent that, in patients with advanced disease, the maximum degree of tumor regression was seen after two courses of DVB, both cycles were given before surgery (Figure 1). Although radiation therapy was originally planned for all patients, this part of the treatment program was changed later so that only patients with T3 tumors (penetration through the esophageal wall), with positive paraesophageal lymph nodes, or with unresectable disease were given post-operative radiation. All patients underwent exploration; 82% had resectable tumor. The operative mortality was 5.6%.

The response rate to chemotherapy alone was substantially higher with the three drug combination, with 57% of patients having major objective tumor regression. Downstaging of the primary lesion (i.e. drop from T2-T1, to T1 or T0) was seen in 30%; three patients had no tumor found in the resected esophagus. However, by our criteria, none had a complete response, as a single focus of microscopic disease was found in lymph nodes in two patients, and, in the third, the tumor had been adjacent to the aorta and so margins could not be guaranteed. The median followup for this study is now 28 months, with a minimum follow-up 17 months. The median survival for the entire group is 16.2 months, with 30% still alive and free of disease. Compared to the historical control group receiving cisplatin-bleomycin alone, there was a significant improvement in long-term survival ($p = 0.023$). A prospective, randomized trial is currently underway to compare the more effective DVB chemotherapy with a 'standard' regimen of pre-operative radiation; this study has only recently started.

In addition to studies at Memorial Hospital, investigators at Wayne State University have used pre-operative chemotheraphy with concurrent radiation therapy [160]. Since both modalities were used simultaneously, the effectiveness of the chemotherapy combination used is not known. The initial program involved the use of mitomycin C and infusion of 5-Flurouracil; the dosage of radiation therapy was 5000-6000 rads. Of 30 patients with potentially curable local-regional tumor who were entered into this study, 23 (76%) came to surgery; all underwent curative or palliative resections. Operative mortality was 13%. More recently, cis-platin has replaced mitomycin-C. [161]. Only 12 patients have been treated to date; all underwent exploration and resection. Mean follow-up for the second study was 6 months. In another trial, 11 patients were treated with a combination of cisplatin, mitomycin-C, bleomycin and prednisone [161]. The objective response rate to chemotherapy was 55%. However, the operative mortality was prohibitively high (45%).

4.4.3. Combined chemotherapy and radiation

Although the data on objective response rates to radiation therapy alone is scanty, it is clear that this conventional modality can cause tumor shrinkage of a greater or lesser extent in 33–50% of patients. Since chemotherapeutic agents have now demonstrated at least some activity, chemotherapy and radiation have been used either concurrently or sequentially. In some cases, the drug combinations used have been chosen on the basis of the responsiveness of other squamous cell carcinomas (such as head and neck or anal epidermoid tumors).

Werner, in South Africa, used methotrexate and radiation therapy before surgery in a group of 93 patients [163]. The dosage of methotrexate was 100mg/m^2/week for 3 doses; radiation therapy, 2000 rads over 5 days, was given immediately following chemotherapy. Tumor regression was not quantitated. Surgery had initially been planned for all patients, but only 59% underwent operation, most frequently because of patient refusal. The average survival for those undergoing surgery was 26 months, and did not appear to be substantially increased, compared to those not undergoing exploration.

Kolaric evaluated the use of bleomycin plus radiation, adriamycin plus radiation and finally a bleomycin-adriamycin combination plus radiation, in three sequential studies. A control arm received chemotherapy alone. The number of patients in each study were quite small (15–20 patients per arm). In each trial, the objective response rate to the radiation-chemotherapy combination was higher than that to chemotherapy alone. Toxicity was however significant, with a particularly high incidence of tracheo-esophageal fistula in the bleomycin-adria-mycin study [149]. The median durations of response for those receiving radiation and chemotherapy ranged from 5 to 9 months.

The ECOG recently compared radiation therapy alone to radiation plus bleomycin in a randomized trial. The radiation dosage was 5000–6000 rads given over 5 to 6 weeks; bleomycin was given daily at 15 units/dose to a total dose of 210 mg. There was no improvement in survival or swallowing function when bleomycin was added to radiation. Objective regressions were not quantitated.

Marcial *et al.* used the combination of methotrexate, bleomycin, 5-FU and vindesine before radiation therapy in a group of 26 patients [164]. These patients appeared to have disease limited to the local-regional area. Following one to two cycles of chemotherapy, patients were assessed for response. 55% had some measure of tumor shrinkage, but whether or not these were major objective regressions is unclear. Following completion of radiation, 66% had 'complete remissions'. The median survival for the whole group was 11 months.

5. Adenocarcinoma of the esophagus

Far more uncommon that epidermoid cancers, this cell type makes up only 5–15% of esophageal carcinomas. Many of theses tumors are actually extensions of adenocarcinomas of the gastroesophageal junction. Surgically, they are treated exactly as are epidermoid cancers. Their response to radiation therapy has not been well established, nor has chemotherapy been well explored. The overall survival appears to be similar to that of epidermoid carcinoma [165–167].

6. Conclusion

In summary, although improvements in surgical technique have increased resectability rates and decreased operative mortality, and radiation therapy toxicities appear to have decreased, the overall prognosis for patients with esophageal cancer is still poor. Advances in systemic chemotherapy, and the introduction of multidisciplinary approaches may represent hope for the future; these trials, however, should still be considered to be investigational. Early diagnosis, allowing improved salvage rates, are probably applicable only to high-risk areas and populations.

References

1. Turnbull A, Rosen P, Goodwer JT, Beattie EJ: Primary malignant tumors of the esophagus other than typical epidermoid cacinoma. Ann Thorac Surg 15: 463–473, 1973.
2. Bosch A, Frias F, Caldwel W: Adenocarcinoma of the esophagus. Cancer 43: 1557–1561, 1979.
3. Haas J, Schottenfeld D: Epidemiology of esophageal cancer. In Recent Concepts in Gastrointestinal Canger. Plenum Press NY: Lipkin and Good, 1978, 145–171.
4. Doll R: The geographical distribution of cancer. Br J Cancer 23: 1–8, 1969.
5. Burrell RJW: Esophageal cancer among Bantu in the Transkei. J Natl Can Inst 28: 495–514, 1962.
6. Yang C: Research on esophageal cancer in China: A review. Cancer Res 40: 2633–2644, 1980.
7. Plowright W, Linsell CA, Peers FG: A focus of rumenal cancer in Kenyan cattle. Br J Cancer 25: 72–80, 1971.
8. Schutte KH: Esophageal tumors in sheep: some ecological observations. J Natl Canc Inst 41: 821–824, 1968.
9. Carter R, Brewer L: Achalasia and esophageal carcinoma. Surg 130: 114–120, 1975.
10. Huang GJ: Early detection and Surgical treatment of esophageal cancer. Japan Surg 11: 399–405, 1981.
11. Segarra MS, Cardus JC: The value of azyography in carcinoma of the esophagus. SGO 141: 248–250, 1975.
12. Murray GF, Wilcox B, Starek P: The assessment of operability of esophageal carcinoma. Annual Thor Surg 23: 393–399, 1977.
13. Guernsey J, Knudsen D: Abdomenal exploration in the evaluation of patients with carcinoma of the thoracic esophagus. J Thoracic Cardiovasc Surg 59: 62–66, 1970.
14. Daffner R: Computer tomography of the esophagus CRC. Critical Reviews in Diagnostic Imaging, p 191–242, 1981.
15. American Joint Committee for Cancer Staging and End Results Reporting Manual for Staging of Cancer, p 65–67, 1977.
16. Wilkins E, Burke J: Colon esophageal bypass, Am. Surg 129: 394–400, 1975.
17. Huguier M, Gordon F, Maillard JN, Lortat-Jawb JL: Results of 117 esophageal replacements SGO 130: 1054–1058, 1970.
18. Postlethwait R, Sealy W, Dillon M, Young W: Colon interposition for esophageal substitution. Ann Thorac Surg 12: 89–109,
19. El-Domeiri A, Martini N, Beattie EJ: Esophageal reconstruction by colon interposition. Arch Surg 100: 358–362, 1970.
20. Steichen F, Ravitch M: Mechanical sutures in esophageal surgery. Ann Surg 191: 373–381, 1980.
21. Wilson SE, Plester WG, Carey JS: Esophagogastrectomy versus radiation therapy for mid-esophageal carcinoma. Ann Thor Surg 10: 195–202, 1970.
22. Ellis FH, Gibbs SP: Esophagogastrectomy for carcinoma. Ann Sug 190: 699–705, 1979.
23. Piccone VA, Ahmed N, Grosberg S, LaVeen H: Esophagogastrectomy for carcinoma of the middle third of the esophagus. Ann Thor Surg 28: 370–377, 1978.
24. Carey J, Plested W, Hughes R: Esophagogastrectomy: Superiority of the combined abdomenal-right thoracic approach. Ann Thor Surg 14: 59–68, 1972.
25. Earlam R, Cunha-Menlo JR: Oesophageal squamous cell carcinoma: A critical review of surgery. Br Surg 67: 381–390, 1980.
26. American Joint Committee: Clinical staging system for carcinoma of the esophagus. CA 25: 50–57, 1975.
27. Angorn IB, Bryer JU, Hegarty MM *et al.*: Carcinoma of the esophagus in Natal Bantu; a local review. In: Silber W (ed), Carcinoma of the Oesophagus. Rotterdam: Balkema, 248–57, 1978.
28. Applequist P: Carcinoma of the oesophagus and gastric cardia. A retrospective study based on statistical and clinical material from Finland. Acta Chir Scand Suppl 430: 1–92, 1972.

29. Belsey R, Hiebert CA: An exclusive right thoracic approach for cancer of the middle third of esophagus. Ann Thoracic Surg 18: 1–15, 1974.

30. Boyd A, Cukhinham R, Engleman A, et al.: Esophagogastrostomy. J Thor Cardiovasc Surg 70: 817–825, 1975.

31. Buck BA, Fletcher WS: Esophageal cancer: results of therapy in an indigent population. J Surg Oncol 5: 101–11, 1973.

32. Cederquist C, Nielsen J, Berthelsen A, et al.: Cancer of the esophagus II. therapy and outcome. Acta Chir Scand 144: 233–40, 1978.

33. Coordinating group for research on esophageal cancer: Early diagnosis and surgical treatment of esophageal cancer under rural conditions. Chin Med J 2: 113–16, 1976.

34. Drucker M, Mansour K, Hatcher J, Symbas P: Esophageal cancer: an aggressive approach. Ann Thorac Surg 28: 133–138, 1979.

35. Gary-Bobo J, Pujol H, Solassol C et al.: Le traitement radio-chirurgical du cancer del-'oeso-phagus thoracique. A propos de 143 cases. J Radiol Electrol Med Nucl 59: 343–5, 1978.

36. Giuli R, Gignoxx B: Treatment of carcinoma of the Esophagus. Ann Surg 192: 44–52, 1980.

37. Hambraeus G, Mercke C, Hammar E, et al.: Surgery alone or combined with radiation therapy in esophageal carcinoma. Cancer 48: 63–68, 1981.

38. Hankins JR, Cole FN, Ward A, et al.: Carcinoma of the esophagus. The philosophy for palliation. Ann Thorac Surg 14: 189–197, 1972.

39. Hunt JA: An integrated approach to the treatment of squamous oesophageal cancer in S.A. black patients. In: Silber W: Carcinoma of the Oesophagus. Rotterdam: Balkema, p 17–43, 1978.

40. Jackson JW, Cooper DKC, Guvendik C, et al.: The surgical management of malignant tumours of the oesophagus and cardia: a review of the results in 292 patients treated over a 15-year period (1961–1975). Br J Surg 66: 98–104, 1979.

41. Just-Viera JO, Silva JE: Long-term survival of patients with carcinoma of the oesophagus in Puerto Rico. Am Surg 42: 62–5, 1976.

42. Kelsen D, Ahudja M, Hopfan S: Combined modality therapy of esophageal carcinoma. Cancer 48: 31–37, 1981.

43. Leverment JN, Mearns Milne D: Oesophagogastrectomy in the treatment of malignancy of the thoracic oesophagus and cardia. Br J Surg 61: 683–688, 1974.

44. Lortat-Jacob JL: Surgical treatment of esophageal cancer. Record of 23 years of experience. Bull Acad Nat Med (Paris) 153: 17–22, 1969.

45. Lowe WC: Survival with carcinoma of the esophagus. Ann Intern Med 77: 915–918, 1972.

46. Marks RD, Schruggs HJ, Wallace KM: Pre-operative radiation therapy for cancer of the esophagus. Cancer 38: 84–89, 1976.

47. McKeown KC: Carcinoma of the oesophagus. Ann R Coll Surg Engl 60: 301–303, 1978.

48. Milne DM: Experiences with oesophagogastrectomy in the treatment of cancer of the oesophagus. In: Silber W: Carcinoma of the Oesophagus. Rotterdam: Balkema, p 428–438, 1978.

49. Mohahsingh MP: Mortality of oesophageal surgery in the elderly. Br J Surg 63: 579–580, 1976.

50. Nakayama K: Surgical treatment of esophageal malignancy. In: Bockus HL: Gastroenterology, 3rd ed. Philadelphia: Saunders, p 307–318, 1974.

51. Parker EF, Gregoire HB: Carcinoma of the esophagus. Long-term results. JAMA 235: 1018–1020, 1976.

52. Pelletier LC, Bruneau J, Cholette JP et al.: Cancer of the esophagus: therapeutic results. Can J Surg 15: 30–36, 1972.

53. Picconi VA, LeVeen HH, Ahmed N et al.: Reappraisal of esophagogastrectomy for esophageal malignancy. Am J Surg 137: 32–38, 1979.

54. Rambo VB, O'Brien PH, Miller MC et al.: Carcinoma of the esophagus. J Surg Oncol 7: 355–365, 1975.

55. Ross WM: Radiotherapy if carcinoma of the oesophagus. Proc R Soc Med 67: 395–398, 1974.

56. Rossetti M: Erfahrungen bei der chirurgischen Behandlung des Oesophaguscarcinoma. Chirurg 43: 489–493, 1972.

57. Roussel A, Gignoux M, Verwaerde JC, et al.: Esophageal cancer in Western France. Retrospective analysis of 1400 cases. Bull Cancer (Paris) 64: 61–66, 1977.

58. Sanfelippo PM, Bernatz PE: Celestin tube palliation for malignant esophageal obstruction. Surg Clin North Am 53: 921–926, 1973.

59. Segol P, Verwaerde JC, Borel B et al.: Traitement radiochirurgical du cancer limite de l'oesophage. Chirurgie 103: 791–797, 1977.

60. Seitz HD, Kohnlein HE: Clinical aspects and therapy of esophageal carcinoma. Zentralbl Chir 98: 721–731, 1973.

61. Skinner DB: Esophageal malignancies, experience with 110 cases. Surg Clin North Am 56: 137–147, 1976.

62. Smith FS, Gibson P, Nicholls TT: Carcinoma of the oesophagus: preoperative irradiation followed by planned resection for lesions in the middle and lowe thirds. An interim report. Aust NZ J Surg 45: 176–178, 1975.

63. Stoller JL, Toppin DI, Flores AD: Carcinoma of the esophagus; a new proposal for the evaluation of treatment. Can J Surg 20: 454–459, 1977.

64. Stone R, Rangel DM, Gordon HE, et al.: Carcinoma of the gastroesophageal junction. A ten year experience with esophagogastrectomy. Am J Surg 134: 70–76, 1977.

65. Takita H, Vincent RG, Caicedo V, et al.: Squamous cell carcinoma of the esophagus. A study of 153 cases. J Surg Oncol 9: 547–554, 1977.

66. Van Houtte P: Radiotherapy of oesophagus cancer. A review of 136 cases treated at the Institut Bordet. Acta Gastroenterol Belg 40: 121–128, 1977.

67. Wahlers B and Kopperfels R: Radiotherapy of esophageal neoplasms. Strahlentherapie 149: 252–261, 1975.

68. Webb JN, Busuttil A: Adenocarcinoma of the oesophagus and of the oesophagogastric junction. Br J Surg 65: 475–479, 1975.

69. Heit H, Johnson L, Siegel S, Boyce H: Palliative dilation for dysphagia in esophageal carcinoma. Annals Internal Medicine 89: 629–631, 1978.

70. Sanfelippo P, Bernat P: Celistin-tube palliation for malignant esophageal obstruction. Surg Clinics NA 53: 921–926.

71. Das SK, John HJ: Oesophageal intubation in obstruction lesions of the esophagus. Br J Surg 60: 403–406, 1973.

72. Holden MP, Wooler GH, Ionescu MI: Mosseau-Barbin tubes for the treatment of carcinoma of the lower twothirds of the oesophagus. Br J Surg 60: 401–402, 1973.

73. Postlethwait RW: Carcinoma of the esophagus. Current Problems in Cancer 11: 6–44, 1978.

74. Cassidy DC, Nord HJ, Boyce HW: Management of malignant esophageal strictures role of esophageal dilation and personal prostheses (abstract) Am J Gastroent 76: 173, 1981.

75. Pearson JG: Radiotherapy for esophageal carcinoma. World J Surg 5: 489–497, 1981.

76. Kelsen DP, Heelan R, Coonley C, Bains M, Martini N, Hilaris B, Golbey RB: Clinical and pathologic evaluation of response to chemotherapy in patients with esophageal carcinoma. Am J Clin Oncol 6: 539–546, 1983.

77. Kolaric K, Marcicic Z, Dujmovic L, Roth A: Therapy of advanced esophageal cancer with Bleomycin, irridiation, and combination of Bleomycin with irridiation. Tumori 62: 255–262, 1976.

78. Van Andel J, Dees J, Dijkhvix C, et al.: Carcinoma of the esophagus: Results of treatment. Ann Surg 190: 684–689, 1979.

79. Wara W, Mauch P, Thomas A, Phillips T: Palliation for carcinoma of the esophagus. Radiology 121: 717–720, 1976.

80. Earle J, Gelber R, Moertel C, Hahn R: A controlled evaluation of combined radiation and

Bleomycin for squamous cell carcinoma of the esophagus. Int J Radiation Oncology Bio Phys 6: 821–826, 1980.

81. Elkon D, Lee Myouk-Sook, Hendrickson F: Carcinoma of the esophagus: sites of recurrence and palliative benefits after definitive radiotherapy. Int J Rad Onc Bio Phy 4: 615–620, 1978.

82. Earlam R, Cunha-Melo JR: Oesophageal squamous cell carcinoma: A critical review of radiotherapy. BJ Surg 67: 457–461, 1980.

83. Applequist P: Carcinoma of the oesophagus and gastric cardia. A retrospective study based on statistical and clinical material from Finland. Acta Chir Scand Suppl 430: 1–92, 1972.

84. Buschke F: Surgical and radiological results in the treatment of esophageal carcinoma. Am J Roentgenol Radium Ther Nucl Med 71: 9–24, 1954.

85. Cederquist C, Nielsen J, Berthelsen A, et al.: Cancer of the esophagus II. Therapy and outcome. Acta Chir Scand 744: 233–240, 1978.

86. Cossu F: Clinico-statistical report of cases of cancer of the esophagus treated at the Instituto O. Alberti' from 1950 to 1965. Radiol Med (Torino) 53: 356–372, 1967.

87. Eberhardt HJ: Experiences with telecobalt irradiation of malignant esophageal tumors. Treatment results in 124 patients in the years 1958–1968. Radiobiol Radiother (Berl) 11: 121–127, 1970.

88. Eichhorn HJ, Lessel A: Studies of three different radiotherapy methods in esophageal carcinoma. Zentralbl Chir 99: 1549–1557, 1974.

89. Gary-Bobo J, Pujol H, Solassol C, et al.: Le traitement radio-chirurgical du cancer de l'oesophage thoracique. A propos de 143 cases. J Radiol Electrol Med Nucl 59: 343–345, 1978.

90. Gunderson LL: Cancer of the GI tract. Radiation therapy: results and future possibilities. Clin Gastroenterol 5: 743–776, 1976.

91. Gynning I, Lindgren M: Roentgen rotation therapy of oesophageal cancer. Acta Chir Scand Suppl 356: 130–136, 1965.

92. Hankins JR, Cole FN, Ward A, et al.: Carcinoma of the esophagus. The philosophy for palliation. Ann Thorac Surg 14: 189–197, 1972.

93. Heinze HG, Klein U, Jirza Z: Megavolt therapy of esophageal carcinoma. Strahlentherapie 145: 504–512, 1973.

94. Holsti LR: Clinical experience with split-course radiotherapy. Radiology 92: 591–596, 1969.

95. Humphrey CR, Cliffton EE: Carcinoma of the distal part of the esophagus and cardia of the stomach. Surg Gynecol Obstet 127: 737–743, 1968.

96. Krishnamurthi S: Cobalt-60 beam therapy in cancer of thoracic esophagus. Ind J Cancer 2: 115–117, 1965.

97. Kuttig H, Schnabel K, Bark R: Pendulum irradiation of the middle part of the esophagus with rapid electrons and ultrahard X-rays. Strahlentherapie 153: 533–537, 1977.

98. Lawler MR, Gobbel WG, Jun, Killen DA, et al.: Carcinoma of the esophagus. J Thorac Cardiovasc. Surg 58: 609–613, 1969.

99. Lawrence W Jun: Surgical management of gastrointestinal cancer. Clin Gastroenterol 5: 703–742, 1976.

100. Leborgne R, Leborgne F, Jun, Barlocci I: Cancer of the oesophagus. Results of radiotherapy. Br J Radiol 36: 806–811, 1963.

101. Lederman M: Carcinoma of the oesophagus, with special reference to the upper third. I. Clinical considerations. Br J Radiol 39: 193–197, 1966.

102. Leon W, Strug LH, Brickman ID: Carcinoma of the esophagus. A disaster. Ann Thorac Surg 11: 583–592, 1971.

103. Levit SH, Frazier AB, James KW: Split-course radiotherapy in the treatment of carcinoma of the esophagus. Radiology 94: 433–435, 1970.

104. Lewinsky BS, Annes GP, Mann SG, et al.: Carcinoma of the esophagus: an analysis of results and of treatment techniques. Radiol Chir (Basel) 44: 192–204, 1975.

105. Marcial VA, Tome JM, Ubinas J: The role of radiation therapy in esophageal cancer. Radiology 87: 231–239, 1966.

106. Marks RD, Jun, Scruggs HJ, Wallace KM: Preoperative radiation therapy for carcinoma of the esophagus. Cancer 38: 84–89, 1976.
107. Martinez I: Cancer of esophagus in Puerto Rico mortality and incidence analysis, 1950–1961. Cancer 17: 1278–1288, 1964.
108. Meynard JM, Tournerie J: A propos of 110 cases of telecobalt therapy for cancer of the esophagus. Arch Fr Mal Appar Dig 54: 1263–1268, 1965.
109. Millburn L, Faber P, Hendrickson FR: Curative treatment of epidermoid carcinoma of the esophagus. Am J Roentgenol Radium Ther Nucl Med 103: 291–299, 1968.
110. Miller C: Carcinoma of thoracic oesophagus and cardia. A review of 405 cases. Br J Surg 49: 507–522, 1961.
111. Moor NG: Preliminary report of survey conducted by the Johannesburg Group of Hospitals on cancer of the oesophagus in the African; aims, policies and results. S Afr Med J 42: 892–894, 1968.
112. Moseley RV: Squamous carcinoma of the esophagus. Surg Gyencol Obstet 126: 1242–1246, 1968.
113. Mustard RA, Ibberson O: Carcinoma of the esophagus. A review of 381 cases admitted to Toronto General Hospital 1937–1953 inclusive. Ann Surg 144: 927–940, 1956.
114. Nakayama K, Orihata H, Yamaguchi K: Surgical treatment combined with preoperative concentrated irradiation for esophageal cancer. Cancer 20: 778–788, 1967.
115. Pearson JG: Present status and future potential of radiotherapy in the management of oesophageal cancer. In: Silber W (ed): Carcinoma of the Oesophagus. Rotterdam: Balkema, p 334–339, 1978.
116. Pelletier LC, Bruneau J, Cholette JP, et al.: Cancer of the esophagus: therapeutic results. Can J Surg 15: 30–36, 1972.
117. Pierquin B, Wambersie A, Tubiana M: Cancer of the thoracic oesophagus: two series of patients treated by 22 Me V betatron. Br J Radiol 39: 189–192, 1966.
118. Robertson R, Coy P, Mokkavesa S: The results of radical surgery compared with radical radiotherapy in the treatment of squamous carcinoma of the thoracic esophagus. J Thorac Cardiovasc Surg 53: 430–440, 1967.
119. Ross WM: Radiotherapy of carcinoma of the oesophagus. Proc R Soc Med 67: 395–398, 1974.
120. Skinner DB: Esophageal malignancies. Experience iwth 110 cases. Surg Clin North Am 56: 137–147, 1976.
121. Stoller JL, Toppin DI, Flores AD: Carcinoma of the esophagus: a new proposal for the evaluation of treatment. Can J Surg 20: 454–459, 1977.
122. Takita H, Vincent RG, Caicedo U, et al.: Squamous cell carcinoma of the esophagus. A study of 153 cases. J Surg Oncol 9: 547–554, 1977.
123. Vanhoutte P: Radiotherapy of oesophagus cancer. A review of 136 cases treated at the Institut Bordet Acta Gastroenterol Belg 40: 121–128, 1977.
124. Verhaeghe M, Rohart J, Adenis L, et al.: Possibilities and results of radiotherapy in the cancer of the esophagus: 300 cases in 10 years. Presse Med 79: 236, 1971.
125. Voutilainen A, Koulumies M: Radiation therapy of esophageal cancer and its results. Ann Chir Gynaecol Fenn 56: 126–129, 1967.
126. Wahlers B, Kopperfels R: Radiotherapy of esophageal neoplasms. Strahlentherapie 149: 252–261, 1975.
127. Walker JH: Carcinoma of the esophagus. Cobalt-60 teletherapy. Am J Roentgenol 92: 67–76, 1964.
128. Watson TA: Radiation treatment of cancer of the esophagus. Surg Gynecol Obstet 117: 346–354, 1963.
129. Watson WL, Goodner JT: Oesophagus. In: Pack GT, Ariel IM (ed), Treatment of Cancer and Allied Diseases. New York: Harper & Row, IV; p 591–599, 1960.
130. Anderson L, Lad T: Autopsy findings in squamous cell carcinoma of the esophagus. Cancer 50: 1587–1590, 1982.

131. Attah E, Hadju S: Benign and malignant tumors of the esophagus at autopsy. Jour Thor Cardiovasc Surg 55: 396–404, 1980.
132. Bosch A, Frias Z, Caldwell W, Jaeschke W: Autopsy findings in carcinoma of the esophagus. Acta Radio Oncol 18: 103–112, 1979.
133. Ravry M, Moetel CG, Schutt AJ, et al.: Treatment of advanced squamous cell carcinoma of the gastrointestinal tract with Bleomycin (NSC 125066). Cancer Chemotherapy Rep 57: 493–495, 1973.
134. Clinical Screening Group. Study of the clinical efficiency of Bleomycin in the treatment of esophageal carcinoma. Cancer Treat Rep 62: 1041–1046, 1978.
135. Rancini G, Bajetta E, Bonadonna G: Terapia con bleomycin da sola o in associazione con methodtrexate nel carcinoma epidermoide dell' esofago. Tumori 60: 65–71, 1974.
136. Ezdinli E, Gelber R, Desai D, Falkson G, Moertel C, Hahn R: Chemotherapy of advanced esophageal carcinoma: Eastern Cooperative Oncology Group experience. Cancer 46: 2149–2153, 1980.
137. Kolaric K, Maricic Z, Roth A, Dujmovic I: Adriamycin alone and in combination with radiotherapy in the treatment of inoperable esophageal cancer. Tumori 63: 485–491, 1977.
137. Engstrom P, Lavin P: Mitomycin versus Cisplatin in esophageal cancer. Proceed ASCO 1: 100a, 1982.
138. Desai P, Borges E, Vohrs V, et al.: Carcinoma of the esophagus in India. Cancer 23: 979–989, 1969.
139. Falkson G: Methyl-GAG (NSC 32946) in the treatment of esophageal cancer. Cancer Chemotherapy Rep 55: 209–212, 1971.
140. Knight WA, Livingston RB, Fabian C: Phase I-II trial of methyl-GAG: a Southwest Oncology Group pilot study. Cancer Treat Rep 63: 1933–1937, 1979.
141. Kelsen DP, Chapman R, Bains M: Phase II study of Methyl-GAG in the treatment of esophageal carcinoma. Cancer Treatment Reports 66: 1427–1429, 1982.
142. Kelsen DP, Bains MS, Cvitkovic E, Golbey R: Vindesine in the treatment of esophageal carcinoma: a phase II study. Cancer Treat Rep 63: 2019–2021, 1979.
143. Panettiere F, Leichman L, O'Bryan R, Haas C, Fletcher W: Cis-diamminedichloride platinum (II), an effective agent in the treatment of epidermoid carcinoma of the esophagus: A preliminary report of an ongoing Southwest Oncology Group Study. Cancer Clin Trials 4: 29–32, 1981.
144. Davis S, Shanmugathasa M, Kessler W: Cis-dichloridiammine platinum (II) in the treatment of esophageal carcinoma. Cancer Treat Rep 64: 709–711, 1980.
145. Coonley C, Bains M, Kelsen DP: VP-16-213 in the treatment of esophageal cancer: A phase II trial. Cancer Treat Rep 67: 397–398, 1983.
146. Kelsen DP, Citkovic E, Bains M, et al.: Cisdiammine dichlros platinum (11) and bleomycin in the treatment of esophageal carcinoma. Cancer Treat Rep 62: 1041–1046, 1978.
147. Coonley C, Kelsen DP, Hilaris B, et al.: Cisplatin and Bleomycin in the treatment of esophageal cancer. Final Report Cancer (in press).
148 Kelsen DP, Hilaris B, Coonlcy C, et al.. Cisplatin, Vindesine, and Bleomycin chemotherapy of coast regional and advanced esophageal carcinoma. Amer J Med 75: 645–652, 1983.
149. Kolaric K, Maricic Z, Roth A, et al.: Combination of Bleomycin and Adriamycin with and without radiation in the treatment of inoperable esophageal cancer. Cancer 45: 2265–2273, 1980.
150. Ladd TE: Platinum, mitomycin, and bleomycin chemotherapy of esophageal carcinoma Proceed ASCO and AACR 21: 419a, 1980.
151. Vogel S, Greenwald E, Kaplan B: Effective chemotherapy for esophageal cancer with methotrexate, bleomycin, and cis-diamminedichlorsplatinum (11). Cancer 48: 2555–2558, 1981.
152. Fiorentino M: Personal communication.
153. Akakura I, Nakamura Y, Kakegawa T, Nakayama R, et al.: Surgery of carcinoma of the esophagus with preoperative radiation. Chest 57: 47–57, 1970.

154. Nakayama K, Kinoshita Y: Surgical treatment combined with preoperative concentrated irradiation. JAMA 227: 178–181, 1974.
155. Parker E, Gregorie H, Ariants J, Ravevel J: Carcinoma of the esophagus. Ann Surg 171: 746–750, 1970.
156. Marks R, Scrugs H, Wallace K: Preoperative radiation therapy for carcinoma of the esophagus. Cancer 38: 84–89, 1976.
157. Guernsey J, Doggett RLS, Mason G, Kohatsu S, Oberhelman H: Combined treatment of cancer of the esophagus. Am J Surg 117: 157–161, 1979.
158. Kelsen DP, Ahudja M, Hopfan S, *et al.*: Combined modality therapy of esophageal carcinoma. Cancer 48: 31–37, 1981.
159. Lannois B, Delarue D, Campion J, *et al.*: Preoperative radiotherapy for carcinoma of the esophagus. Surg Gyenc Obstet 153: 690–692, 1981.
160. Steiger Z, Franklin R, Wilson R, *et al.*: Complete eradication of squamous cell carcinoma of the esophagus with combined chemotherapy and radiotherapy. American Surgeon 47: 95–98, 1981.
161. Steiger Z, Franklin R, Wilson R: Eradication and palliation of squamous cell carcinoma of the esophagus with chemotherapy, radiotherapy, and surgical therapy. J Thorac Cardiovasc Surg 82: 713–719, 1981.
162. Kukla L, Ladd T, McGuire W, Thomas P: Multimodality therapy of squamous carcinoma of the esophagus. Proceed ASCO and AACR 22: 449, 1981.
163. Werner ID: Multi-disciplinary approach in the management of squamous carcinoma of the oesophagus. Front Gastrointest Rep 5: 130–135, 1979.
164. Marcial V, Velez-Garcia E, Cintron J, *et al.*: Radiotherapy preceded by multi-drug chemotherapy in carcinoma of the esophagus. Cancer Clin Trials 3: 127–130, 1980.
165. Bosch A, Frias Z, Caldwell W: Adenocarcinoma of the Esophagus. Cancer 43: 1557–1561, 1979.
166. Poleynard G, Marty A, Burnbaum W, *et al.*: Adenocarcinoma in the columnar-lined (Barrett Esophagus). Arch Surg 112: 907–1000, 1977.
167. Lortant-Jawb J, Maillarn J, Richard C: Primary esophageal adenocarcinoma: report of 16 cases. Surgery 64: 535–543, 1968.

7. Large bowel cancer: restorative rectal surgery

DAVID A. ROTHENBERGER, SANTHAT NIVATVONGS, VENDIE H.
HOOKS III, ERIC S. ROLFSMEYER and STANLEY M. GOLDBERG

1. Introduction

The term restorative rectal surgery is applied to operations for carcinoma of the
rectum with first eliminate the cancer and secondly restore or preserve anorectal
function where the alternative is total excision of the rectum with permanent
colostomy. Lesions located sufficiently proximal that there is no question of the
need for total rectal excision are excluded from consideration here. This chapter
will discuss the theoretical basis for restorative surgery of cancer of the rectum,
delineate the options available, review the results of the various operative techniques and outline the authors' approach to carcinoma of the rectum.

2. Historical perspective

A brief review of the evolution of operations for carcinoma of the rectum is
instructive (Fig. 1). Kraske [1] described a technique of sacral excision of the
rectum in 1885. By removal of the coccyx and lower sacrum, access to the rectum
above the levators was obtained. Either the entire rectum and anal canal was
excised or a sleeve of rectum containing the cancer was excised with establishment of end-to-end continuity. Sacral excision became the most popular method
of operation for cancer of the rectum in Germany and Austria. In a 1929 report
from Vienna, 984 patients underwent sacral excision with an immediate mortality
of 11.6% and a five-year survival rate of 30% [2].

Meanwhile, the technique of an extended perineal excision as popularized by
Lockhart-Mummery [3] became the most common operation for rectal cancer in
the early 1900's in England. First, an exploratory laparotomy was performed to
assess the operability of the growth, to determine the presence of distant spread,
and to construct a sigmoid colostomy. The distal bowel was cleansed daily until
the perineal phase was performed about two weeks later. An average of 23 cm of
rectum and distal sigmoid was resected. At St. Mark's Hospital, 370 cases were

J.J. DeCosse and P. Sherlock (eds), Clinical Management of Gastrointestinal Cancer.
© *1984, Martinus Nijhoff Publishers, Boston. ISBN 0-89838-601-2. Printed in The Netherlands.*

treated by perineal excision in the early 1900's with an 11.6% immediate mortality and a 40% five-year survival [4].

Ernest Miles' [5] investigations of rectal cancer lead to the conclusion that lymphatic spread developed in three directions: 1) upwards along the superior rectal and inferior mesenteric vessels to the paraaortic chain; 2) laterally in the tissue between the levators and pelvic peritoneum to end in the internal iliac nodes on the pelvic side wall; and 3) downwards through the sphincter muscles, the perineal skin, ischiorectal fat and eventually to the inguinal nodes. He believed that even with a carcinoma at the rectosigmoid junction, all three zones of spread were often involved. Thus, in 1908, he described his technique of an abdominoperineal excision, the first widely accepted procedure to primarily approach rectal carcinoma via the abdomen [6]. He excised the rectum and anal canal, the sphincters and considerable parts of levator ani muscles, the ischiorectal fat, the pelvic peritoneum, the sigmoid colon, its mesocolon and vessels. He reported the use of this procedure in 61 patients with an operative mortality of 36% [7]. Dukes [8] reported a comparative study of the late results of extended perineal and combined abdominoperineal excision performed at St. Mark's Hospital (Table 1).

There was no significant difference in survival for the two operations in cases without lymphatic metastases (Dukes A and B) but a clear cut difference when lymphatic spread had occurred (Dukes C). It was clear that the main inadequacy of the perineal or sacral routes was in dealing with the important superior zone of lymphatic spread. As abdominal surgery became safer, the Miles' abdomino-perineal excision which provided for proximal lymphovascular pedicle ligation became the accepted operation for carcinoma of the rectum in England and America. It remains the 'gold standard' by which the results of all other operations for rectal cancer must be compared.

The pioneering efforts of Kraske, Lockhart-Mummery, Miles and others early in this century laid the groundwork for the modern operative management of carcinoma of the rectum. Over ensuing decades, many surgeons, anatomists and physiologists contributed to a better understanding of the routes of spread of rectal cancer and of the mechanisms of anal continence. This new information stimulated the development and acceptance of the currently available restorative

Table 1. Five year survival rate after excision of the rectum (operation deaths excluded)

Dukes stage	Perineal Excision %	Combined Exicions %
A	82.2	83.9
B	61.7	62.3
C	17.9	31.0
Total	44.9	47.1

St. Mark's Hospital Statistics: Dukes [44].

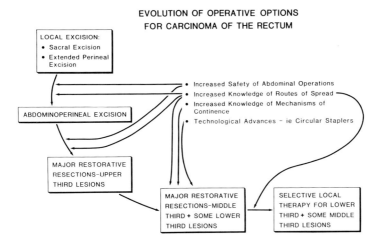

EVOLUTION OF OPERATIVE OPTIONS
FOR CARCINOMA OF THE RECTUM

Figure 1. Over the past century, the operative approach to carcinoma of the rectum has changed dramatically such that preservation of anal sphincter function is now often possible.

procedures as alternatives to abdominoperineal excision (Fig. 1). The next two sections will briefly review this information which is a prerequisite to a discussion of the proper operative approach to rectal carcinoma.

3. Spread of rectal carcinoma

Rectal adenocarcinoma begins as an in situ epithelial mucosal lesion, usually, though perhaps not always, arising within an adenoma [9]. At this stage it is entirely localized without ability to metastasize and thus is totally curable by local measures. The term 'invasive' is used when the cancer has penetrated the muscularis mucosa since as it reaches the submucosa, it has access to lymphatics and veins and thus the capacity for distant metastasis.

3.1. Direct spread

A rectal carcinoma spreads directly in three dimensions within the bowel wall: 1) circumferentially around the lumen of the bowel; 2) longitudinally both proximally and distally; and, 3) transversely through the bowel wall. The extent of circumferential spread has correlated with survival [10, 11]. Quer *et al.* [12] based on a study of 91 operative specimens stretched to conform to the operative measurements of length, reported that retrograde intramural spread beyond the lowest palpable or visible edge of the carcinoma was distinctly unusual for low grade malignancies. There was no spread in 86 specimens, spread less than 1.5 cm in two, and spread beyond 1.5 cm in only three specimens. Two of the latter three patients had obvious metastases at the time of operation. Grinnell [13], in a study of 76 operative specimens found that direct upwards or downwards spread beyond the visible borders of the lesion was unusual unless the tumor was a poorly differentiated carcinoma. There was no spread in 67, spread less than 1.0 cm in six and spread more than 1.0 cm in three patients, two of whom had a poorly differentiated carcinoma.

As the tumor grows and penetrates transversely through the bowel wall, it gains access to the lymphatics and veins in the submucosa and thus the capacity for distant metastasis [9]. Deeper invasion into the muscularis propria results in a greater incidence of lymphatic and venous dissemination [14]. As the tumor enlarges and penetrates transversely through the serosa, direct extension into the adjacent fat, mesentery and contiguous viscera such as prostate, vagina or bladder occurs. In addition, greater access to lymphatic and venous channels occurs as the tumor penetrates the full thickness of the bowel wall. Thus, it is not surprising that survival correlates with the depth of penetration of the cancer [9].

3.2. Lymphatic spread

Miles' concepts of the three directional lymphatic spread of rectal cancer were accepted for several decades. In the 1930's, several studies failed to confirm Miles' findings in two important respects [15, 16, 17, 18]. First, they found that the upward spread of cancer cells in lymphatics was usually embolic with an orderly progression from the regional pararectal nodes to the superior rectal nodes to the inferior mesenteric nodes and finally to the paraaortic nodes. Crossover with lymphatic drainage from other viscera was possible [18]. Second, lateral or downward spread was unusual unless the superior zone lymphatics were plugged with tumor. More recent studies confirm these conclusions.

3.3. Venous spread

The growing lesion first gains access to intramural veins as it penetrates the muscularis mucosa and invades the submucosa. Even then, the presence of intravenous tumor plugs attached to the intimal lining occurs rarely, being demonstrated in only 3% of patients with less than complete penetration of the bowel wall [19]. Once the tumor has penetrated through the entire bowel wall, such venous invasion is more common and is found in up to 50% of the specimens [20]. Venous spread occurs even more commonly in those with lymphatic metastases. The demonstration of such venous invasion with attached tumor plugs correlates negatively with survival. On the other hand, the presence of free tumor cells in the venous effluent of colorectal cancers which is well documented, does not correlate with survival. Venous spread can ultimately result in hepatic, pulmonary, adrenal, renal, bone, brain, and other metastases.

3.4. Other routes of spread

Some studies suggest that perineural extension can occur as far as 10 cm from the primary and may account for some degree of local recurrence independent of other factors [21, 22]. Implantation of tumor into the peritoneal cavity or at the anastomosis may also account for some recurrences, though this is rare.

4. Anatomy and physiology of continence

Hertz [23] in 1911, suggested that the sensation of fullness and the feeling of impending evacuation was due to rectal distention which was detected by receptors in the rectal wall. Goligher and Hughes [24] in 1951, stressed the importance of preserving at least 6–8 cm of anorectal stump during sphincter-saving excision if 'sensory incontinence' was to be avoided. These concepts have slowly changed in recent decades with new knowledge providing the anatomic and physiologic basis for modern restorative rectal operations.

The major resections described below allow one to resect the rectum above the levator ani while leaving undisturbed the anorectum below. The reservoir function of the curved compliant rectum is lost since it is replaced by a straight colon but the anal sphincter reflexes are maintained, suggesting that the receptors for the reflexes lie outside the rectum, most likely in the pelvic floor [25]. Urgency, a frequent complaint in these patients, is probably due to the loss of reservoir function to accommodate the entry of stool. Another frequent finding in these patients is impairment of sensation which is probably caused by damage of the nerve supply to the anorectum during dissection or from postoperative infection. These defects are usually temporary and improve with time, usually within six months [26]. It is now clear that normal or near normal continence can be obtained if the pelvic muscles and the sphincter muscles are preserved. The rectum itself is not essential for the appreciation of impending evacuation or for the sphincter inhibitory reflexes.

5. Major restorative resections

The awareness that the primary route of spread of rectal cancers is upwards, that it is not essential to preserve a long rectal cuff to achieve continence and that abdominal surgery could be safely performed kindled an interest in operations which: 1) allowed proximal lymphovascular pedicle ligation and clearance of the primary and its potential routes of spread; and 2) restored continuity. Operations were developed in the middle decades of this century to accomplish these two goals. The abdominal phase of these operations was similar but differences in means of achieving restoration of bowel continuity distinquish the techniques.

5.1. Operations available

In the 1930's and 1940's, Dixon and associates at the Mayo Clinic and Wangensteen of the University of Minnesota, promoted an anterior approach to rectal cancers through the abdominal cavity with a sutured anastomosis [27, 28]. This so called anterior resection was initially reserved for cancers of the rectosigmoid and intraperitoneal rectum. It was found that anterior resection for such lesions resulted in long-term cure equal to that provided by abdominoperineal excision [29, 30, 31]. This fact, coupled with surgeons' increased ability to reliably suture lower colorectal anastomosis, lead to the use of anterior resection for some cancers of the extraperitoneal rectum. Still, this technique was a demanding one and in obese patients with a narrow pelvis, hand-sutured low anostomoses were sometimes impossible to construct. The technical limitations of anterior resections promoted development of operations which enabled a lower colorectal or coloanal anastomosis to be performed. Thus, pull-through operations, abdominosacral resection, abdominotranssphincteric resection, and an endo-anal approach with coloanal anastomosis were promoted by a variety of surgeons as alternative to abdominoperineal resection. The introduction of the end-to-end anastomosis (EEA) stapling device in 1978, provided the means to perform lower, more reliable anterior anastomoses than had been possible previously with hand-sewn end-to-end anastomoses [32]. Anterior resection has now been extended to mid and even some lower third rectal cancers.

It is useful to arbitrarily subdivide anterior resection into three categories: 1) high anterior resection; 2) low anterior resection; and 3) extended low anterior resection (Table 2). Technical demands are greater, complications are more frequent, and functional results are less acceptable with each of these subdivisions as shorter anorectal stumps are preserved. For most surgeons, anterior resection is the primary alternative to abdominoperineal resection. Abdominosacral resection, abdominotranssphincteric resection, pull-through operations, or abdominotransanal resection with coloanal anastomosis are options applied by a relatively small number of surgeons whose familiarity with the techniques allows them to achieve satisfactory results.

5.2. Abdominal phase

The abdominal dissection attempts first to clear the tumor and its potential routes of spread and second to mobilize sufficient colon proximally to ensure a well vascularized anastomosis without tension. A mechanical and oral intraluminal antibiotic bowel prep with pre-operative systemic intravenous antibiotics for wound prophylaxis are administered routinely. For anterior resection, pull-through operations or endoanal anastomosis, the patient is placed in a modified lithotomy position. This position provides exposure for both the abdominal and perineal operators. For an abdominosacral resection, the patient is placed in the right lateral position whereas in the transsphincteric procedure, the patient undergoes the abdominal phase in the supine position and then is turned to the prone jackknife position for the anastomosis.

5.2.1. Controversies in extent of resection

The abdominal phase of an abdominoperineal resection or of any of the major restorative resections can be identical in terms of extent of proximal and lateral dissection (Fig. 2). The only mandatory differences is in the extent of resection of the rectum and extrarectal tissues distal to the tumor. The exact conduct of the abdominal dissection will vary depending on the surgeon's training and interpretation of several controversial aspects of rectal cancer surgery. A full discussion of these issues is beyond the scope of this chapter. Suffice it to say, that controversy persists regarding: 1) the optimal level of proximal lymphovascular pedicle ligation and extent of proximal nodal dissection; 2) the optimal extent of lateral and circumferential clearance at the level of the cancer; 3) the value of concomitant visceral resections; and 4) the optimal distal margin beyond the

Table 2. Anterior resection of rectosigmoid carcinoma*

I.	*High anterior Resection*
	A. Partial Mobilization of Rectum
	B. Anastomosis to Rectum Partly Devoid of Peritoneum
II.	*Low anterior resection*
	A. Complete Mobilization of Rectum
	1. Pelvic Peritoneum Opened Completely
	2. Mobilized Posteriorly to Coccyx
	3. Lateral Ligaments Divided Completely
	4. Mobilized Anteriorly to Pubis
	B. Anastomosis to Rectum Devoid of Peritoneum
III.	*Extended low anterior resection*
	A. Low Anterior Resection Plus
	B. Additional Anterior Mobilization to Levators
	1. Division of Denonvillier's Fascia
	2. Mobilization of Rectovaginal Septum or Rectum from Seminal Vesicles-Bladder Base and Prostate.

* Authors' suggested, though admittedly arbitrary, classification of anterior resection. Technical demands are greater, complications are more frequent, and functional results are less acceptable as shorter anorectal stumps are preserved.

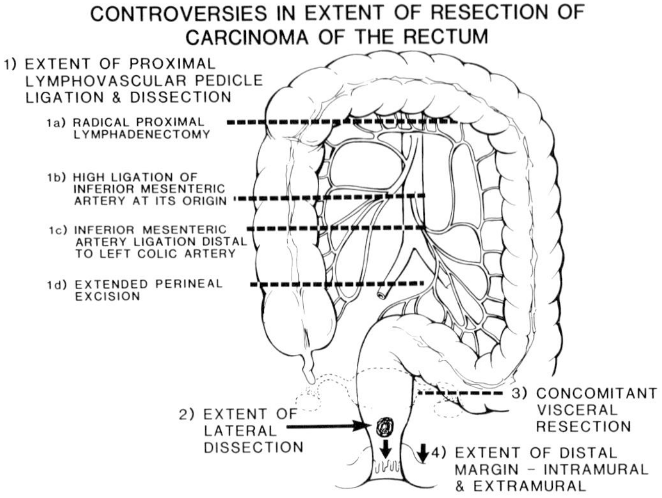

CONTROVERSIES IN EXTENT OF RESECTION OF
CARCINOMA OF THE RECTUM

1) EXTENT OF PROXIMAL
   LYMPHOVASCULAR PEDICLE
   LIGATION & DISSECTION

   1a) RADICAL PROXIMAL
       LYMPHADENECTOMY

   1b) HIGH LIGATION OF
       INFERIOR MESENTERIC
       ARTERY AT ITS ORIGIN

   1c) INFERIOR MESENTERIC
       ARTERY LIGATION DISTAL
       TO LEFT COLIC ARTERY

   1d) EXTENDED PERINEAL
       EXCISION

2) EXTENT OF
   LATERAL
   DISSECTION

3) CONCOMITANT
   VISCERAL
   RESECTION

4) EXTENT OF DISTAL
   MARGIN – INTRAMURAL
   & EXTRAMURAL

Figure 2. The four major areas of controversy regarding the ideal extent of resection for carcinoma of the rectum are depicted. Lockhart-Mummery's extended perineal excision ligated the superior rectal vessels 5 to 7.5 cm below the sacral promontory. (1d) Miles' abdominoperineal resection improved survival of patients with Dukes C lesions by extending the proximal dissection to the level of the inferior mesenteric artery just distal to the left colic artery. (1c) More proximal ligation at the level of the origin of the inferior mesenteric artery (1b) or more proximal dissection along the aorta and vena cava (1a) are techniques of unproven value. Whether the lateral dissection should include hypogastric lymphadenectomy is debated (2). The efficacy of concomitant visceral resection of grossly uninvolved viscera remains open to question (3). The ideal distal margin remains controversial (4).

primary. No prospective comparative trials exist and most of the literature consists of retrospective reviews without sufficient data to totally resolve these controversies.

The controversy regarding the optimal distal margin of resection is especially critical to a discussion of restorative rectal operations. Unfortunately, no standard definition of 'distal margin' exists. Some authors measure distal margin *in situ* prior to mobilization of the rectum while others use a stretched, fresh specimen and still others use a fixed, nonpinned specimen. Some use only gross measurements while others use microscopic measurements [33]. The lack of uniformity in the use of this term makes it very difficult to compare one report with another. The data regarding extent of distal intramural and extramural lymphatic spread in operative specimens has been presented. (See Section 3.1. and 3.2.). One of the best recent studies regarding distal margins is that of Tonak *et al.* [33]. They reported that in 98 patients with carcinoma of the middle rectum who underwent anterior resection with a distal margin of less than 3.0 cm as determined by the pathologist in a fresh specimen without tension, the incidence of local recurrence was 33% (32/98). If the distal margin was more than 3.0 cm, the incidence of local recurrence was 13% (8/64).

5.2.2. Abdominal dissection – authors' technique

Exposure is gained via an infraumbilical transverse incision, a midline incision or other appropriate incision. Thorough exploration of the abdominal cavity is then performed to: 1) exclude significant concomitant disease states; 2) stage the involvement of abdominal viscera; and 3) confirm proper positioning and functioning of the nasogastric tube and urinary Foley catheter. For rectal carcinomas, it is usually impossible to assess local resectability until some of the dissection has been performed. Certainly, no determination as to feasibility of restorative anastomosis can be made for a mid or low rectal cancer until full mobilization of the rectum is completed. Intent and extent of resection is then determined based on size of the primary, the fixation of the mass, and the involvement of adjacent structures.

The sigmoid colon is mobilized by incising the lateral peritoneal reflection (white line of Toldt). This incision is carried cephalad to the distal descending colon and caudad parallel to the rectum. The left spermatic or left ovarian vein can be easily identified. At the level of the iliac crest, the ureter is usually just medial to this vein. The vein, ureter and retroperitoneal areolar tissue are pushed aside with a stick sponge so that a fan-shaped flap of sigmoid mesentery is created. The peritoneum on the medial side of the sigmoid is incised and the incision carried down to the pelvis. The inferior mesenteric artery is identified and it is clamped, divided, and doubly ligated just distal to the take-off of the left colic artery. The inferior mesenteric vein is ligated at the corresponding level. By drawing the rectum taut, a plane of areolar tissue behind the rectum, at the level just above the promotory of the sacrum, is identified and easily entered with blunt and sharp dissection to the S_3 and S_4 level, where the rectosacral fascia is encountered. This fascia, which varies from a thin fibrous band to a thick ligament is cut with a long, heavy scissors and mobilization to the level of the coccyx is achieved.

Anterior mobilization of the rectum is achieved by incising the peritoneum at the retrovesical reflection. Next, by pulling the rectum taut with one hand, placing the four fingers of the other hand behind the rectum and sweeping laterally while the thumb is placed anteriorly in the midline and swept laterally, the lateral ligaments containing the accessory middle rectal vessels are exposed, clamped, divided and ligated. Care is taken to identify and avoid the ureters during this manuever. Mobilization is continued distally in the plane between the seminal vesicles in men or vagina in women and Denonvillier's fascia to the level of the pubis symphysis. The pelvis is irrigated and absolute hemostasis achieved. Only at this point in the operation when the rectum is fully mobilized can a decision be made as to the feasibility of restorative anastomosis and the type of anastomosis that will be performed.

5.3. Anastomotic techniques

The major restorative resections are distinquished by the method of reconstituting bowel integrity.

5.3.1. Abdominosacral resection [34]
This technique is a logical extension of Kraske's sacral resection and has been used since the 1930's. The sacral phase involves excision of the coccyx and division of Waldeyer's fascia to expose and retrieve the previously mobilized rectosigmoid. Following resection, a direct anastomosis between the sigmoid colon and distal rectum is performed.

5.3.2. Abdominotranssphincteric resection [58]
Instead of exposing the rectum through the bed of the sacrum and coccyx, the external anal sphincter and levator ani muscles are divided via a posterior wound to expose the lower rectum. After mobilization, a resection is performed at the level of the internal sphincter. Following an anastomosis, the levator ani and external sphincter are reconstructed.

5.3.3. Pull-through operations
A variety of pull-through operations have been developed, all of which restore continuity by pulling the proximal bowel through the rectal stump with union of the cut ends of bowel achieved by adhesions or by anastomosis outside the anus. A critical and technically difficult step in these operations is to gain enough length to bring well vascularized bowel well beyond the anus. The perineal phase of the operation varies according to the technique utilized.

5.3.3.1. Bacon technique [35].
The mucosa lining the preserved anorectal stump is stripped and the anal sphincter divided posteriorly. The proximal divided colon is drawn through the bared anal canal to protrude 5.0 cm beyond. A rubber tube is tied into the stump and not removed until the first bowel movement. The sphincters are sutured around the emerging colon. After adhesive union forms between the proximal colon and anal canal, the redundant colon is excised.

5.3.3.2. Black technique [36].
The rectal mucosa, sphincter muscles and levator ani muscles are not disturbed in this technique. The proximal bowel is pulled through the intact rectal stump to protrude beyond the anus. Union can thus take place only between the cut upper edge of the anorectal stump and the serosal surface of the colon. Later, protruding colon is excised.

5.3.3.3. Maunsell-Weir technique [37, 38].
The short, intact anorectal stump left after resection of the cancer during the abdominal phase is everted by the perineal operator. The divided proximal colon is drawn through the everted anorectal

stump so that the cut edges of both stumps lie opposite one another outside the anus where they can easily be anastomosed. Next, the anastomosis is placed back in the pelvis.

5.3.3.4. Turnbull-Cutait technique [39, 40]. This technique, which combines some features of Black's operation with the Maunsell-Weir technique was divised independently by Turnbull and Cutait in 1961. The rectosigmoid colon is pulled through the rectal stump which is everted outside the anus. The extrusion of the sigmoid colon beyond the everted stump is amputated 7–10 days later and sutures are applied around the adhesive union. The anastomosis gradually recedes through the anus into the pelvis.

5.3.4. Abdominotransanal resection with coloanal anastomosis
This operation developed by Parks [41] shares many concepts and technical details with the pull-through operations. The abdominal phase, performed in a modified lithotomy position, is similar to that of all the major resections. During the perineal phase of the operation, the rectal mucosa and submucosa are excised leaving the bared sphincter muscles intact (Fig. 3). The proximal colon is drawn through the denuded rectal stump and an end-to-end hand-sutured coloanal anastomosis performed. Parks routinely adds a temporary, proximal transverse colostomy.

5.3.5. Anterior resection
If a high resection is performed for a tumor located sufficiently proximal so that the proposed site of anastomosis is readily exposed, a handsutured one or two-layer anastomosis can be reliably performed. Alternative techniques of a stapled anastomosis either with the TA or GIA stapling devices have been described [42]. The intraluminal circular staplers were designed to facilitate anterior ana-stomoses but we would caution that insertion of these devices into a non-mobilized rectum may produce an inadvertant rectal tear which can be difficult to recognize or repair. A recent modification of the EEA-stapler replaces the straight shaft with a curved one and is useful in this setting. Some surgeons suggest using the circular staplers via a proximal colotomy but this has the disadvantage of producing an additional suture or staple line, albeit a small one.

Fow low or extended low anterior resections, the circular staplers (EEA-stapler manufactured by US Surgical Corporation or the intra-luminal stapler-ILS-manufactured by Ethicon Corporation) inserted via the anus have been found to create a secure, two-layer inverted anastomosis deep in the pelvis at levels where it is technically very difficult to hand-suture a secure anastomosis [43]. The site of proposed resection is identified distal to the rectal tumor. The rectal wall is exposed and mesorectum cleared for a 2.0 to 3.0 cm length. An assistant inserts a proctoscope to irrigate the rectum prior to transection and to confirm the adequacy of the proposed distal margin. The abdominal surgeon

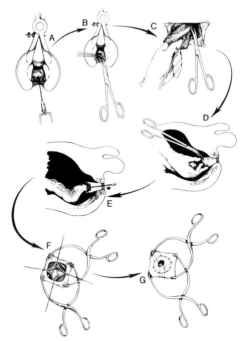

Figure 3. Coloanal anastomosis technique: A) Injection of dilute epinephrine solution to elevate the mucosa and submucosa from the internal sphincter; B) and C) Rectal mucosectomy with preservation of the anus; D) Completion of the rectosigmoid resection; E) Advancement of the mobilized proximal colon through the preserved muscular cuff; F) and G) Completion of the coloanal anastomosis.

places a right angle bowel clamp across the bowel wall just proximal to the intended line of resection. Stay sutures or Babcock clamps are used to control the rectal stump and provide exposure for placement of the pursestring in an open fashion (Fig. 4). Alternatively, a transabdominal pursestring suture is placed in a closed fashion (Fig. 4). For the short rectal stump or when anatomic considerations such as obesity and a narrow, deep pelvis are present, this can be difficult. For such cases, several maneuvers to aid in placement of the pursestring have been developed (Fig. 4). Some have advocated stapling the rectal stump closed with the TA instrument and then inserting a circular stapler without the anvil to create an end-to-side colorectal anastomosis (Fig. 4). In our experience, it has been awkward to place the TA stapler across a truly short rectal stump and the other techniques have worked better. In addition, this technique crosses two staple lines which could be a disadvantage.

Next, the site of proximal sigmoid or descending colon resection is readied for anastomosis by clearing the mesentery for 2.0 to 3.0 cm. If there is any question regarding tension at the proposed anastomosis in the pelvis, the descending colon and splenic flexure are mobilized entirely. The bowel is then transected between clamps and a 2-0 Prolene®, fullthickness pursestring suture is placed approx-

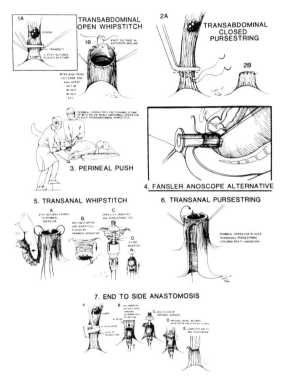

Figure 4. Techniques for management of the rectal stump prepatory to anterior anastomosis. The preferred approach is to place the pursestring by transabdominal approach with an open whipstitch (1a and 1b) or a closed pursestring (2a and 2b). The perineal push method in which the assistant applies pressure to the perineum thus bringing the rectal stump into view for the abdominal operator, can facilitate pursestring placement (3). A Fansler anoscope can be used in a similar fashion to push the rectal stump upward so the abdominal operator can place an open whipstitch (4). Alternatively, the rectum can be everted and the perineal operator can then place a whipstitch before reinverting the rectum (5). The pursestring can be placed on a short rectal stump via the transanal approach (6). Another alternative is to close the rectal stump, insert the stapler without the anvil, and then construct an end-to-side anastomosis (7).

imately 2 to 3 mm from the cut edge with bites taken 4 to 5 mm apart.

Once the pursestring sutures are properly placed, the correct instrument is selected and assembled. In general, for colorectal anastomosis, the EEA-31 or the ILS-29 or 32 cartridges are used. Proper assembly is critical. The cartridge should be checked to assure the presence of staples and the circular knife and the anvil checked for the plastic and metal rings. The lubricated stapler is inserted into the rectum in a closed position with the handle up and the safety on. The abdominal operator protects the rectum by placing his hand posteriorly and directs the perineal operator as he gently advances the instrument until the anvil screw is protruding through the rectal lumen. The stapler is opened fully. Normally, the rectal pursestring is tied first, thus securing the rectum around the shaft

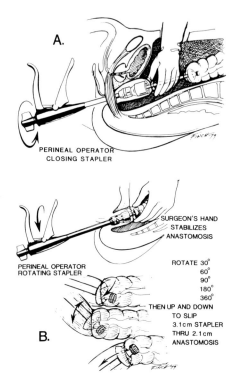

Figure 5. A) Closing the gap of the EEA stapling instrument: the rectosigmoid has been resected, proximal and distal pursestring sutures placed, and the two limbs of bowel tied around the central rod of the stapler which has been inserted through the anus. As the perineal operator closes the gap by turning the wing-nut, the abdominal operator keeps the gap free of extraneous tissues. B) Removal of the EEA stapling instrument: The stapler has been closed completely, the safety catch released, and the handle compressed to create an inverted, two-layer end-to-end anastomosis. The stapler is removed by turning the wing-nut three complete revolutions to open the gap and by rotating the stapler gently. Next, the stapler is gently rocked up and down to slip the anvil through the anastomosis.

of the instrument. Next, the proximal stump is placed over the anvil and its pursestring tied securely. For a low anastomosis, it is more convenient to pass the entire cartridge up through the rectal stump, secure the proximal bowel on the anvil and then withdraw the cartridge to the level of the rectal pursestring which is tied last. The stapler is closed fully while the abdominal operator keeps the viscera, mesentery, and other tissues out of the gap (Fig. 5). The stapler is fired and then removed by turning the wing nut three revolutions, rotating the stapler gently, and then gently rocking and withdrawing the instrument from the anus (Fig. 5).

The perineal operator checks to be certain all staples have fired and determines the completeness of the rings of tissue incorporated by the tied pursestrings and resected as the stapler fires. Next, a proctoscope is inserted and the anastomosis is visualized to check for gaps, bleeding or other abnormalities. The anastomotic level is noted. The procotoscope is withdrawn several centimeters and after the abdominal operator has filled the pelvis with saline, air is insufflated to check for an air leak. The abdominal operator meanwhile, has tried to visualize the anastomosis and makes a final check regarding its vascularity and tension. If there is tension, additional proximal mobilization is performed. If technical problems with the anastomosis are found, they must be remedied.

The abdomen is irrigated and a final check made for hemostasis. Abdominal closed suction drains placed deep in the pelvis are occasionally used for 24–72 hours postoperatively, but most often are not needed. The lateral gutter and mesenteric defect are left open. The abdomen is closed in layers.

Postoperatively, the patient receives two additional doses of systemic intravenous antibiotics. The nasogastric tube is removed when bowel function returns. The Foley catheter is removed 3 to 5 days postoperatively.

5.4. Results

Analysis of the outcome of the major restorative resections must include comparison of mortality rates, morbidity, functional results and assessment of recurrence and survival data. The results of restorative resections must be viewed in the perspective of results obtained with abdominoperineal excision.

5.4.1. Mortality
As noted in Table 3, mortality for any of the major restorative resections is similar to that reported after abdominoperineal excision. In general, mortality rates of 2–10% are typical of large series of cases, with an average of approximately 5%. Mortality rates are usually significantly higher when palliative resections are performed [44]. Mortality is also higher after restorative resection of low-lying lesions since fatal complications arising from anastomotic leaks are more common [45, 46]. Surgical inexperience is likely to result in high mortality as well with most surgeons noting a decrease in mortality as their experience grows [47, 48]. Our own mortality rate is 0.6% (2/309 patients) for anterior resection and 0.4% (1/247 patients) for abdominoperineal resection.

5.4.2. Morbidity
The incidence of bladder dysfunction, impotency, inadvertant operative injury of other viscera, and major cardiopulmonary complications is similar for all of the major resections. As compared to abdominoperineal excision, the primary risk of all restorative procedures relates to anastomotic disruption which can occur because of inadequate vascularity, tension or faulty suture techniques. Contamination or inadequate hemostasis may result in infected pelvic hematomas which secondarily drain through the anastomosis.

Goligher [49] has pointed out the very high subclinical leak rate found in 70% of low and 40% of high hand-sewn anterior anastomoses. Conflicting results have been reported in two randomized trials comparing the security of one-layer with two-layer suture techniques [50, 51]. The modern circular staplers have decreased the clinical leak rate as judged by fecal fistula or local abscess to very low levels. In our personal series of 391 stapled anastomoses, clinical leaks occurred in only 13 patients (3%). High anterior anastomoses rarely disrupt since 12 of the 13 leaks occurred in the 251 patients who underwent a low or an extended low stapled anastomosis.

The incidence of pelvic abscess and fecal fistula after pull-through operations in most series ranges from 10 to 30% often resulting from necrosis of the pulled-through colonic stump which occurs in 5 to 22% of cases [52, 53, 54, 55]. Cutait [40] reported that use of two stages and the delayed anastomosis decreased the disruption of the anastomosis from 31.5% to 2.5%.

In a recent series of 76 patients who underwent a coloanal anastomosis, pelvic sepsis developed in ten patients (13%) and anastomotic disruption in two patients (3%) [56]. Localio [57] reports that peritonitis developed in 4% and fecal fistula in 12% of patients treated by abdominosacral resection. When compared to

Table 3. Mortality of major resections for rectal carcinoma

Procedure	Author	Date	No. pts	Mortality
Abdominoperineal Resection	Mayo *et al.* [105]	1951	689	4.1%
	Abel [106]	1957	188	5.3%
	Gabriel [47]	1957	1223	9.2%
	Lloyd-Davies [48]	1957	1090	8.6%
	Morgan [107]	1965	615	3.1%
	Authors' Series	1979	247	0.4%
	McDermott *et al.* [72]	1982	107	5.6%
Anterior Resection	Deddish & Stearns [46]	1961	189	5.3%
	Vandertoll & Beahrs [45]	1965	1766	4.2%
	Morgan [107]	1965	251	4.4%
	Lockhart-Mummery *et al.* [29]	1976	751	4.2%
	Authors' Series	1982	309	0.6%
Pull-Through Resection	Waugh & Turner [52]	1958	268	3.4%
	Bacon [108]	1960	673	4.3%
	Black [36]	1967	157	3.2%
	Kennedy *et al.* [53]	1970	158	4.5%
Endoanal Resection	Parks & Percy [56]	1982	76	4.0%
	Keighley & Matheson [64]	1980	8	12.5%
Abdominosacral Resection	Localio *et al.* [57]	1978	100	2.0%

anterior resection and abdominoperineal resection, the abdominosacral resection was associated with an increased anastomotic leak rate in younger men. Localio therefore, recommends a proximal colostomy for this age group. Mason [58] reports pelvic sepsis in 18% after his transsphincteric operation.

5.4.3. Functional results

As noted earlier, anal continence can be preserved with only a short anorectal stump. The rectal reservoir function is lost, however, and frequency and urgency of defecation result, putting greater than normal demands on the anal sphincters. If the sphincters were inadequate pre-operatively, or damaged during the conduct of the operation, incontinence may result.

The pull-through procedures are the least satisfactory in achieving satisfactory functional results. Bacon found only 3 of 145 patients wore perineal pads because of incontinence but 61% of the patients required irrigations because of problems with defecation [59]. Waugh and Turner [52] found that only 10% of patients had perfect control following the Bacon procedure. Black [36] reported normal continence in 70%, partial incontinence in 17%, and total incontinence in 13% in his series of 157 patients. He also noted troublesome strictures at the union site in many patients. Approximately 25% of patients have perfect continence after the Turnbull-Cutait procedure, though tolerable function is achieved in about 90% [53, 55, 60, 61].

Of the 76 patients treated by a coloanal anastomosis in Parks' [56] series, 39 had normal bowel function; 30 were normal except for 3–4 bowel movements per day; six were moderately impaired, and one was incontinent. Detailed physiologic studies of 12 of these patients revealed they were no different than normal people [62]. Rudd [63] reports excellent continence after coloanal anastomosis whereas Keighley and Matheson [64] reported disappointing functional results after endoanal anastomosis in eight patients and noted that very low anterior resection with circular staplers produced superior functional results. Localio [65] reports that all 100 patients treated by abdominosacral operation were continent for flatus and stool. Mason [58] similarly reports good results with 60% of patients having normal function and 30% slight impairment only after transsphincteric resection.

High anterior resection has minimal effect on bowel habits or continence [66]. After low and especially after extended low anterior resections, staining of underwear may occur in 20% and difficulty controlling flatus in about 10% [55]. Frank fecal incontinence is rare and has occurred only once in our series of 309 anterior resections. Frequency and urgency increase as the distal rectal stump becomes shorter. Function usually improves during the first few months after a low anterior resection and for most patients becomes very acceptable.

5.4.4. Recurrence and survival

Much of the controversy regarding restorative resections relates to the question 'do they offer the same opportunity for cure that abdominoperineal excision does?' As noted earlier, the abdominal dissection can be the same in restorative procedures and total excision with one exception – the extent of dissection distal to the tumor.

A comparison of survival rates after restorative procedures versus abdominoperineal excision can be misleading since surgeons tend to treat more favorable lesions with restorative procedures and more unfavorable lesions with abdominoperineal excision [29, 67, 68]. The five-year survival of proximal rectal cancers is about 10% greater than that of distal rectal cancers [69]. Upper lesions are obviously more amenable to treatment by restorative resections. Distal third cancers whether resected by abdominoperineal excision or restorative resection fare the worst in terms of survival and pelvic recurrences [70]. Thus, it is not surprising that many studies note a 7–20% greater five-year survival after anterior resection of rectal cancers when compared to abdominoperineal excision [29, 30, 31].

In several studies, authors have compared lesions at the same level treated by abdominoperineal resection or restorative resection. Localio [57] reviewed his 10 year experience with anterior resection, abdominoperineal resection and abdominosacral resection for rectal cancer in patients matched for age, sex, level of lesion, and extent of spread. There was no difference in five-year survival or incidence of pelvic recurrence. Glenn and McSheary [71] found the five-year survival similar after resection of cancers above 10 cm from the anal verge. Many others report a similar result for these upper third lesions. Thus, restorative resections are accepted by almost all surgeons today for such lesions.

More controversial, however, is the role of restorative resection for middle third rectal cancer. McDermott et al. [72] reported their experience with 417 patients with a middle third rectal carcinoma. Between 1950 and 1980, the proportions of these patients treated by restorative resection increased from 26 to 93%. Distribution by age, sex, tumor stage, and histology was similar in both groups of patients. Ten-year survival rates were 60% after restorative resection and 59% after total excision. In another study of 248 patients with carcinoma of the middle third of the rectum treated by anterior resection (176) or by abdominoperineal excision [72] the authors found no evidence of increased local recurrences as long as at least a 3.0 cm distal margin was achieved during anterior resection [33]. They also found no correlation between grade of malignancy and incidence of local recurrence.

The St. Mark's Hospital experience with 42 poorly differentiated cancers of the mid-rectum (8–12 cm from the anal verge) was recently reviewed. Twenty-eight underwent abdominoperineal excision and 14 an anterior resection. They concluded that anterior resection offered as good a prospect of cure as total rectal excision even for these poorly differentiated cancers of the mid-rectum. Our own data supports the conclusion that sphincter preservation for middle third rectal cancers will not lessen survival prospects provided at least a 2.0 to 3.0 cm distal margin is achieved. Parks [56] reported that of 32 patients undergoing a curative resection and coloanal anastomosis, 21 (66%) were alive without sign of recurrence 3 or more years after their procedure. Twelve of 19 patients (63%) were alive without recurrence for five-years [56]. Keighley and Matheson [64], on the other hand, reported pelvic recurrence in three of eight patients 6, 9 and 14 months after resection of rectal cancers 5 to 8 cm from the anal verge with restoration by a coloanal anastomosis.

6. Local treatment

It is interesting that in recent years, treatment for carcinoma of the rectum has come full circle since local therapy is once again being advocated. As opposed to the late 1800's where such therapy was the only approach available, local treatment today is being used in a highly selective way. Current understanding of the development and spread of carcinoma of the rectum has increased our ability to better predict which lesions might be cured with local therapy alone. Similarily, we can better predict which lesions are beyond hope of cure no matter how radical the resection. Both such situations account for the increased use of local therapy for cure or palliation in the modern era [74].

6.1. Selection criteria

Many different sets of criteria for tumor selection for local therapy have been proposed. Mason [75] considers only freely mobile or mobile lesions for local excision. Nichols *et al.* [76], based on a prospective trial comparing pre-operative rectal digital examination with pathologic examinations or final surgical assessment, have suggested a clinical staging system based on mobility, extent of extrarectal spread, presence or absence of tumor ulceration and amount of lumenal circumference involved to aid in selection of patients for local treatment and restorative resection. The difficulties in the selection process can be further illustrated by differing criteria for local excision proposed by Beart, Jagelman, and Salvati in a recent symposium on restorative resection [77]. Beart felt that tumors should be less than 4 cm in size, Grade III or less, and obviously nonannular, where as Jagelman felt the lesion in question should be 3 cm or less in diameter, polypoid, and mobile. On the other hand, Salvati felt local excision should be used only for those cancers arising in a villous adenoma or a tubular adenomatous polyp. All agreed that the tumor should be within 5 to 7 cm of the dentate line and technically it must be possible to remove the entire lesion. These varying sets of criteria are clinical attempts to identify cancers which have not spread to local nodes and are unlikely to recur locally. Such lesions are appropriate for local treatment.

6.2. Options available

Options for local therapy are local excision, electrocoagulation and endocavitary irradiation. Of these, local excision which is in essence a total biopsy, provides pathologic information about the primary lesion whereas, both electrocoagulation and irradiation destroy the evidence and no further pathologic information can be obtained. Electrocoagulation is probably technically the easiest procedure whereas endocavitary irradiation requires very specialized equipment and training. On the other hand, unlike electrocoagulation and local excision, endocavitary irradiation can be performed on an ambulatory outpatient basis and anesthesia is not required. Furthermore, there is almost no risk of bleeding and only a negligible risk of perforation [78]. Both electrocoagulation and irradiation give an 'extra margin' of destruction but unfortunately, it cannot be determined if this is needed or complete on any given patient.

6.2.1. Local excision
The technique of local excision can be accomplished either transanally or by posterior incision using the transsphincteric or transsacral approach with an extremely low mortality even in unfit elderly patients [41, 58, 79]. Regardless of the method of exposing the tumor, a full-thickness excision containing a margin of surrounding normal tissue is necessary. For pedunculated or small sessile lesions confined to the mucosa, diathermy snare excision via an endoscope is appropriate. If during a submucosal excision of a villous tumor, a suspicious area of deeper involvement is encountered, the excision must be deepened to a full thickness. It is essential that the specimen be pinned out for proper orientation and that close communication and cooperation between surgeon and pathologist exist. A potential disadvantage of the Mason or Kraske approaches is that of extensive retrorectal seeding of cancer. Two such instances occurred at Memorial Sloan Kettering Cancer Center making subsequent abdominoperineal resection incomplete. Both patients died of recurrence [80].

Stearns [80] reported a 75% five-year survival in 31 patients with nonpedunculated cancers treated by local excision. Beart [77] in comparing 292 cases treated locally with 494 cases who had abdominoperineal resection for non-annular cancers 4 cm or less in diameter of Grade III or less histology reported a better survival for those having had local treatment. Lock et al. [74] reported a favorable experience in 143 patients with early rectal cancer treated by local excision over a 24 year period at St. Mark's Hospital.

6.2.2. Electrocoagulation
Although initially reported by Byrne [81] in 1889 and reintroduced by Straus [82], electrocoagulation as a method of treatment of rectal cancers received little attention until Madden [83] advocated electrocoagulation as the 'preferred' method of treatment.

Various methods of electrocoagulation have been described using different types of electrical units and electrodes. This is not an office procedure, but instead patients should be hospitalized and the procedure performed in an operating room setting under either spinal or general anesthesia. The patient should have both a mechanical and antibiotic bowel prep as though undergoing surgical resection. Proper illumination, exposure and effective suction are essential. A large operating proctoscope is highly desirable. Crile and Turnbull [84] have described several helpful observations as follows. When tumor is destroyed by electrocoagulation, it crumbles and can be wiped away. Muscle chars to the consistency of leather, and fat is recognized both by its color and by the sizzling that is produced when it is heated. Posteriorly, electrocoagulation can be quite radical but anteriorly more caution must be exercised. Fixation of the tumor to the rectovaginal septum is a contraindication to electrocoagulation because destruction of such tumors results in a rectovaginal fistula.

Eisenstat et al. [81] have found that if more than three electrocoagulation sessions are necessary, then abdominoperineal resection should be considered. One should not persist when it become obvious that the procedure is failing to control the tumor.

It is impossible to accurately assess the efficacy of electrocoagulation since no specimen is available for analysis. Nonetheless, the number of five-year survivals reported by several authors is impressive [84, 85]. Salvati and Rubin [86] reported a comparison of survival in 47 patients treated by electrocoagulation and 37 treated by abdominoperineal resection. The one to ten year survival for electrocoagulation was 48% and the one to eight year survival for the abdominoperineal resection group was 46%. Eisenstat et al. [81] reported a five-year survival of greater than 70% in 24 patients with lesions involving one third or less of the rectal circumference. Furthermore, in patients requiring conversion to abdominoperineal resection the five-year survival was 26%. This compares favorably to the overall five-year survival in Dukes' C lesions where abdominoperineal resection is employed [52].

6.2.3. Endocavitary irradiation

Papillon [78] introduced the technique of endocavitary contact irradiation delivering a total of 10,000 to 15,000 rads to the tumor in 3 to 5 short applications during an overall treatment time of 4 to 6 weeks. In a series of 207 cases, he reported a five-year survival of 74%. Sischy [87] in this country has had a similar experience to that of Papillon. These are highly selected cases.

7. Clinical assessment

Accurate clinical assessment optimizes the choice of treatment for a select patient and a select tumor and minimizes intraoperative misadventures and postoperative morbidity and mortality.

7.1. Cancer status

Local factors such as the precise location from the anal verge, size, percent of fixation, and histologic grade of the primary are best determined by thorough rectal and pelvic examinations and rigid proctoscopy with biopsy [76]. Computerized tomography may be of value in determining the extent of local spread, though Nichols *et al.* [76] found rectal digital examination to be the most accurate (and cheapest) test available. A preoperative biopsy is useful to confirm the diagnosis of adenocarcinoma of the rectum. Early studies suggested that biopsy correlated well with the final histologic grading but recent studies suggest that preoperative biopsy is not totally accurate in assessing histologic grade [73, 78].

Synchronous lesions in the colon must be excluded. Between 2 and 5% of patients with cancer of the rectum have a synchronous carcinoma and up to 20 to 30% have synchronous neoplastic polyps [89]. Copeland *et al.* [90] found a synchronous cancer in 14.6% of patients who had multiple colonic polyps. Preoperative total colonic evaluation with colonoscopy or air contrast barium enema should detect these lesions, the presence of which may greatly affect the type of operative intervention to be performed. If complete or high grade obstruction is present, these studies are impossible. A more concentrated effort to closely examine the remaining bowel at laparotomy is made in such cases and after full recovery from the rectal cancer surgery, total colonic evaluation must be obtained.

The presence of distant metastases may influence the choice between local therapy or major resection. Pulmonary metastases are best screened by a routine chest xray with any suspicious areas checked further by fluoroscopy or tomography. Screening for liver metastases is more difficult. Radionucleotide scans and ultrasound have little use in routine screening because of the lack of reliability of these tests and the expense incurred [91]. Finlay and McCardle [92] reported that CT scanning detected 'occult' liver metastases in 11 of 35 patients who had recently undergone apparent curative resection.

Only 9% of those patients with occult liver metastases detected by CT scan survived 30 months as compared to 88% survival for 30 months for patients with normal CT scans. The CT scan thus seems valuable in predicting prognosis but whether this justifies its expense on a routine basis remains open to question. If effective adjuvant therapy for such liver metastases is developed, then routine screening for 'occult' liver metastases would be reasonable. Certainly, if the presence of liver metastases would change the operative approach, CT scanning is worth pursuing. Percutaneous, directed needle biopsy or laparoscopic biopsy may also be useful in this setting. Obviously, the surgeons' assessment of the liver at the time of laparotomy may also influence his choice of procedures. Screening for bone, cerebral, adrenal or other sites of distant metastases is not performed in the absence of specific, suspicious symptoms or findings. The role of the carcinoembryonic antigen is controversial. In select patients, it may play a role in follow-up in which case a preoperative level is useful as a baseline [93].

7.2. General health status

The ability of a given patient to undergo major surgery influences choice of treatment. The pre-operative examination and routine laboratory tests should be aimed at identifying correctable problems such as anemia, malnutrition, or fluid and electrolyte imbalance as well as defining concomitant disease states. Age per se should not dictate therapy.

Whenever a restorative resection is contemplated for a rectal cancer, the surgeon must assess the state of the anal sphincters. It would be tragic to perform a restorative procedure in a patient whose sphincters are incapable of maintaining continence. The possibility that a stoma, either temporary or permanent, may be necessary should be discussed with the patient pre-operatively. Some patients may have impairments such as severe arthritis, hemiplegia or blindness which would make a stoma almost impossible to live with. In such cases, local therapy may be a better choice of treatment. A pre-operative consultation with a qualified enterostomal therapist is invaluable whenever the possibility of a stoma is considered.

7.3. Technical details

The pre-operative preparation of the patient should include a complete mechanical and antibiotic bowel preparation regimen. The efficacy of such preparations has been validated in several trials. Though more controversial, perioperative systemic intravenous antibiotics do seem to decrease the incidence of wound infection.

We find a pre-operative intravenous pyelogram of value in demonstrating the course and number of ureters and the presence of any genitourinary anomalies. This is especially true in patients who have had prior pelvic or distal colonic surgery, previous diverticulitis, prior pelvic irradiation, and in those with large, bulky rectal tumors. Ureteral catheters are considered in such patients to help avoid or at least to aid recognition of ureteral injuries [94].

8. Special situations

The question of whether an anastomosis can be safely performed after irradiation is increasingly relevant to clinical practice. Palliative resections, unfortunately, continue to constitute a significant percentage of operations for carcinoma of the rectum and they pose some special considerations. Obstruction and perforation almost never occur with rectal cancer and are not considered here.

8.1. Restorative resection in irradiated bowel

Although preoperative irradiation in carcinoma of the rectum has not been shown to improve the five-year survival to a statistically significant level, there appears to be a reduction in lymph node invasion, local recurrence, and distant metastases [95]. In most studies, preoperative irradiation was used in low-lying lesions, followed by abdominoperineal resections. The operative and postoperative complications did not appear to be high [95, 96, 97]. Information regarding resections and anastomosis in irradiated bowel is indeed limited. Photopulos *et al.* [98] reported a series of 17 patients who underwent bowel resection and anastomosis using GIA and TA staplers after having received 4000–6000 rads for gynecologic cancers. There were no anastomotic complications.

In Pilepich's *et al.* [97] series with preoperative irradiation of 5000 rads, seven patients underwent an anterior resection with primary anastomosis and complementary colostomy without leaks. In Stevens *et al.* [96] series, 13 patients with carcinoma of the rectum and sigmoid colon, with the lower margin of the tumors below 12–20 cm, received preoperative irradiation of 5000 rads. They subsequently underwent an anterior resection with a primary anastomosis. Four patients had complementary colostomies. Six patients developed post-operative complications: small bowel obstruction-2, anastomotic leak-2, anastomotic stenosis-1, and abdominal wound dehiscence-1. Prospective studies of the effects of low-dose and high-dose preoperative irradiation on low anterior anastomoses in dogs were reported by Schauer *et al.* [99] and Bubrick *et al.* [100]. The dogs received irradiation equivalent to 2000 rads and 4000 rads respectively. A secure low anastomosis was achieved in both studies. The data also suggested that the staplers produced a more secure anastomosis then a hand-sewn anastomosis.

It thus appears that a low anterior resection can be performed with reasonable safety in both low-dose and high-dose preoperative irradiation. However, more specific data is needed. Every attempt should be made to use the descending colon proximally and the rectum well below the lesions, since these two areas are exposed to a lesser amount of irradiation. Although a complementary colostomy does not prevent anastomotic leak, it may save lives and make the management easier should anastomotic dehiscence occur. This should be considered particularly if high-dose irradiation was given pre-operatively.

8.2. Palliative resection

A palliative resection for carcinoma of the rectum is reasonable to relieve symptoms, prevent obstruction, and improve the patients' well-being, if it can be done with an acceptable morbidity and mortality [101]. Removal of the primary lesion, in most cases, relieves the symptoms, particularly of pain, obstruction, and bleeding and restores health and well-being at least for a short period of time

[102, 103]. The operative morbidity and mortality are similar to curative resections in some studies but significantly higher in others [101]. Patients over the age of 75 years with a previous history of cardiovascular disease seem especially at high risk to undergo resection [103].

The choice between a low anterior resection or an abdominonperineal resection for palliation is based largely on one's ability to clear the pelvis of tumor and safely restore continuity. One should keep in mind that after an extended low anterior resection, the palliative value may be lost by a prolonged hospital stay or a prolonged struggle to regain anal continence. In such a circumstance, resection with a well constructed end-colostomy will be more valuable. Similarily anterior resection with residual tumor in the pelvis invites early, symptomatic recurrence but a colostomy without excision of the tumor affords no worthwhile palliation. One cannot expect irradiation or chemotherapy to be effective. Spurious diarrhea with passage of blood and mucus still persists [44]. For unresectable tumors of the lower- and middle-third of the rectum, electrocoagulation may temporarily control the symptoms [104].

9. Authors' approach

Our personal approach to carcinoma of the rectum is guided by several principles. First, one must keep in mind that some cancers of the rectum are curable by very simple local therapy while others are incurable no matter how radical the operative approach. Long-term survival after resection of carcinoma of the rectum, stage for stage, has not changed significantly in several decades. Second, the surgeon's role is to intervene in the natural history of carcinoma of the rectum in the hopes of providing long-term cure whenever possible, but this must be done without excessive mortality and morbidity. A critical analysis and long-term follow-up of most reports suggesting that more radical operations will cure more patients usually reveals no improvement in survival or improvement in survival only if one ignores the increased mortality associated with the more radical operations. At present, an approach which keeps operative mortality at less than 5% is mandatory. Third, preservation of anal continence is worth an 'all out' effort. Some restorative procedures are technically easy but many are difficult and demanding. A team approach with at least two and sometimes three surgeons present to assist in restoration of continence is critical, and can make the difference between preserved continence or a permanent stoma. Fourth, some patients are best served by an abdominoperineal resection and well constructed colostomy. We now have the technical capability to restore continence after resection of many lesions of the lower rectum. We must carefully judge which lessions and which patients are suited for restorative procedures.

Lesions of the upper third of the rectum are almost all treated by anterior resection. Even elderly, frail patients tolerate this procedure quite well. An

182

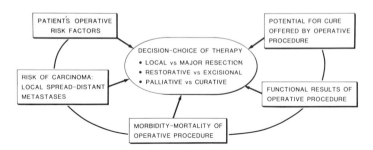

Figure 6. The surgeon must balance five factors to properly select the ideal operative procedure for a patient with carcinoma of the rectum.

extremely high risk patient may be treated by a transanal excision or fulguration of the lesion if technically possible. Alternatively, a transsphincteric approach could be used to effect local excision.

Lesions of the middle third of the rectum in good risk patients are treated by major resection. It is almost always possible to restore continuity with a low anterior anastomosis using the circular staplers. Occasionally, a coloanal anastomosis is provided. Rarely, an abdominoperineal excision is necessary. For poor risk patients, lesions of the middle third of the rectum can be managed by local transanal excision or fulguration. The transsacral or transsphincteric approaches are rarely used.

Lesions of the lower third of the rectum in good risk patients are generally treated by major resection. If technically feasible and if a 3.0 cm distal margin is obtained, an extended low anterior anastomosis or a coloanal anastomosis is performed. Often, abdominoperineal resection is necessary. We are impressed with some of the data suggesting that fulguration is the preferred method of treatment of such lesions but to date, we have used this method only for palliation or in high risk patients.

Summary

Surgical management of carcinoma of the rectum has evolved over the past century to the point that the modern surgeon has multiple options of therapy available to him. Of the major resections, abdominoperineal resection or anterior resection are the most commonly used. Pull-through procedures because of their technical demands and variable functional results are rarely performed today. The abdominosacral resection, abdominotranssphincteric resection and the abdominotransanal resection with coloanal anastomosis are options used routinely by a few surgeons but only in selective situations by most surgeons. Local treatment is being increasingly performed today though its exact role is not completely defined.

Current knowledge of the routes of spread of rectal cancer and of the mechanisms of anal continence coupled with the increased safety of abdominal operations and the technological advances such as the circular staplers have brought us to the point where most cancers of the mid-and upper rectum can be resected by an abdominal approach and continuity restored. Most cancers of the lower third of the rectum are best treated by abdominoperineal excision but some can be treated locally with preservation of sphincter function. The dilemma today is to achieve the proper matching of five variables: 1) the patient's operative risk factors; 2) the risks posed to the patient by his rectal cancer; 3) the risk inherent to the proposed operation; 4) the potential for cure offered by the proposed operation; and 5) the functional results of the proposed operation (Fig. 6). The debate over what constitutes optimal therapy for rectal cancer cannot ignore any of these variables.

References

1. Kraske P, cited in Goligher JC: Treatment of Carcinoma of the Rectum. In: Surgery of the Anus, Rectum and Colon. 4th Edition. Bailliere Tindall, London, 1980, p 502–666.
2. Mandl F, cited in Goligher JC: Treatment of Carcinoma of the Rectum. In: Surgery of the Anus, Rectum and Colon. 4th Edition. Bailliere Tindall, London, 1980, p 502–666.
3. Lockhart-Mummery JP: Resection of the rectum for cancer. Lancet 1: 20–24, 1920.
4. Gabriel WB: The end results of perineal excision and of radium in the treatment of cancer of the rectum. Br J Surg 20: 234–48, 1932.
5. Miles WE: The radical abdomino-perineal operation for cancer of the rectum and of the pelvic colon. Br Med J 2: 941–3, 1910.
6. Miles WE: A method of performing abdominoperineal excision for carcinoma of the rectum and of the terminal portion of the pelvic colon. Lancet 2: 1812–13, 1908.
7. Miles WE, cited in Goligher JC: Treatment of Carcinoma of the Rectum. In: Surgery of the Anus, Rectum and Colon. 4th Edition. Bailliere Tindall, London, 1980, p 502–666.
8. Dukes CE, cited in Gabriel WB: Principles and Practice of Rectal Surgery. 4th Edition. HK Lewis, London, 1948, p 50–61.
9. Morson BC: Adenomas and Adenoma-Carcinoma Sequence. Morson BC, Dawson IMP (ed). Chapter 38. In: Gastrointestinal Pathology, 2nd Edition. Blackwell Scientific Publications, Oxford, 1979, p 630–37, 654, 665–9.
10. Coller FA, Kay EB, MacIntyre RS: Regional lymphatic metastases of carcinoma of the colon. Ann Surg 114: 56–67, 1941.
11. Grinnell RS: Spread of carcinoma of the colon and rectum. Cancer 3: 641–52, 1950.
12. Quer EA, Dahlin DC, Mayo CW: Retrograde intramural spread of carcinoma of the rectum and rectosigmoid. Surg. Gynecol Obstet 96: 24–30, 1953.
13. Grinnell RS: Distal intramural spread of carcinoma of the rectum and rectosigmoid. Surg Gynecol Obstet 99: 421–30, 1954.
14. Cohen AM, Wood WC, Gunderson LL, Shinnar M: Pathological studies in rectal cancer. Cancer 45: 2965–8, 1980.

15. Dukes CE: Spread of cancer of the rectum. Br J Surg 17: 643–8, 1930.

16. Gabriel WB, Dukes CE, Bussey HJR: Lymphatic spread in cancer of the rectum. Br J Surg 23: 395–413, 1935.

17. Westhues H, cited in Goligher JC: Incidence and Pathology of Carcinoma of the Colon and Rectum. In: Surgery of the Anus, Rectum and Colon. 4th Edition. Bailliere Tindall, London, 1980, p 392–406.

18. Wood WQ, Wilkie DPD: Carcinoma of the rectum: An anatomical pathological study. Edinb Med J 40: 321–43, 1933.

19. Dukes CE, Bussey HJR: The spread of rectal cancer and its effect on prognosis. Br J Ca 12: 309–11, 1958.

20. Talbot IC, Ritchie S, Leighton MH, Hughes HO, Bussey HJR, Morson BC: The clinical significance of invasion of veins by rectal cancer. Br J Surg 67: 439–42, 1980.

21. Seefeld PH, Bargen JA: The spread of carcinoma of the rectum: Ivasion of lymphatics, veins and nerves. Ann Surg 118: 76–90, 1943.

22. Spratt JS Jr, Spjut HJ: Prevalence and prognosis of individual clinical and pathological variables associated with colorectal carcinoma. Cancer 20: 1976–85, 1967.

23. Hertz AF, Oxon MD: The sensibility of the alimentary canal in health and disease. Lancet 1: 1119–1124, 1911.

24. Goligher JC, Hughes ESR: Sensibility of the rectum and colon. Lancet 1: 543–48, 1951.

25. Cortisini C: Anorectal reflex following sphincter-saving operations. Dis Col Rectum 23: 320–26, 1980.

26. Suzuki H, Matsumato K, Amano S, Fujioko M, Honsumi M: Anorectal pressure and rectal compliance after low anterior resection. Br J Surg 67: 655–57, 1980.

27. Dixon CF: Surgical removal of lesions occurring in the sigmoid and rectosigmoid. Am J Surg 46: 12–17, 1939.

28. Wangensteen OH: Primary resection (closed anastomosis) of rectal ampulla for malignancy with preservation of sphincter function. Surg Gynecol Obstet 81: 1–24, 1945.

29. Lockhart-Mummery HE, Ritchie JK, Hawley PR: The results of surgical treatment from carcinoma of the rectum at St. Mary's Hospital from 1948 to 1972. Br J Surg 63: 673–7, 1976.

30. Mayo CW, Fly OA: Analysis of a five-year survival in carcinoma of the rectum and rectosigmoid. Surg Gynecol Obstet 103: 94–100, 1956.

31. Whittaker M, Goligher JC: The prognosis after surgical treatment for carcinoma of the rectum. Br J Surg 63: 384–8, 1976.

32. Ravitch MM, Steichen FM: A stapling instrument for end-to-end inverting anastomoses in the gastrointestinal tract. Ann Surg 189: 791–97, 1979.

33. Tonak J, Gall FP, Hermanek P, Hager TH: Incidence of local recurrence after curative operations for cancer of the rectum. Aust NZ J Surg 52: 23–7, 1982.

34. Localio AS, Stahl WM: Simultaneous abdominosacral resection and anastomosis for mid-rectal cancer. Am J Surg 117: 282–89, 1969.

35. Bacon HE: Evolution of sphincter muscle preservation and re-establishment of continuity in the operative treatment of rectal and sigmoid cancer. Surg Gynecol Obstet 81: 113–27, 1945.

36. Black BM: Combined abdominoendorectal resection: Reappraisal of a pull-through procedure. Surg Clin N Am 47: 977–82, 1967.

37. Maunsell HW: A new method of excising the two upper portions of the rectum and the lower segment of the sigmoid flexure of the colon. Lancet 2: 473–6, 1982.

38. Wier RF: An improved method of treating high-seated cancers of the rectum. J Am Med Ass 37: 801–03, 1901.

39. Turnbull RB, Cuthbertson A: Abdominorectal pull-through resection for cancer and for Hirschsprung's disease. Cleveland Clin Quarterly 28: 109–14, 1961.

40. Cutait DE, Figlialini FJ: A new method of colorectal anastomosis in abdominoperineal resection. Dis Col Rectum 4: 335–42, 1961.

41. Parks AG: Transanal technique in low rectal anastomosis. Proc R Soc Med 65: 975–6, 1972.
42. Ferguson EF, Houston CH: Simplified anterior resection: Use of the TA stapler. Dis Col Rectum 18: 311–18, 1975.
43. Rothenberger DA, Goldberg SM: Staplers in operations for large bowel cancer. In: Large Bowel Cancer. DeCosse JJ (ed). Churchill Livingstone, New York, 1981, p 94–112.
44. Goligher JC: Surgery of the Anus, Rectum and Colon. 4th Edition. Bailliere Tindall, London, 1980, p 502, 639.
45. Vandertoll DJ, Beahrs OH: Carcinoma of the rectum and low sigmoid: Evaluation of anterior resections of 1766 favorable lesions. Arch Surg 90: 793–8, 1965.
46. Deddish MR, Stearns MW: Anterior resection for carcinoma of the rectum and rectosigmoid area. Ann Surg 154: 961–66, 1961.
47. Gabriel WB: Discussion on major surgery in carcinoma of the rectum, with or without colostomy, excluding the anal canal and including the rectosigmoid. Proc R Soc Med 50: 1041–47, 1957.
48. Lloyd-Davis OV: Discussion on major surgery in carcinoma of the rectum, with or without colostomy, excluding the anal canal and including the rectosigmoid. Proc R Soc Med 50: 1047–50, 1957.
49. Goligher JC, Graham NG, DeDombal FT: Anastomotic dehiscence after anterior resection of rectum and sigmoid. Br J Surg 57: 109–117, 1970.
50. Everett WG: A comparison of one layer and two layer techniques for colorectal anastomosis. Br J Surg 62: 135–40, 1975.
51. Goligher JC, Lee PWR, Simpkins KC, Lintott DJ: Controlled comparison of one and two layer techniques of suture for high and low colorectal anastomoses. Br J Surg 64: 609–14, 1977.
52. Waugh JM, Turner JC: Abdominoperineal resection with preservation of the anal sphincter for cancer of the mid-rectum. Surg Gynecol Obstet 107: 777–83, 1958.
53. Kennedy JT, McOmish D, Bennett RC, Hughes ESR, Cuthbertson AM: Abdomino-anal pull-through resection of the rectum. Br J Surg 57: 589–95, 1970.
54. Black BM, Bothan RJ: Combined andomino-perineal resections for lesions of the mid and upper parts of the rectum. Arch Surg 76: 688–96, 1958.
55. Goligher JC, Duthie HL, DeDombal FT, Watts JM: The pull through abdominoanal excision for carcinoma of the middle third of the rectum: A comparison with low anterior resection. Br J Surg 52: 323–35, 1965.
56. Parks AG, Percy JP: Resection and sutured colo-anal anastomosis for rectal carcinoma. Br J Surg 69: 301–4, 1982.
57. Localio AS, Eng K, Gauge TH, Ranson JHC: Abdominosacral resection for carcinoma of the mid rectum: Ten year experience. Ann Surg 188: 475–80, 1978.
58. Mason YA: Transsphincteric exposure for low rectal anastomosis. Proc R Soc Med 65: 974, 1972.
59. Bacon HE: Abdominoperineal proctosigmoidectomy with sphincter preservation. Five year and ten year survival after pull-through operations for cancer of the rectum. J Am Med Ass 160: 628–34, 1956.
60. Bennet RC, Hughes ESR, Cuthbertson A: Long-term review of function following pull-through operations of the rectum. Br J Surg 59: 723–5, 1972.
61. Kirwan WO, Turnbull RB, Fazio VW, Weakley FL: Pullthrough operation with delayed anastomosis for rectal cancer. Br J Surg 65: 695–8, 1978.
62. Lane RHS, Parks AG: Function of the anal sphincters following colo-anal anastomosis. Br J Surg 64: 596–99, 1977.
63. Rudd WWH: The transanal anastomosis: A sphincter-saving operation with improved continence. Dis Col Rectum 22: 102–5, 1979.
64. Keighley MRB, Matheson D: Functional results of rectal excision and endo-anal anstomosis. Br J Surg 67: 757–61, 1980.

65. Localio SA, Eng K: Sphincter-saving operations for cancer of the rectum. N Eng J Med 300: 1028–30, 1979.

66. Goligher JC: The functional results after sphincter-saving resections of the rectum. Ann R Coll Surg Eng 8: 421–23, 1951.

67. Jones PF, Thompson HJ: Long term results of a consistent policy of sphincter preservation in the treatment of carcinoma of the rectum. Br J Surg 69: 564–68, 1982.

68. Slanetz CA, Herter FP, Grinnell RS: Anterior resection versus abdominoperineal resection for carcinoma of the rectum and rectosigmoid. Am J Surg 123: 110–26, 1972.

69. Gilchrist RK, David VC: A consideration of pathological factors influencing five year survival in radical resection of the large bowel and rectum for carcinoma. Ann Surg 126: 421–38, 1947.

70. Morson BC, Vaughan EG, Bussey HJR: Pelvic recurrences after excision of the rectum for carcinoma. Br J Surg 2: 13–5, 1963.

71. Glenn F, McSherry CK: Carcinoma of the distal bowel in 32 year review of 1026 cases. Ann Surg 163: 838–49, 1966.

72. McDermott F, Hughes E, Pihl E, Milne BJ, Price A: Long term results of restorative resection and total excision for carcinoma of the middle third of the rectum. Surg Gynecol Obstet 154: 833–37, 1982.

73. Elliot MS, Todd IP, Nichols RJ: Radical restorative surgery for poorly differentiated carcinoma of the mid-rectum. Br J Surg 69: 273–4, 1982.

74. Lock MR, Cairns DW, Ritchie JK, Lockhart-Mummery HE: The treatment of early colorectal cancer by local excision. Br J Surg 65: 346–9, 1978.

75. Mason YA: Selective surgery for carcinoma of the rectum. Aust NZ J Surg 46: 322–9, 1976.

76. Nichols RJ, Mason YA, Morson BC, Dixon AK, Fry IK: The clinical staging of cancer. Br J Surg 69: 404–08, 1982.

77. Beart RW, Jagelman DG, Salvati EP: Symposium: Sphincter saving operations for rectal cancer. Cont Surg 21: 59–62, 1982.

78. Papillon J: Rectal and Anal Cancers: Conservative treatment by irradiation – An alternative to radical surgery. Springer-Verlag, New York, 1982, p 24–33.

79. Christiansen J: Excision of mid-rectal lesions by the Kraske sacral approach. Br J Surg 67: 651–2, 1980.

80. Stearns MW, Steinberg SS, DeCosse JJ: Local Treatment of Rectal Cancer. In: Large Bowel Cancer, Vol. I. DeCosse, JJ (ed). Churchill Livingstone, New York, 1981, p 144–53.

81. Eisenstat TE, Deak ST, Rubin RJ, Salvati EP, Greco RS: Five year survival in patients with carcinoma of the rectum treated by electrocoagulation. Am J Surg 143: 127–32, 1982.

82. Strauss SF, Crawford RA, Strauss HA: Surgical diathermy of carcinoma of rectum, its clinical end results. J Am Med Ass 104: 1480–84, 1935.

83. Madden JL, Kandalaft S: Electrocoagulation: A primary and preferred method of treatment for cancer of the rectum. Ann Surg 166: 413–19, 1967.

84. Crile G, Turnbull RB: The role of electrocoagulation in the treatment of carcimona of the rectum. Surg Gynecol Obstet 135: 391–96, 1972.

85. Madden JL, Kandalaft S: Electrocoagulation in the treatment of cancer of the rectum: A continuing study. Ann Surg 174: 530–40, 1971.

86. Salvati EP, Rubin RJ: Electrocoagulation as a primary therapy for rectal carcinoma. Am J Surg 132: 583–6, 1976.

87. Sischy B, Remington JH: Treatment of carcinoma of the rectum by intracavitary irradiation. Surg Gynecol Obstet 141: 562–4, 1975.

88. Sugarbaker PH: Current Problems in Surgery. Year Book Medical Publishers, 1982, p 765–80.

89. Ekelund GR, Pihl B: Multiple carcinomas of the colon and rectum. Cancer 33: 1630–34, 1974.

90. Copeland EM, Jones RS, Miller LD: Multiple colon neoplasms. Prognosis and therapeutic implications. Arch Surg 98: 115–9, 1969.

91. Read DR, Hambrick E, Abcariam H, et al.: The preoperative diagnosis of hepatic metastasis in

cases of colorectal carcinoma. Dis Col Rectum 20: 101–06, 1977.

92. Finlay IG, McCardle CS: The identification of patients of high risk following curative resection for colorectal carcinoma. Br J Surg 69: 583–84, 1982.

93. Goslin R, Steele G Jr, MacIntyre R, Sugarbaker P, Cleghorn K, Wilson R, Samcheck N: The use of preoperative plasma CEA levels for the stratification of patients after curative resections of colorectal cancers. Ann Surg 192: 747–51, 1980.

94. Leff EI, Groff W, Rubin RJ, Einestat TE, Salvati EP: Use of ureteral catheters in colonic and rectal surgery. Dis Col Rectum 25: 457–60, 1982.

95. Roswit B, Higgins GA Jr, Keehn RJ: Preoperative irradiation for carcinoma of the rectum and rectosigmoid colon: Report of a national Veterans Administration randomized study. Cancer 35: 1597–1602, 1975.

96. Stevens KR Jr, Allen CV, Fletcher WS: Preoperative radiotherapy for adenocarcinoma of the rectosigmoid. Cancer 37: 2866–72, 1976.

97. Pilepich MV, Munsenrider JE, Tak WK, Miller HH: Preoperative irradiation of primarily unresectable colorectal carcinoma. Cancer 42: 1077–81, 1978.

98. Photopulos GJ, Delgado G, Fowler WC Jr, Walton LA: Intestinal anastomoses after radiation therapy for surgical stapling instruments. Surg Gynecol Obstet 54: 515–8, 1979.

99. Schauer RM, Bubrick MP, Feeney DA, Johnson GR, Rolfsmeyer ES, et al.: Effects of low-dose preoperative irradiation on low anterior anastomoses in dogs. Dis Col Rectum 25: 401–5, 1982.

100. Bubrick MP, Rolfsmeyer ES, Schauer RM, Feeney DA, Johnson GR, et al.: Effects of high-dose and low-dose preoperative irradiation on low anterior anastomoses in dogs. Dis Col Rectum 25: 406–15, 1982.

101. Johnson WR: McDermott FT, Pihl E, Barrie JM, Price AB, Hughes ESR: Palliative operative management in rectal carcinoma. Dis Col Rectum 24: 606–9, 1981.

102. Lockhart-Mummert HE: Surgery in patients with advanced carcinoma of the colon and rectum. Dis Col Rectum 2: 36–9, 1959.

103. Joffe J, Gordon PH: Palliative resection for colorectal carcinoma. Dis Col Rectum 24: 355–60, 1981.

104. Fritsch A, Seidl W, Walzel C, Maser K, Schiessel R: Palliative and adjunctive measures in rectal cancer. World J Surg 6: 569–77, 1982.

105. Mayo CW, Lee MJ, Davis RM: A comparitive study of operations for carcinoma of the rectum and rectosigmoid. Surg Gynecol Obstet 92: 360–4, 1951.

106. Abel AL: Discussion on major surgery in carcinoma of the rectum, with or without colostomy excluding the anal canal and including the rectosigmoid. Proc R Soc Med 50: 1035–41, 1957.

107. Morgan CN: Carcinoma of the rectum. Ann R Coll Surg Eng 36: 73, 1965.

108. Bacon HE: Major surgery of the colon and rectum: Rehabilitation and survival rate in 2,457 patients. Dis Col Rectum 3: 393–402, 1960.

8. Large bowel cancer: utility of radiation therapy

LEONARD L. GUNDERSON, TYVIN A. RICH, JOEL E. TEPPER,
DANIEL E. DOSORETZ, ANTHONY H. RUSSELL,
and R. BRUCE HOSKINS

1. Introduction

For 1982, both the expected incidence (114,000) and expected number of deaths
(52,000) for adenocarcinoma of the large bowel ranked second only to carcinoma
of the lung [1]. The male/female incidence ratio is essentially equal. Studies done
during the last decade have shown a proximal shift of lesion incidence within the
large bowel (i.e., rectal cancers have become less common and colon cancers
more frequent). The cause for this is uncertain.

Survival rates for colorectal carcinoma have improved slightly over the past 25
to 30 years. Such improvements, however, have been the results of an increase in
operability with little improvement by stage of disease in those patients who have
survived a 'curative resection.'

Recent developments have led to marked interest in a combined modality
approach for initial treatment of rectal and selected colonic carcinomas: 1) Local
failure or recurrence (LF) within the operative field has been identified as a
significant problem in various operative series in spite of potentially curative
surgery [2–11]. 2) Although significant palliation of 75 to 85% of such failures can
be obtained with radiation alone or in combination with chemotherapy, the
duration of palliation is often limited, the curative potential is 5% or less in most
series, and therefore, prevention of local recurrence is a necessity. 3) Data is
accumulating to indicate the curative potential of radiation for patients with
residual or unresectable disease (10 to 30%) or those who refuse abdominoperineal resection [12–18]. Radiation dose levels required to accomplish such
results (6000 to 7000+ rads) can, however, result in significant complications in
surrounding dose-limiting tissues and organs unless many precautions are applied
[15, 19]. Conventional supervoltage irradiation, therefore, is not a competitive
alternative to operation for lesions which are resectable. A preferred method is to
combine more moderate radiation doses of 4500 to 5000 rad with potentially
curative surgery when high risk of local recurrence exists.

The intent of this manuscript is to discuss information concerning large bowel

J.J. DeCosse and P. Sherlock (eds), Clinical Management of Gastrointestinal Cancer.
© *1984, Martinus Nijhoff Publishers, Boston. ISBN 0-89838-601-2. Printed in The Netherlands.*

cancer that is pertinent not only to the radiation oncologist but also to all oncologists. For instance, the brief section on diagnostic evaluation is not intended to be complete but annotates those studies that are pertinent to good radiation therapy.

2. Anatomy and pathways of tumor spread

2.1. Colon and rectum

With colorectal cancer, the four standard mechanisms of tumor spread exist (direct extension, lymphatic, hemotgenous, and surgical implantation), but in addition, transperitoneal spread may be possible. Extension within the bowel wall (intramural spread) is rare and usually only for short distances. In a series by Black and Waugh [20], only 4 of 103 patients had microscopic intramural spread greater than 0.5 cm from the gross lesion (maximum 1.2 cm). Since primary venous and lymphatic channels originate in submucosal layers of the bowel, lesions limited to the mucosa are at little risk for either venous or lymphatic dissemination. Transperitoneal spread is rare for the rectum since most of the rectum is below the peritoneal reflection, but with colonic lesions there can be direct extension to the serosal or peritoneal surface.

Lymph node involvement is found in nearly 50% of patients and is usually orderly and predictable. Skip metastasis or abnormal spread occurs in only 1 to 3% of node-positive patients but according to Grinnell [21], is usually due to lymphatic blockage. The major spread through lymphatic channels is in a cephalad direction except for lesions 8 cm or less above the anal verge when both lateral and distal (caudad) flow can occur. In female patients, this latter pattern of flow places the posterior vaginal wall at risk [22].

2.2. Rectum

The rectum is surrounded by a fibro-fatty network in its lower two-thirds and by a number ot organs and structures which can be involved by direct extension. Although the uterus and portions of vagina or small bowel can be removed with minimal morbidity, the risks are increased with prostate or base of bladder involvement. The surgeon may have to leave residual disease when tumor involves those organs or pelvic side wall structures such as vessels, nerves, muscle, or bone.

Lymphatic drainage of lesions limited to the rectum is by two main routes. The upper rectum drains via the inferior mesenteric system and the mid and lower rectum can, in addition, drain directly to internal iliac and presacral nodes. Lesions which extend to the anal canal can spread to inguinal nodes, and lesions which extend beyond the rectal wall spread via the lymphatic system of the invaded tissue and/or organ.

2.3. Colon

Anatomically, the ascending and descending colon as well as splenic and hepatic flexures are similar to the rectum. They are relatively immobile structures which lack a true mesentery and usually don't have a peritoneal covering (serosa) on the posterior and lateral surfaces. Lesions that extend through the entire bowel wall have the potential, as with rectal carcinoma, of compromised operative margins – especially with posterior or lateral extension. Unless lesions are on the anterior wall and extend through the entire serosa, peritoneal seeding may not be a major risk.

The transverse and sigmoid colon have a complete mesentery and serosal covering and are freely mobile except for their proximal and distal segment. For lesions that involve the mobile portion of either organ, extension completely through the wall to the serosal surface does not necessarily imply narrow circumferential margins or involvement of surrounding structures, and the risk of peritoneal seeding may be as great as or greater than the risk of local recurrence. In these bowel locations, the risk of inadequate operative removal is probably the greatest when there is tumor adherence to or invasion of surrounding organs or tissues, or when the lesion originates in the proximal or distal portions of each where gross extra-colonic extension can result in reduced operative margins. The cecum is between these extremes, having a variable mesentery.

Lymphatic drainage is via the mesenteric system (inferior for the left colon and superior on the right) unless adjacent organs or structures are involved. If sigmoid, cecal, or descending colon lesions involve pelvic organs or structures, the iliac systems may be at risk. Whan abdominal colon lesions involve the posterior abdominal wall, direct spread to para-aortic lymph nodes can occur, and if the anterior abdominal wall is involved, inguinal nodes are also at risk.

3. Diagnostic evaluation

Studies which evaluate the local extent of disease include digital exam, proctoscopy and/or colonoscopy, barium enema including cross table lateral views, computed body tomography (CT), and an intravenous pyelogram (IVP). When lesions are palpable, one should note the inferior extent relative to the anal verge and whether the lesion is clinically mobile or fixed. In all sites it is helpful to describe the lesion's position on the bowel wall, the degree of circumference involved, and whether the lesion is exophytic or ulcerative. If hematuria is present or findings on CBT or IVP suggest possible bladder involvement, preoperative cytoscopy should be performed.

Workup for systemic spread involves a combination of laboratory and radiographic studies. Lab evaluation should include liver and renal function studies and a baseline CEA. While LDH is considered by some to be a nonspecific study, we and others find it and CEA to be the most commonly elevated laboratory studies in early metastatic liver disease. Preoperative radiographs should include chest films and, if liver function tests are abnormal, a liver scan.

4. Pathology

4.1. Prognostic features

Although a large number of pathologic features have been previously analyzed, the best prognostic indicators are status of nodes and extent of the primary lesion. Lymph node involvement per se is not as important as the area [23] and number [21, 24] of involved nodes. Prognosis is also related to the degree of direct tumor extension within the bowel wall (confined to vs beyond mucosa) [2, 24] as well as the amount of extra-rectal or extra-colonic extension [2, 3, 9, 11, 23]. The solitary finding of either involved lymph nodes or complete wall penetration is not as ominous as the presence of both [2, 3, 9, 11, 24].

4.2. Staging systems

A comparison of common staging systems [2, 5, 6, 23, 25, 26] is shown in Table 1. A modification [5, 6] of the Astler-Coller rectal system [2] applicable to all carcinomas of the digestive tract, is preferred in analyzing data because it reflects more accurately the influence that initial extent of disease has on later patterns and incidence of failure as well as survival rates. In the past, the Dukes' staging system [23, 25] has long been useful because of its ability to predict the outcome of survival after surgery, but it is less useful in distinguishing subpopulations of patients at greatest risk for local failure. The modified system differentiates by degree of extra-rectal or extra-colonic involvement in the B2 and C2 group be it macroscopic only (m), gross or macroscopic extension confirmed at microscopy (m&g), or adherence to or invasion of surrounding organs or structures (B3 or C3). This system has been used to analyze the patterns of recurrence after potentially curative surgery and indicates that within each Dukes' stage (B and C) there are subgroups of patients with significantly different risks for local failure [7, 9] (see also Chapter 2).

5. General management

5.1. Operative considerations

For resectable lesions, operation remains the main treatment of choice. The need for adjuvant preoperative or postoperative treatment should be determined by extent of disease. The objective of surgery is to remove the tumor and primary nodal drainage with as wide a margin around both as is technically feasible and safe [27–29]. If adjacent organs are involved, they should be removed en bloc with the specimen. Exceptions to this are when tumor is adherent to prostate or base of bladder since the side effects of pelvic exenteration are excessive. A preferable alternative would be preoperative irradiation to shrink the lesion, remove the lesion with organ sparing techniques, and boost areas of adherence with additional irradiation intraoperatively or postoperatively.

Combined abdominoperineal resection (Miles' operation-APR) and anterior resection are the main operative procedures applied for rectal cancer with factors in choice being clinical level of lesion, operative findings, and the surgeon's individual preference and training. When adjuvant radiation may play a role, consideration should be given to some of the following items. Whenever feasible, the pelvic floor should be reconstructed to minimize the amount of small bowel within the true pelvis. If abdominoperineal resection needs to be performed, some form of primary or partial closure of the perineum should be considered to speed healing (2 to 6 weeks vs 2 to 3 months) and decrease the interval to postoperative radiation or chemotherapy. Anatomic location of the bowel pri-

Table 1. Staging systems for colorectal carcinoma. Comparison of Dukes' scheme with TNM and a modification of the Astler-Coller system by Gunderson and Sosin

Staging system			
Dukes'	Modified Ast-Col	TNM+	
A	A	T_1N_0	Nodes negative; lesion limited to mucosa
	B_1	T_2N_0	Nodes negative; extension of lesion through mucosa but still within bowel wall
B	B_2 *	T_3N_0	Nodes negative; extension through the entire bowel wall (including serosa if present)
C	C_1	T_2N_1	Nodes positive; lesion limited to bowel wall
	C_2 *	T_3N_1	Nodes positive; extension of lesion through the entire bowel wall (including serosa)

* Separate notation is made regarding degree of extension through the bowel wall: microscopic only (m); gross extension confirmed by microscopy (m&g); adherence to or invasion of surrounding organs or structures ($B_3 + C_3$; TNM system − T_5).
+ By definition M_0 or no evidence of metastases.
Modified from Gunderson LL, Current Prob Cancer 1: 40, 1976.

mary should be precisely noted. Small clips should be placed around areas of adherence and residual disease for the purpose of boost field radiation. It would also be helpful if clips were placed around the tumor bed in adjuvant cases so that shrinking field techniques of irradiation can be considered.

For the purpose of postoperative irradiation, anterior resection, when feasible, is preferable to abdominoperineal resection in mid and high rectal lesions. This is due to several factors: 1) less small bowel in the pelvis postoperatively; 2) fewer technical and physical problems during irradiation as the perineum doesn't need to be included; and 3) faster rate of healing if a perineal wound is not necessary.

Low anterior resections are technically feasible and produce survival rates similar to abdominoperineal resections in the large group of patients with lesions from 8 to 15 cm above the anal verge [30]. Low anterior resections are being done with increasing frequency for lesions 6 to 8 cm above the verge due to the wide availability of the EEA stapling device. Since distal intramural spread is possible with this latter group of patients, one may have to consider small field adjuvant postoperative irradiation when distal margins are ≤2 cm, even if nodes are negative, and the lesion is confined to the wall.

When deciding which operative procedure is possible and adequate, the surgeon and pathologist commonly refer to the distal bowel margin (amount of resected normal bowel below the primary lesion), but both need to pay more attention to nodal and circumferential margins. When lesions extend through the entire bowel wall, the real surgical problem is often the inability to get sufficient lateral and anterioposterior margins due to anatomical limitations. When perirectal nodes are involved, there is an increased risk of nodal involvement near the surgeons' mesenteric ligature or in internal iliac or presacral nodes. However, the surgeon rarely removes or even biopsies the latter two node groups, and the pathologist rarely examines the former.

Following moderate doses of preoperative irradiation (4500 to 5000 rad), only abdominoperineal resections used to be recommended due to a possible increase in anastomotic leaks. On the basis of published data by Stevens et al. [31] and unpublished data from others, it has been shown that such doses do not preclude anterior resection and primary anastomosis. An unirradiated loop of large bowel should be used for the proximal limb of the anastomosis with temporary diverting colostomies done only on the basis of operative indications.

5.2. Operative failure after 'curative resection'

5.2.1. Rectal cancer
As shown in Tables 2 and 3, the risk of local recurrence after 'curative resection' is a double pathologic prognostic factor related to disease extension beyond the bowel wall as well as to nodal involvement [2, 3, 9, 11, 24]. Local recurrence in the group with nodal involvement but tumor confined to the wall (i.e., CI) is 20 to

25% which is actually less than in the group with nodes negative but extending through the wall (i.e., B2 ± B3) where the risk is 30 to 35% (Table 2). The group that has both bad prognostic factors, nodal involvement and extension through the wall (i.e., C2 ± C3), has nearly an additive risk of local recurrence varying from 50 to 65% in the clinical series and 70% in the reoperative series.

In the MGH series [9], the incidence of both total and local failure in the node-

Table 2. Colorectal cancer – extent of disease vs later local failure (LF). Varied series – after curative resection

Modified* A-C Stage	Clinical Series U Florida (Colo-rectum)		Portland, Me (Rectum-cAPR)		MGH (Rect-R Sig)		Re-Op'n U Minn (Rectum-cAPR)	
Within Wall								
A	0/30	–	0/1	–	0/3	–	–	–
B_1	3/20	(15%)	6/42	(14.3%)	3/36	(8.3%)	–	–
C_1	4/19	(21.1%)	1/5	–	2/4	–	4/17	(23.5%)
Through Wall								
B_2 ($\pm B_3$)	29/106	(27.4%)	13/37	(35.1%)	18/59	(30.5%)	–	–
C_2 ($\pm C_3$)	33/64	(51.6%)	24/37	(64.9%)	20/40	(50%)	28/40	(70%)
Totals	69/239	(28.9%)	44/122	(36.1%)	43/142	(30.3%)	–	–

* See Table 1 re-definition of extent.
Modified from Gunderson LL, Alimentary Tract Radiology III. Ed Margolis and Burhenne p. 395, 1979.

Table 3. Extent of tumor vs later failure & survival – MGH. 142 rectal-rectosigmoid patients – 'curative resection'

Initial extent*	Total failure		Pelvic recurrence (LF)	
LN (−)				
A [mucosa only]	0/3	–	0/3	–
B_1 [beyond mucosa; within wall]	7/36	(19%)	3/36	(8%)
B_2 (m) [through wall, micro]	4/12	(33%)	2/12	(17%)
B_2 (m&g) [through wall, macro]	14/32	(44%)	8/32	(25%)
B_3 [adjacent organ or structure]	10/15	(67%)	8/15	(53%)
LN (+)				
C_1 [within wall]				
C_2 (m) [through wall, micro]	6/11	(55%)	4/11	(36%)
C_2 (m&g) [through wall, macro]	20/27	(74%)	14/27	(52%)
C_3 [adjacent organ or structure]	5/6	(83%)	4/6	(67%)

* Modified Astler-Coller Stage.
Modified from Rich T, Gunderson L, Galdabini J, *et al.,* Cancer 52: 1317–1329, 1983.

negative group increased with each degree of extension beyond the wall (Table 3). The incidence of pelvic recurrence for the B3 group was double that of the B2 (m&g) subgroup and three times higher than the B2(m) subgroup. In the node-positive group, although the number of patients in each subgroup was small, there were also suggestive differences. As shown in Table 4, Withers *et al.* [11] had larger subsets of node-positive patients. A definite increase in local recurrence was found when difficulty was encountered in the surgical dissection or there was operative adherence (S), and with pathologic involvement of surrounding structures (P). Therefore, even in the node-positive group, the degree of extra-rectal extension appears to be an independent factor influencing the risk of local recurrence.

Although the risk of local recurrence should be markedly diminished with the addition of adequate adjuvant irradiation, this will not ensure an increased cure rate. Prevention of early demise from pelvic recurrence may allow development of subclinical or occult systemic disease. As shown by Gilbert, however, if we do nothing more than prevent the tremendous symptomatic problem of local recurrence, we have accomplished a great service.[4]

5.2.2. Colon cancer

Increasing data is being accumulated in autopsy [32], clinical [4, 33–35], and reoperative series [36] to indicate that local recurrence is a significant problem after resection of colonic as well as rectal lesions (Tables 5–7). Clinical series can, however, underestimate the incidence of local failures, in view of silent tumor bed failures and may place excess emphasis on liver only failures. Although data from clinical series [33] suggest that one-third of failures occur solely in the liver,

Table 4. Rectal cancer - local failure vs extent of disease. (MD Anderson Hospital)

Extent*		Total pts	LF (%)
LN (−)			
B₁		149	3%
B₂			
a)	No unusual problems	146	12%
b)	Adherance or difficult dissections (S)	52	22%
B₃ – Adjacent structure (P)		11	31%
LN (+)			
C₁		12	32%
C₂			
a)	No unusual problems	92	28%
b)	Adherance or difficult dissection (S)	23	70%
C₃ – Adjacent structure (P)		11	45% } 62%

* Modified Asther Coller Stage   S = surgical   P = pathological.
Modified from Withers R, *et al.* (1982) Raven Press pp 351-362.

autopsy (Table 5) [32] and reoperative series [36] suggest that this may be less than 10%.

In the University of Washington series [35], 186 of 550 patients with colon cancer had later evidence of failure. Within the failure group, 64 of the 186 had a reoperation at some interval (symptomatic look in 54). As shown in Table 6, in the group with reoperation, one could accurately divide abdominal failures into a retroperitoneal nodal component of disease versus peritoneal seeding. In addition, a much higher percentage of patients were found to have a local component of failure.

A total of 230 patients had reoperative procedures following curative resection of colorectal cancer at the University of Minnesota [36], and failures were defined in 152. Since this was a select high-risk group with a majority of patients having nodal involvement alone or in combination with extension beyond the bowel wall at the time of the initial procedure, data in this series cannot be compared directly with other series. Failures in the tumor bed ± nodes were most common with rectal lesions but were not uncommon with primaries at other bowel sites (Table

Table 5. Colorectal cancer – patterns of failure, MGH

	Clinical + Autopsy*		Autopsy†		
	Sigmoid + Rectum	Proximal to Sigmoid	Proximal to Sigmoid	Sigmoid	Rectum
Pelvis					
Alone	30%	–	–	11%	12%
Component	45%	10%	9%	27%	41%
Abdomen					
Alone	7%	24%	–	–	–
Component	23%	48%	–	–	–
Any Component					
Peritoneal	–	–	31%	41%	25%
Regional Nodes	–	–	49%	57%	59%
Liver					
Alone	13%	30%	5%	2%	2%
Component	45%	61%	67%	68%	48%
Lung					
Alone	4%	4%	–	–	5%
Component	32%	27%	31%	43%	52%
Any Component					
Bone	7%	3%	7%	7%	16%
Brain	6%	3%	7%	4%	5%

* Percentage are of 177 patients with clinical or pathological proof of tumor failure (74% of patients had biopsy or autopsy tissue confirmation).

† Percentages are of 145 patients with autopsy proof of tumor failure (sigmoid 44, rectum 56, proximal to sigmoid 45).

7). Peritoneal seeding was least common with rectal primaries which are less accessible to the peritoneal cavity. The incidence of hematogenous failures was similar for all sites although the distribution differed. With rectal primaries, hematogenous failures were fairly evenly divided between liver and lung due to venous drainage via both the mesenteric and internal iliac routes; with colon primaries, initial hematogenous failures were usually in the liver.

5.2.3. Rectum and colon

Other factors, in addition to extent of disease, that may influence local failure after curative resection include the location of tumor, blood vessel invasion and histological grade [9]. The relative importance of each of these varies by series.

5.3. Chemotherapy

At present, the results of either single or combined agent chemotherapy for advanced disease or in an adjuvant setting have been disappointing [37]. Three agents of drugs have been documented to have consistent but not outstanding activity: fluorinated pyrimidines (5-FU, 5-FUDR), nitrosoureas, and mitomycin C. For single agent chemotherapy of advanced disease, 5-FU has an accepted 15 to 20% response rate and accepted rates for the other two agents are the same or slightly less.

6. Adjuvant irradiation

Differences of opinion exist regarding the preferred sequence of combining

Table 6. Extrapelvic colon patterns of failure (U Washington)

Failure any component	Total group*			Reoperation†	
	# %		(%)	#	%
Local failure	54 – 29		(9.8)	29/61	(47.5%)
Abdominal failure	73 – 39		(13.3)		
Retroperit. LN	– –		–	13/38	(34%)
Peritoneal seeding	– –		–	28/64	(44%)
Liver metastasis	74 – 40		(13.5)	18/54	(33.5%)

* Open % are of 186 pts. with failure and ( ) % of total group of 550.
† 54 of 64 had symptomatic reoperation.
Failure by stage: A 1/58 (1.5%); B_1 9/106 (8.5%); B_2 63/200 (31.5%); B_3 14/23 (61%); C_1 9/20 (45%); C_2 75/126 (59.5%) C_3 15/17 (88%).
From Russell et al. (1984) Cancer (in press).

surgery and irradiation (XRT). In summary, the major advantage of preoperative XRT is the potential damaging effect on cells that may be spread locally or distantly at the time of operation. The major advantage of postoperative treatment is the ability to subselect out groups of patients at high risk for local recurrence on the basis of operative and pathologic findings and delete patients with advanced but undiagnosed metastatic disease before exploration or those at low risk for local recurrence. A well-designed combination of preoperative and postoperative XRT (sandwich technique) could, in fact, combine the theoretical advantages of each.

6.1. Preoperative adjuvant irradiation

A number of centers have applied preoperative irradiation for resectable rectal ± rectosigmoid lesions with a variety of dose and portal arrangements [16, 31, 38–41]. All have demonstrated proof of tumoricidal responsiveness at the time of surgery either by partial or total regression of the primary or the finding of a lower incidence of lymph node involvement than would ordinarily have been anticipated.

In two prospective randomized low-dose series (Princess Margaret Hospital [16] 500 rad × 1 or VA Hospital [39, 40] 2000 to 2500 rad in 2 to 2 1/2 weeks vs operation alone), survival was statistically better in some irradiated patient groups. In the VAH series of 700 patients, local recurrence and distant metastases were also decreased in an autopsy subgroup, but both were still unacceptably high at 29% and 40% respectively. In the high-dose, nonrandomized Oregon series [31, 41], (5000 to 6000 rad 6 to 7 weeks), only 1 of 45 patients (2.3%) with subsequent curative resection was proven to have later pelvic recurrence. This

Table 7. Patterns of failure – colorectal. U Minnesota Reoperation series

Site of Primary	Failure total	Component of failure*								
		LF-RF			PS			DM		
		#	%	(%)	#	%	(%)	#	%	(%)
Extrapelvic										
Transverse	3/8	3 –	100	(38)	1 – 33		(13)	2 – 67		(25)
Cecum	26/37	18 –	69	(49)	6 – 23		(16)	10 – 38		(27)
Asc., Desc.										
Flexures	29/46	23 –	79	(50)	14 – 48		(30)	17 – 59		(37)
Pelvic										
Rectum	52/74	48 –	92	(65)	3 – 6		(4)	26 – 50		(35)

Open % are of failure group and ( ) % of total subgroup at risk.
* LF-RF (local-regional Failure); PS (peritoneal seeding); DM (hematogenous).
From Gunderson and Sosin. Submitted for publication.

latter data suggests that adequate doses of preoperative XRT in combination with surgery may make a major impact on local recurrence (29% vs 2.3% in VAH vs University of Oregon data).

6.2. Postoperative adjuvant irradiation

Three major prospective but nonrandomized postoperative series applied similar dose levels of 4500 to 5500 rad in 5 to $6^{1}/_{2}$ weeks and treated only those patients at high risk for local recurrence [5, 10, 11, 42, 43]. Table 8 compares local recurrence rates after curative resection alone or in combination with XRT. For equivalent total groups (B2–3, C2–3 ± C1), local recurrence decreased from 37% to 48% with operation alone to 6% to 8% in the XRT series. Similar decreases were seen for each extent of disease. In the B2–3 subgroup, the reduction was nearly ten-fold from 30 to 35% down to around 5% and in the C2–3 subgroup, from 45 to 65% down to 10 to 12%.

Distant failures in the three nonrandomized series continued to be a problem in 25 to 30% of patients in spite of the improvement in local control. As shown in

Table 8. Extent of disease vs later local failure (LF).

Clinical Series After Curative Resection of Colorectal Cancer				
Extent of disease	Operation alone	Operation + Postop XRT		
	U Florida, MDAH, MGH, Maine	MDAH[1] (rectal)	LDS-SLC[2] (colorectal)	MGH[4] (rectal)
Within Wall LN+ (C_1)	20 to 30%	0/3	0/2	1/9 (11%)
Through Wall LN− ($B_2 \pm B_3$)	25 to 35%	1/18 (5.5%)	0/10	2/36 (5.5%)
LN+ ($C_2 \pm C_3$)	45 to 65%	3/33 (9.1%)	2/16[3] (12.5%)	5/50[5] (10%)
LN−, LN+ ($B_3 + C_3$)	–	1/8 (12.5%)	–	–
LN Status unknown (B_{2-3} vs C_{2-3})	–	–	0/4	–
Totals	35 to 50%	5/62 (8.1%)	2/34 (6%)	8/95[5] (8.4%)

[1] Aug 77 analysis.
[2] June 78 analysis – minimum 2 year F/U.
[3] Both had deviation in planned dose/time scheme – received ≃4500/5 wk.
[4] June 81 analysis – minimum 2 year F/U and 66% with minimum 3 year F/U.
[5] Marginal recurrence in 1 additional patient (6/50 or 12% $C_2 + C_3$ and 9/95 or 9.5% of total group).

Table 9, hematogenous failures are much more common than peritoneal except for the C3 group where the peritoneal failure incidence was 50% (5/10) in the MGH series [43].

Local recurrence was compared in nonrandomized but sequential series for operation alone (103 patients) versus operation and postoperative irradiation (95 patients) in the the MGH analysis [43]. Since one cannot fairly compare overall local recurrence rates as one group is at risk for a longer time period, both groups were analyzed at the three-year period postoperatively. As shown in Table 10, there was a statistically significant reduction in local recurrence at nearly each stage level in the groups who received adjuvant postoperative irradiation (B2[g], B3, C1 + C2[m], C2[g]).

In a randomized trial from the Gastrointestinal Tumor Study Group [44], patients were randomized to a surgical control arm versus treatment arms of postoperative irradiation, postoperative chemotherapy, or a combination thereof. In radiation alone arm, patients received either 4000 or 4800 rad and in the radiation plus chemotherapy arm, either 4000 or 4400 rad. The disease-free survival of all three treatment arms was superior to surgery alone at the interval of 130 to 156 weeks. The difference between the combined arm of chemotherapy plus irradiation versus surgery alone is statistically significant (P<.03 to .05 dependent on method of analysis). The combined arm did not, however, result in a decrease in the incidence of distant metastases but rather a decrease in local recurrence when patterns of first site of failure were analyzed (Table 11). This suggests that the effect of the chemotherapy was not a systemic effect but rather a local effect as a radiopotentiator. In spite of the improvement in disease-free survival in both arms with irradiation, the local recurrence rate with radiation alone was too high with a minimum of 7 of 47 or 15% at latest analysis (may be higher as only first patterns of failure have been published).

The 6 to 8% incidence of local recurrence in the three nonrandomized but prospective postoperative series previously discussed was only approximately

Table 9. Rectal cancer patterns of failure – MGH. 32 of 97 Pts. (33%) – Failure after XRT

Pattern	Only Failure	Any Component
LF	4 (4.2%)[1]	8 (8.4%)[1]
DM	20 (21.1%)[2]	29 (30.5%)
PS	3 (3.2%)[3]	8 (8.4%)

See Table 7 re terminology.

[1] One additional patient had a marginal miss (perineal scar underdosed – 5/95 or 5.3%; 9/95 or 9.5%).

[2] Extrapelvic LN failure alone in 1 pt (RF).

[3] All had a pelvic component (PS ± LF) – Incidence by stage: B_2 (m)(g) + B_3 + C_1 + C_2 (m) 0/51; C_2 (g) 3/34 (8.8%); C_3 5/10 (50%).

From Hoskins B, Gunderson L, *et al.* (1984) Cancer (in press).

one half that of the GTSG study treating similar patient subgroups. This is perhaps due to the fact that the minimum dose within the boost field of the nonrandomized series was usually 5000 rad, whereas approximately 50% of the patients in the GTSG radiation alone arm received only 4000 rad.

6.3. Pre- ± postoperative irradiation

In rectal-rectosigmoid cancer, the concept of using low-dose preoperative irradiation to be followed by selective postoperative treatment in patients at high risk for local recurrence was instituted independently at Massachusetts General Hospital (MGH) [45] and Thomas Jefferson University Hospital (TJUH) [46, 47] in 1976. Both used preoperative doses of 500 rad × 1 with operation the same or following day, and MGH also used 1000 rad in 5 fractions with operation in 1 to 3 days (preferably the following day to allow less tumor cell repopulation). Postoperatively, both institutions usually delivered 4500 rad in 25 fractions over 5 weeks to patients with the following indications: 1) extension through the wall, nodes negative (MGH deleted some patients with only focal microscopic extension and good circumferential margins-preferably ≥1.5–2 cm); 2) nodes positive but confined to the bowel wall (patients with only 1 to 2 adjacent nodes were deleted at MGH if 15 to 20 were examined); or, 3) nodes positive and extension through the wall. The recent analyses of both series [45, 47] suggest that one can safely select patients who do not require the postoperative component of irradiation and yet achieve excellent local control and good survival rates. Such an approach may be preferable to high dose preoperative irradiation for resectable lesions.

Table 10. Rectal Cancer – pelvic failure at 3 years, MGH

Modified A-C stage	Surgery alone		Adjuvant post-op XRT	
B$_2$ (m)	(12)	8.3%	(6)	18.2%
B$_2$ (m&g)	(32)	25%	(23)	0%[1]
B$_3$	(15)	57.6%	(7)	0%[1]
C$_1$				
C$_2$ (m) }	(11)	43.2%	(15)	7.2%[1]
C$_2$ (m&g)	(27)	52.8%	(34)	8.9%[1]
C$_3$	(6)	100%	(10)	30.5%
	(103)		(95)	

[1] Significant at P≤.05.
 #'s in parentheses = total #pts at risk; Open #'s = % with pelvic failure.
 From Hoskins B, Gunderson L, *et al.* (1984) Cancer (in press).

6.4. Criteria for patient selection

For lesions that are definitely resectable, we prefer the use of low-dose preoperative irradiation and the addition of postoperative treatment only when indicated. The advantage over full-dose preoperative XRT is that ≃50% of patients do not require the entire sequence of treatment. The relative merits of this selective 'sandwich' technique will ultimately require comparison with full-dose preoperative and postoperative XRT in randomized trials. Patients who are candidates for postoperative irradiation are those with nodal involvement, gross extension of tumor beyond the bowel wall, or a combination thereof in whom expected local recurrence rates after operation alone are high. We prefer full-dose preoperative irradiation mainly in those patients who have disease fixation to structures or organs that cannot be resected safely.

7. Radiation – residual, recurrent, or unresectable disease

Although it appears that significant gains can be achieved with the addition of irradiation in an adjuvant setting, the job becomes more difficult if residual disease has been left behind after resection or if patients present with unresectable disease since the radiation dose levels required are increased in magnitude. In the residual disease subgroups from MGH [12] and Albert Einstein [14], the

Table 11. Rectal cancer – patterns of initial failure. (Randomized GITSG Study)

Site of initial failure	Treatments				
	Control	Chemo	XRT	XRT + CT	Total
Local/Regional	8	7	7	2	24
Distant (Only)	17	9	10	9	45
Liver	5	1	1	5	12
Other	8	4	5	3	20
Liver + Other	4	4	4	1	13
Local + Distant	3	3	0	0	6
Site Unconfirmed	0	0	0	0	0
Total Failure/Total at Risk	28/57 (49.1%)	19/49 (38.8%)	17/47 (36.2%)	11/39 (28.2%)	75/192 (39%)
Local Failure Component	11/57 (19.3%)	10/49 (20.4%)	7/47 (14.9%)	2/39 (5.1%)	30/192 (15.6%)
Distant Failure Component	20/57 (35.1%)	12/49 (24.5%)	10/47 (21.3%)	9/39 (23.1%)	51/192 (26.6%)

Modified from Mittleman, *et al.* (1981) Green and Stratton pp 547-557.

incidence of local recurrence after external beam irradiation varied by the amount of residual disease being 50% to 54% (AE – 9/18; MGH – 13/24) if there was gross residual versus 15 to 26% (AE – 2/13; MGH – 8/31) if there was only microscopic residual. In the MGH analysis, a possible dose-response correlation was seen in the group with microscopic residual with an 11% LF risk (1/9) if the boost was ≥6000 rad and 33% (7/21) if the boost dose was ≤5500 rad (Table 12). In the patients with gross residual, a dose-response correlation could not be discerned.

In patients with disease that is unresectable for cure due to tumor fixation, a number of institutions have given preoperative radiotherapy in an attempt to shrink the lesion, allow resection, and possibly improve local control and survival [38, 41, 48–50]. The resectability rate after doses of 4500 to 5000 rad has varied from 50% to 75% by series (Table 13). Even in those patients who were resected, the incidence of local recurrence has been excessive at 36 to 45%.

Although combinations of external beam radiation and surgery do seem to decrease pelvic recurrence and improve survival in the subgroups with residual disease (postoperative XRT) or initially unresectable disease (preoperative XRT), local recurrence is still unacceptably high, and survivial could be improved. In view of this, pilot studies were instituted at Massachusetts General Hospital in which 32 patients received the standard previous treatment of external beam irradiation and surgery, but in addition had an intraoperative electron beam boost of 1000 to 1500 rad to the remaining tumor or tumor bed at the time of surgical resection after preoperative XRT of initially unresectable disease or at

Table 12. Residual disease of colorectum – dose VS LF, MGH. Dose in rad vs LF (External Beam)

Amount of residual	≤5000	5000–5999	6000–6499	≥6500	Totals
Gross	2/3	4/11	5/6	2/4	13/24 (54%)
Microscopic	0/1[1]	7/21 (33%)	1/9 (11%)		8/31 (26%)

[1] Early death due to PS.
From Allee P, Gunderson L, Munzenrider J.
ASTR Proceedings, Int J Rad Oncol 7:1208, 1981.

Table 13. Unresectable rectal cancer: pre-op radiation

Series	Resectability rate	LF after resection
U Oregon	20/40 (50%)	45%
MGH	18/25 (72%)	43%
Tufts	33/44 (75%)	36%

re-exploration if residual disease was left [15, 51–53]. For the 16 patients who presented with unresectable primary lesions, the addition of intraoperative radiotherapy has yielded survival rates which are statistically better than the previous group treated with only external beam irradiation and surgical resection [48, 52, 53]. There have not been any local recurrences with a minimum 20-month follow-up in the group with all three treatment modalities. In the group with residual disease, again there have not been any local recurrences in the seven patients that received all treatment modalities versus 54% and 26% for the group with gross and microscopic residual treated with only external beam techniques. The remaining nine patients presented with unresectable recurrent lesions.

8. Primary irradiation

8.1. Endocavitary irradiation (Papillon technique)

8.1.1. Philosophy and principles
Treatment of carefully selected patients with low and mid rectal lesions by a technique of low kilovoltage endocavitary irradiation is one of the acceptable sphincter saving options available. When the technique was initiated by Papillon [54, 55], many of his patients were not good candidates for operative procedures (40% of the initial 106 patients were poor-risk patients who were fragile, elderly, or had cardiovascular, hepatic, or respiratory disease). Indications have been extended as good results were reported. Treatment selection is now based on both tumor and equipment factors as discussed in detail by Papillon as well as Sischy and Remington [56]: 1) lesion ≤12 cm above anal verge; 2) maximum size 3×5 cm; 3) exophytic and mobile; and 4) moderate or well differentiated.

Patients are treated on an outpatient basis using a Phillips 50 KV superficial x-ray unit with rapid output (1000 to 2000 rad per minute). The treatment proctoscope is inserted after gradual dilation of the anus (Fig. 1). Patients receive 2500 to 4000 rad per treatment to a total maximum dose of 8000 to 15,000 rad (treatment fractions usually separated by 2 to 3 weeks). By the third treatment, visualization of the original lesion is often difficult. While the total dose seems excessive, it should be realized that at a depth of 6.25 mm only 50 percent of surface dose is delivered (doses are calculated as maximum surface dose). Therefore, the first one or two treatments are essentially absorbed in the exophytic portion of the tumor to cause shrinkage so that the last one to two treatments can treat the tumor bed and rectal wall.

This technique remains a useful alternative of treatment for appropriate lesions in all patient populations including the elderly and fragile. It has some potential advantages over fulgeration: 1) ambulatory outpatient treatment; 2) colostomy or anesthesia not required; 3) minimal risk of fistulae or perforation; 4) no induration and, therefore, easier to evaluate in follow-up; and 5) poor surgical risks are

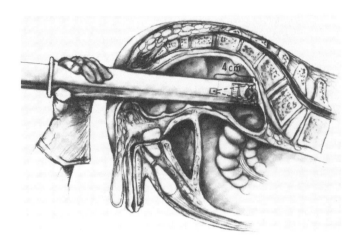

Figure 1. Endocavitary treatment proctoscope in position for purpose of localized irradiation of early rectal cancer. (From Sischy and Remington Surg. Gynecol. Obstet. 141: 562–564, 1975).

still candidates. In the authors' experience, the knee chest position is sometimes difficult to achieve in the fragile elderly patient. With posterior wall lesions, patients can be treated in the lithotomy position in stirrups, and for lesions in other locations they can be treated while lying on their side. If low anterior resections and procedures including colo-anal anastomoses have acceptable morbidity and become more routine, this procedure will have fewer indications in patients who are medically operable.

8.1.2. Results

The largest experience with endocavitary irradiation is that of Papillon in France. In his latest publication, 186 cases had been treated with curative intent with endocavitary XRT alone or in combination with implant [55]. The overal local failure rate was only 7.5%. Of 133 patients at risk for 5 years, 104 (78%) were alive and free of disease, and only 12 (9%) had died from their malignancy. Local recurrence had occurred in 11 (8.3%), and surgical salvage was possible in 6 patients.

Sischy (radiotherapist) and Remington (surgeon) have applied endocavitary techniques in the US since July 1973. In their most recent publication, 39 patients had been treated with curative intent through December 1978 (56). Local recurrence occurred in only two patients (5.1%). One who initially had an anaplastic lesion required an APR for recurrence ten months after endocavitary treatment and is alive and NED five years later. The second was an elderly patient with a large lesion who was retreated with endocavitary XRT with 5000 rad in 25 fractions. Minimum follow-up in the first 25 patients was 18 months. In summary, the superb results of the larger Papillon series have been paralleled in the smaller US series by Sischy and Remington and support the need for evaluation of this approach in other US institutions.

8.2. External beam irradiation

Although results with radiation seem to be better in most series in those patients with inoperable (surgical or medical) and/or residual carcinoma as opposed to those with recurrence, there is need for improvement. Wang and Schulz [18] obtained cures in 12.5% (2 of 16) of the inoperable group and 22% (2 of 9) of the group with partial resection. Sklaroff [17] treated ten elderly patients (age range 61 to 84) who were medically inoperable. At the time of his report, five were alive and without disease from 6 months to 9 years, and an additional patient died at 10 months without evidence of disease.

The best results with primary irradiation were reported by Rider [16] in a series of 229 patients treated at the Princess Margaret Hospital with five-year survival of 10% for the total group. A 'curative attempt' with doses starting as low as 3500 rad was undertaken in 65 patients. Seventy percent were referred due to inoperability (tumor fixation – 60%; medical inoperability – 10%) and the remainder due to distant metastases (5%) or patient or physician refusal of operative intervention (potentially operable). Three-year survival was approximately 42% and five-year was 29% (11 of 38). Doses of 4500 to 5000 rad in 20 fractions over 4 weeks yielded the best results. Some of their patients had slow regression of the lesion following radiation with clinical and histologic persistence at a time period of one year or occasionally longer, but with freedom of disease within the treated field at the three-year period.

A more recent analysis from the Princess Margaret Hospital in 1981 showed that a group of 123 patients had been treated with radical external beam irradiation from 1970 to 1977 [13]. In this paper, an important change was made in data analysis in that patients with mobile lesions were considered separately from those with fixation. In the 67 patients who presented with tumor fixation, local control was achieved in only 6 of 67 (9%), and five-year actuarial survival was 8%. Of 56 patients who presented with mobile lesions, local control was achieved in 21 of 56 (38%), and five-year actuarial survival was 40% (relative 5-year survival 55%).

Although primary radiation [13, 16, 18] produces superb palliation and occasional cure with fixed lesions and decent local control and cure with mobile lesions ($\simeq$40%), the results do not compare favorably to the use of combined surgery and irradiation [7, 42]. Primary irradiation should probably be reserved for the patient who is a poor medical candidate for resection or refuses the procedure.

9. Radiation treatment factors

9.1. Therapeutic ratio

It does little good to accomplish adequate local control if it's achieved with a high incidence of complications. A suitable therapeutic ratio between local control and complications is achieved only with close interaction between the surgeon and the radiotherapist. Major surgical considerations include both use of clips to mark areas at high risk as well as the use of pelvic reconstruction techniques whenever possible. There are also things that should be done from a radiation standpoint including the use of: 1) lateral fields to avoid as much small bowel as possible while still including the area at risk; 2) shrinking or boost field techniques; and 3) treatment with bladder distension.

The incidence of small bowel obstruction requiring reoperation varies when applying parallel opposed versus multiple field techniques with external beam doses of 4500 to 5500 rad in an adjuvant setting. In the M.D. Anderson series which used parallel opposed techniques, an incidence of 17.5% occurred in irradiated patients in contrast to 5% with surgery alone [11]. When the superior extent of the radiation field was shifted from the L-2 to L-3 region down to L-5, the incidence of operative intervention decreased to 10 to 12%. This is similar to the incidence in the LDS Hospital series with paralleled opposed techniques [5, 42]. In the MGH series [43] with multiple field techniques, use of bladder distension, etc., the incidence of small bowel obstruction requiring operative intervention is essentially equal in the group receiving irradiation (4%) as compared with operation alone (5%). The minimum follow-up in the irradiated group in the MGH series was 24 months and greater than two-thirds of patients were at risk for 3 or more years.

9.2. Radiation techniques

9.2.1. Rectum and colon

Preoperative and postoperative techniques should not differ that markedly except for the need to cover the perineal structures in the postoperative rectal group. The intent of both approaches is to include the primary tumor or tumor bed with margin as well as nodal areas that are either not removed by the surgeon or cannot be removed with 'no-touch' technique and may result in tumor dissemination.

Total abdominal techniques have been applied in some institutions for all colon lesions [14, 57]. Such fields are probably warranted on a theoretical basis only when the risk of peritoneal seeding is high due to tumor extension to a peritoneal surface. Even then the therapeutic gain is uncertain due to the large treatment volume. At present, our preference with extrapelvic colon lesions is to identify fields that cover the tumor bed with adequate margin. We include unremoved nodal chains only if nodes are involved near the surgeon's vascular ligature since that portion of the field includes much additional small bowel. In view of borderline chemotherapy and the optimistic results of total abdominal radiation plus pelvic boost for resected Stage II and early Stage III ovarian cancer at Princess Margaret Hospital [58], one cannot overlook the potential future application of combining total abdominal radiation with a tumor bed and possibly nodal boost for appropriate lesions. However, there is a major difference in patterns of failure, since the liver is rarely at risk with ovarian cancer but is at high risk with large bowel cancer. Accordingly, for colon cancer, a more aggressive treatment approach may be required for the liver.

9.2.2. Nodal coverage

The inferior mesenteric (IM) system is, in our opinion, the surgeon's domain for left-sided bowel lesions, as essentially four levels of nodes can be removed without manipulation. For right colon lesions, removal of the superior mesenteric system is adequate but less inclusive than the IM resection due to the need to spare the iliocolic branches to the small bowel. In most institutions, internal iliac and presacral LN dissections are not a standard part of rectal cancer surgery due to limited gain [29] and should probably be included in the initial irradiation volume. External iliac nodes are not a primary nodal drainage site and are not included unless pelvic organs with primary external iliac drainage are involved by direct extension (i.e., sigmoid lesion with bladder involvement; rectal cancer with involvement of bladder, prostate, cervix or vagina).

9.2.3. Rectum

The value of delineating necessary tumor bed and nodal volumes is demonstrated most vividly for cancer of the rectum. Since most tumor bed failures are in the posterior one-half to two-thirds of the true pelvis and the internal iliac and presacral LN have a posterior location relative to external iliac nodes, lateral treatment portals can spare a substantial volume of anteriorly located normal tissues (Fig. 2B, D).

Although exact field arrangements are dependent in part on the precise location of the primary tumor, presence or absence of adjacent organ involvement, area and number of nodes involved, etc., some generalizations can be made. The width of AP:PA ports (Fig. 2A, C) should be sufficient to cover the pelvic inlet with margin around the desired internal or external iliac nodes. Lateral margins extending 1 to 2 cm beyond the widest port of the bony pelvis are usually sufficient depending on treatment energy and penumbrum. The superior margin should usually be at least 1–2 cm above the level of the sacral promontory (occasionally mid L-5 to L-4 and infrequently, para-aortic coverage to L-1 or T-12) and may depend on the extent of mesenteric and/or iliac nodal involvement which is not usually known preoperatively. The inferior extent is again somewhat variable.

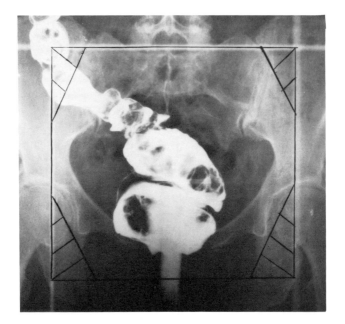

2a

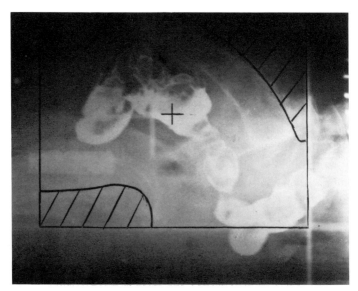

2b

Figure 2. Postoperative radiation therapy 4 field techniques after surgical resection of rectal cancers – patients are in prone treatment position (A, B) PA:AP and lateral fields after anterior resection with contrast in the rectum, a BB in the anal verge and a tampon in the vagina. (C–E) PA:AP fields in a male patient (C) and lateral fields and port films in a female patient (D, E) after abdominoperineal resection (Both patients had 4 field setups). Films C & D demonstrate the use of BB's to mark the entire perineal scar in both male and female patients – the posterior extent of the scar is often more posterior than the sacrum and posterior fall off of the field may be necessary, as shown on the port film (E).

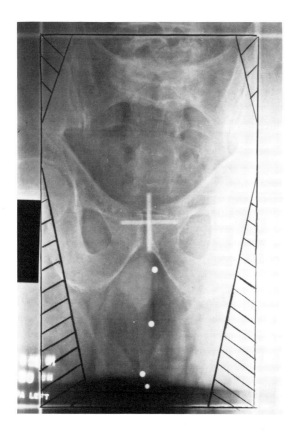

2c

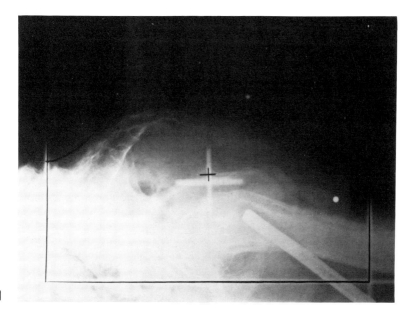

2d

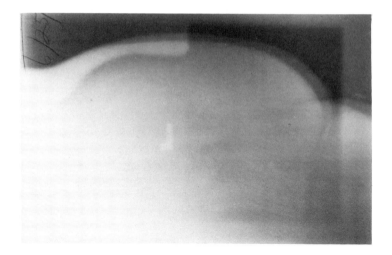

2e

For both preoperative radiation and postoperative radiation following anterior resection, the usual intent is coverage of at least the obturator foramina although this may occasionally be more extensive than necessary. The minimal extent should usually be 2 to 5 cm below the gross tumor (preoperative) or below the most inferior extent of dissection or mobilization of the distal limb (postoperative) which ideally would be marked with surgical clips. With low anterior resections, the inferior field extent may be at or near the anal verge.

When *lateral portals* are applied (Fig. 2B, D), treatment in the prone position is preferred as it allows one to visualize the sacrum and can cause positional shifts in small bowel [59]. If patients are treated in supine position, the pelvis should be raised off the table top by styrofoam or similar material to allow delineation of bony structures and field margins. The posterior field margin is vital since the rectum and perirectal tissues lie just anterior to the sacrum and coccyx. Accordingly, dependent on treatment energy, the posterior field margin should be a minimum of $1^1/_2$ to 2 cm behind the anterior bony sacral margin to allow for some daily patient movement and can be shaped with cerrobend or similar blocks to spare posterior muscle and soft tissues. We prefer individual cerrobend blocks over movable corner blocks as the latter are difficult to position precisely due to distortions in shin markings resulting from sloping contours of the posterior portion of the pelvis. The anterior margin can sometimes be shaped to reduce the amount of irradiation to the femoral head and bladder inferiorly and, when external iliac LN need to be included, to decrease the amount of small bowel superiorly.

Following abdominoperineal resection, the *perineum* with its anteroposterior and inferolateral aspects of operative dissection must be included along with the tumor bed-nodal volumes or marginal recurrence due to implantation may occur. [5, 7, 42] Lead shot or wire should be used to mark the entire extent of the perineal scar when localization films are obtained, both AP:PA and laterally

(Fig. 2C–E). The inferior (caudad) and posterior field edges should be $1^{1}/_{2}$ to 2 cm beyond the scar as marked. Anteriorly, the lower one-third of the rectum abuts the posterior vaginal wall and prostate, and these structures should be included. In female patients, adequate coverage of the vagina is assured if a contrast soaked gauze pad or tampon is placed therein during treatment planning. Inferolaterally, the margin should be the lateral aspect of the ischial tuberosities. Bolus material is necessary during the PA treatment to prevent underdosage of the scar surface. If the buttocks are taped together to achieve a bolus effect, this produces more intergluteal skin reaction than use of bolus materials and often necessitates a treatment break. If parallel opposed anteroposterior ports are used for an entire sequence of adjuvant treatment (definitely not our recommendation), this may produce unacceptable acute perineal and genital reactions and undesirable chronic sequelae in both male and female depending upon the energy of the beam used, thickness of the patient, and total dosage employed. Use of angled AP:PA portals for a portion of treatment can help minimize the above problem.

We prefer a combination of the previous techniques to achieve an adequate perineal dose with acceptable morbidity. The perineum is included to a dose level of 4500 rad in five weeks without difficulty in most patients by using multiple field techniques including laterals, taping the buttocks appart while using controlled thickness and width of bolus over the perineal scar, and having male patients elevate the penis and scrotum cephalad behind the sumphysis during the PA treatment. Because of skin reactions, patients occasionally require a 7- to 10-day rest during treatment and the use of sitz baths, aquaphor ointment, and/or steroid cream. Most finish on schedule, and limited skin reactions resolve within 1 to 2 weeks of completion.

9.3. Dose – large and boost field

The dose delivered to the extended tumor bed-nodal portal should be the institution or individuals standard subclinical nodal dose [60] – approximately 4500 to 5000 rad in 5 to 6 weeks (usually 2 or more fields per day 5 days per week). Following this, strong consideration should be given to a boost field portal to the primary tumor bed and immediately adjacent nodes, especially if the large field dose is in the 4500 rad range. Our usual total dose in the boost field with both preoperative and postoperative cases is 5000 to 5500 rad in 6 to $6^{1}/_{2}$ weeks. Boost fields are defined by barium enema studies or clip placement and should usually be 10×10 cm or 12×12 cm to ensure adequate coverage to at least the 5000 rad level.

For *extrapelvic lesions*, treatment of the tumor bed and/or paraaortic nodes with the patient on his side (lateral decubitus position) rather than supine can markedly shift the position of small intestine [15, 19]. Such treatment position is used for about 1000 or 2000 rad of the planned adjuvant sequence.

9.4. Dose, aims, and XRT techniques – residual, recurrent, unresectable

When doses above 5000 rad are contemplated, small bowel films should be obtained to help define dose limits and field shaping. Doses of greater than 5000 rad in 180 rad fractions, 5 days per week, are rarely used unless there is good small bowel mobility or a minimal amount of small bowel within the field. Doses above 6000 rad, in similar daily fractions, are not used unless the small bowel is completely out of the boost field.

For patients with residual, recurrent, or fixed pelvic lesions, a *major difference* in treatment technique is the necessity of *including* the *sacral canal* as *tumor volume* for the initial 4500 to 5000 rad when unresectable or recurrent tumors present with posterior or lateral fixation or residual disease exists in a similar location after resection [15, 19]. This is necessary because of the increased risk of tumor spread along nerve roots. Failure to do so can result in a marginal recurrence in the sacral canal.

Boost fields are usually treated with three-field (PA and lateral) or four-field techniques (lateral and paired posterior obliques). Field shaping of the lateral boost portals is often helpful in deleting additional small intestine anteriorly and superiorly. Bladder distension can also be extremely useful in displacing small bowel loops superiorly and anteriorly out of both large and boost fields. In some elderly patients, bladder catheterization and distension is occasionally necessary [15]. The concept of applying shrinking field techniques to a maximum dose of 6000 to 7000 rad has been used for pelvic colorectal lesions since 1974 by the primary author.

In still other patients, the small bowel films identify patients in whom immobile loops remain in an area at high risk. In such instances, the radiotherapist must limit his dose to conform to small bowel tolerance, or the surgeon must re-explore the patient and reconstruct the pelvis and/or allow the delivery of an intraoperative boost while the small bowel is displaced [15, 51–53].

10. Conclusions and future possibilities

10.1. Adjuvant irradiation

In an adjuvant setting, doses of 5000 rad in $5^1/_2$ to 6 weeks given either pre-operatively or postoperatively in conjunction with resection of all known disease, produces superb local control in most patient subgroups with rectal and rectosigmoid carcinoma. In the subgroup with both node involvement and extension through the wall, the incidence of local recurrence has been reduced from 45 to 65% down to 10 to 12%, but one may ultimately have to increase the radiation dose to 5500 to 6000 rad in this subgroup whenever the volume of small bowel within the boost field is minimal to nonexistent. The complication rate appears to be satisfactory provided multi-field techniques, bladder distension, etc., are applied.

For both colon and rectal cancer, distant failures via either the hematogenous or peritoneal route are too high at a level of 25 to 30%. Whether these can be modified by combining local field radiation with systemic therapy, by applying a radiation technique of low-dose preoperative radiation therapy followed by postoperative when indicated or by the use of whole abdominal or liver treatment in conjunction with tumor bed-nodal irradiation in selected subgroups remains to be seen in subsequent trials. For lesions at high risk for local recurrence but with extension to a peritoneal surface and positive cytology of peritoneal washings [61, 62], it would be of interest to randomize to local irradiation alone versus local XRT + whole abdominal treatment (liver + peritoneal surfaces) and for lesions below or beneath the peritoneal surface to compare local irradiation to local XRT + treatment of the liver. Careful studies will be necessary to determine whether treatment to the peritoneal surfaces should be given with external beam irradiation, intraperitoneal radiocolloids or chemotherapy or a combination thereof, and whether the liver should be treated with external beam irradiation, infusion chemotherapy, or combined methods.

10.2. Lesion resectability

As experience with high resolution computed body tomography (CT) increases, it is possible that preoperative CT studies can be applied in conjunction with physical exam (rectum) or other diagnostic studies to help determine which lesions are unresectable for cure due to adherence to or involvement of technically unresectable structures (i.e., to do a resection would result in cut through and potential spread of disease). Such information could be important in designing future trials that apply either high or low dose preoperative irradiation before exploration and resection in an attempt to alter the incidence of systemic as well as local failure [5, 19, 31, 41, 45–47]. In sites where the risk of peritoneal seeding is high (colon ± upper rectum), the use of minilaps ± peritoneoscopy may be indicated before initiation of the high-dose sequence.

10.3. Unresectable, residual, recurrent

When unresectable or residual disease is treated with a combination of conventional irradiation and resection, local control and long-term survival can be achieved in 30 to 50% of patients. The presence of dose-limiting normal tissues, however, prevents delivery of adequate levels of external beam irradiation in a majority of patients. In early colorectal pilot studies from MGH, the addition of intraoperative electron boosts appeared to significantly improve both local control and survival [51–53]. Even if such results can be duplicated in randomized trials for rectal and rectosigmoid lesions, they may not be able to be achieved in colonic malignancies where systemic failures play a more predominant role. As discussed in the adjuvant section, wide field external beam irradiation may be necessary in addition to the aggressive local approach.

For cases found to be locally unresectable for cure at initial exploration, it would be worthwhile to obtain a baseline CT study, deliver 4500 to 5000 rad, and then restage the patient 3 to 4 weeks later. If the patient is without evidence of metastases and lesion extent is stable or reduced on a repeat CT, it would be justifiable to consider exploration and resection ± an intraoperative or post-operative 'boost' dose of irradiation. This sequence may be preferable to the alternative of resection of such lesions at the initial exploration, since this usually results in disease cut through and may produce an increased incidence of peritoneal or hematogenous failure.

For locally advanced or recurrent colorectal lesions in which the surgeon feels operative resection will never have a role, the combination of external beam irradiation and chemotherapy can achieve useful palliation in 75 to 80% of patients and an occasional cure [5, 15–18, 42]. If lesion size and location are such that intraoperative boosts with electrons, implantation techniques, or ortho-voltage can be safely used to supplement external beam doses, further gains may be possible. Early pilot studies suggest, however, that even with such boost techniques, the addition of radiation dose modifiers (radiation sensitizers, hyperthermia, etc.) may be necessary. When such intraoperative boosts cannot be applied dose levels achievable with external beam irradiation vary depending on location of tumor and normal tissues. For rectal lesions, a boost field can occasionally be carried to 6000 to 6500 rad if small bowel can be deleted. For colonic malignancies, the dose within the boost field is often limited to 5000 to 5500 rad in view of the presence of stomach, liver, or small intestine. At these dose levels, the chance for permanent local control is minimal, and any gains in local control will be achieved with combinations of chemotherapy and irradiation, or the use of radiation dose modifiers (sensitizers, protectors, hyperthermia, etc.).

In summary, it appears that radiotherapy has much to add in the therapeutic management of patients with colorectal malignancies. This can be achieved with a suitable risk of complications only if there is close interaction between the surgeon and the radiotherapist wherein both apply all mechanisms possible to limit dose to organs such as small bowel.

References

1. Silverberg E: Cancer Statistics, 1982. Cancer 32: 15–31, 1982.
2. Astler VB, Coller FA: The prognostic significance of direct extension of carcinoma of the colon and rectum. Ann Surg 139: 846–851, 1954.
3. Cass AW, Million RR, Pfaff FA: Patterns of recurrence following surgery alone for adenocarcinoma of the colon-rectum. Cancer 37: 2861–2865, 1976.
4. Gilbert SB: The significance of symptomatic local tumor failure following abdomino-perineal resection. Int J Rad Oncol Biol Phys 4: 801–807, 1978.
5. Gunderson LL: Combined irradiation and surgery for rectal and sigmoid carcinoma. In: Emerging role of Radiotherapy in Four Selected Areas. Fletcher G (ed.), Current Prob Cancer 1: 40–53, 1976.
6. Gunderson LL, Sosin H: Areas of failure found at reoperation (second or symptomatic look) following 'curative surgery' for adenocarcinoma of the rectum: Clinicopathologic correlation and implications for adjuvant therapy. Cancer 34: 1278–1292, 1974.
7. Gunderson LL, Tepper JE, Dosoretz DE, Kopelson G, Hoskins RB, Rich TA, Russell AH: Patterns of failure after treatment of gastrointestinal cancer. In: Proceedings of CROS-NCI Conference on Patterns of Failure after Treatment of Cancer. Ed. J. Cox. Cancer Treatment Symposia. In press.
8. Moosa AR, Ree PC, Marks JE, Levin B, Platz CE: Factors influencing local recurrence after abdomino-perineal resection for cancer of the rectum and rectosigmoid. Br J Surg 62: 727–730, 1975.
9. Rich T, Gunderson LL, Galdabini J, *et al.* Clinical and pathologic factors influencing local failure after curative resection of carcinoma of the rectum and rectosigmoid. Cancer 52: 1317–1329, 1983.
10. Romsdahl M, Withers HR: Radiotherapy combined with curative surgery. Arch Surg 113: 446–453, 1978.
11. Withers HR, Romsdahl MM, Saxton JP: Elective radiation therapy in the curative treatment of cancer of the rectum and rectosigmoid colon. In: Gastrointestinal Cancer. Strocklein JR, Romsdahl MM, ed. New York: Raven Press, 1981: 351–362.
12. Allee PE, Gunderson LL, Munzenrider JE: Postoperative radiation therapy for residual colorectal carcinoma. ASTR Proceedings. Int J Rad Oncol 7: 1208, 1981.
13. Cummings BJ, Rider WD, Harwood AR, Keane TJ, Thomas GM: External beam radiation therapy for adenocarcinoma of the rectum. Dis Colon Rectum (In Press).
14. Ghossein NA, Samala EC, Alpert S, *et al.*: Elective postoperative radiotherapy after incomplete resection of a colorectal cancer. Dis Colon Rectum 24: 252–256, 1981.
15. Gunderson LL, Cohen AM, Welch CW: Residual, inoperable, or recurrent colorectal cancer: surgical-radiotherapy interaction. Am J Surg 139: 518–525, 1980.
16. Rider WD: Is the Miles operation really necessary for the treatment of rectal cancer? J Can Assoc Radiol 26: 167–175, 1975.
17. Sklaroff D: Radiation as primary therapy for rectal carcinoma. Am Fam Physician 8: 81–85, 1973.
18. Wang CC, Schulz MD: The role of radiation therapy in the management of carcinoma of the sigmoid, rectosigmoid, and rectum. Radiology 79: 1–5, 1962.
19. Gunderson LL, Meyer JE, Sheedy P, Munzenrider JE: Radiation Oncology. Part XVIII. In: Alimentary Tract Radiology, 3rd Edition. Margolis AR, Burhenne HJ, eds. St. Louis: CV Mosby, 1983: 2409–2446.
20. Black WA, Waugh JM: The intramural extension of carcinoma of the descending colon, sigmoid and rectosigmoid: a pathologic study. Surg Gyn Obst 87: 457–464, 1948.
21. Grinnell RS: Lymphatic block with atypical and retrograde lymphatic metastasis and spread in carcinoma of the colon and rectum. Ann Surg 163: 272–280, 1966.
22. Enquist IF, Block IR: Rectal cancer in the female: selection of proper operation based upon

anatomic studies of rectal lymphatics. Prog Clin Cancer 2: 73–85, 1966.
23. Dukes CE: The pathology of rectal cancer. In: Cancer of the Rectum, C. Dukes, ed. Edinburgh: E & S Livingston, 1960: 59–68.
24. Copeland EM, Miller LD, Jones RS: Prognostic factors in carcinoma of the colon and rectum. Am J Surg 116: 875–881, 1968.
25. Gabriel WB, Dukes C, Bussey HJR: Lymphatic spread in cancer of the rectum. Br J Surg 23: 395–413, 1935.
26. Wood DA: Clinical staging and end results classification. TNM system of clinical classification as applicable to carcinoma of the colon and rectum. Cancer 28: 109–13, 1971.
27. Enker WE: Surgical treatment of large bowel cancer. In Carcinoma of the Colon and Rectum. Enker WE, ed. Yearbook Medical Publishers, 93–106, 1978.
28. Enker WE, Kemeny N, Shank B, Rotstein L: Defining the needs for adjuvant therapy of rectal and colonic cancer. Surg Clin N Amer 61: 1295–1309, 1981.
29. Polk HC, Ahmad W, Knutson CO: Carcinoma of the colon and rectum. Curr Prob Surg 1973 Jan, p 1–64.
30. Slanetz CA, Herter FP, Grinell RS: Anterior resection versus abdominoperineal resection for cancer of the rectum and rectosigmoid. Am J Surg 123: 110–117, 1972.
31. Stevens KR, Fletcher WS, Allen CV: Anterior resection and primary anastomosis following high dose pre-operative irradiation for adenocarcinoma of the rectosigmoid. Cancer 41: 2065–2071, 1978.
32. Welch J, Donaldson GA: The clinical correlation of an autopsy study of recurrent colorectal cancer. Ann Surg 89: 496–502, 1979.
33. Welch JP, Donaldson GA: Detection and treatment of recurrent cancer of the colon and rectum. Am J Surg 135: 505–511, 1978.
34. Malcolm AW, Perencevich NP, Olson RM, et al.: Analysis of recurrence patterns following curative resection for carcinoma of the colon and rectum. Surg Gynecol Obstet 152: 131–136, 1981.
35. Russell AH, Tong D, Dawson LE, Wisbeck W: Adenocarcinoma of the proximal colon: sites of initial dissemination and patterns of recurrence following surgery alone. Cancer (In press).
36. Gunderson LL, Sosin H: Adenocarcinoma of the colon: areas of failure in a reoperation series (second or symptomatic looks). (Submitted for publication).
37. Moertel CG: Alimentary tract cancer. In: Cancer Medicine. Holland J, Frei E, eds. Philadelphia: Lea & Febiger, pp 1753–1866, 1982.
38. Kligerman MM, Urdanetta N, Knowlton A, et al.: Preoperative irradiation of rectosigmoid carcinoma including its regional lymph nodes. Am J Roentgenol 114: 498–503, 1972.
39. Roswit B, Higgins GA, Keehn RJ: A controlled study of preoperative irradiation in cancer of the sigmoid colon and rectum. Radiology 97: 133–140, 1970.
40. Roswit B, Higgins GA, Keehn RJ: Preoperative irradiation for carcinoma of the rectum and rectosigmoid colon: report of a National Veteran's Administration randomized study. Cancer 35: 1597–1602, 1975.
41. Stevens KR, Allen CV, Fletcher WS: Preoperative radiotherapy for adenocarcinoma of the rectosigmoid. Cancer 37: 2866–2874, 1976.
42. Gunderson LL: Radiation therapy of colorectal carcinoma. In: Digestive Cancer, vol 9. Thatcher N (ed.), XII International Cancer Congress Proceedings, New York: Permagon Press, pp. 29–38, 1979.
43. Hoskins B, Gunderson LL, Dosoretz D, Galdabini J: Adjuvant postoperative radiotherapy in carcinoma of the rectum and rectosigmoid. Cancer (In press).
44. Mittleman A, et al.: (for GITSG group). Adjuvant chemotherapy and radiotherapy following rectal surgery: an interim report from the gastrointestinal tumor study group (GITSG). In: Salmon SE, Jones SE, eds. Adjuvant therapy of cancer III. New York: Green and Stratton, 1981: 547–557.

45. Gunderson LL, Dosoretz DE, Hedberg SE, *et al.*: Low-dose preoperative irradiation, surgery, and elective postoperative radiation therapy for resectable rectum and rectosigmoid carcinoma. Cancer 52: 446–451, 1983.
46. Mohüiddin M, Dobelbower RR, Kramer S: A new approach to adjuvant radiotherapy in rectal cancer. Int J Rad Oncol Biol Phys 6: 205–207, 1980.
47. Mohüidden M, Kramer S, Marks G, Dobelbower RR: Combined pre- and postoperative radiation for carcinoma of the rectum. Int Rad Oncol Biol Phys 8: 133–136, 1982.
48. Dosoretz DE, Gunderson LL, Hoskins B, *et al.*: Preoperative irradiation for localized carcinoma of the rectum and rectosigmoid: patterns of failure, survivial, and future treatment strategies. Cancer 52: 814–818, 1983.
49. Emami B, Pilepich M, Wilett C, Munzenrider JE, Miller HH: Management of unresectable colorectal carcinoma (preoperative radiotherapy and surgery). Int J Rad Oncol Biol Phys 8: 1295–1299, 1982.
50. Pilepich MV, Munzenrider JE, Tak WK, Miller HH: Preoperative irradiation of primarily unresectable colorectal carcinoma. Cancer 42: 1077–1081, 1978.
51. Gunderson LL, Shipley WU, Suit HD, *et al.*: Intraoperative irradiation: a pilot study combining external beam irradiation with 'boost' dose intraoperative electrons. Cancer 49: 2259–2266, 1982.
52. Gunderson LL, Cohen AM, Dosoretz DD, *et al.*: Residual, unresectable or recurrent colorectal cancer: external beam irradiation and intraoperative electron beam boost ± resection. Int J Rad Oncol 9: 1597–1606, 1983.
53. Gunderson LL, Tepper JE, *et al.*: Intraoperative ± external beam irradiation. In: Current Problems in Cancer. RC Hickey (ed). Chicago: Yearbook Medical Publishers Inc. (741): 1–69.
54. Papillon J: Endocavitary irradiation in the curative treatment of early rectal cancers. Dis Colon Rect 17: 172–180, 1974.
55. Papillon J: Intracavitary irradiation of early rectal cancer for cure. Cancer 36: 696–701, 1975.
56. Sischy B, Remington JH, Sobel SH: Treatment of rectal carcinomas by means of endocavitary irradiation. Cancer 46: 1957–1961, 1980.
57. Turner SS, *et al.*: Elective postoperative radiotherapy for locally advanced colorectal cancer. Cancer 40: 105–108, 1977.
58. Dembo AJ, Van Dyk J, Japp B, *et al.*: Whole abdominal irradiation by a moving strip technique for patients with ovarian cancer. Int J Rad Oncol Biol Phys 5: 1933–1942, 1979.
59. Green N, Ira G, Smith WR: Measures to minimize small intestine injury in the irradiated pelvis. Cancer 35: 1633–1640, 1975.
60. Fletcher GH: Clinical dose-response curves of human malignant epithelial tumors. Br J Radiol 46: 1–12, 1973.
61. Creasman WT, Disaia PJ, Blessing J, *et al.*: Prognostic significance of peritoneal cytology in patients with endometrial cancer and preliminary data concerning therapy with intraperitoneal radiopharmaceuticals. Am J Obstet Gynecol 141: 921–929, 1981.
62. Nakajima T, Harashima S, Hirata M, Kajitani T: Prognostic and therapeutic value of peritoneal cytology in gastric cancer. Acta Cytol 22: 225–229, 1978.

9. Treatment of squamous cell cancer of the anus

NORMAN D. NIGRO*

1. Introduction

Squamous cell cancer of the anus is a rare lesion comprising less than 5% of all rectal cancers. As Gabriel suggested in 1941 [1], these tumors are best divided into two distinct groups according to the site of origin. They are anal margin cancers, which develop primarily in the perianal skin, and anal canal cancers which arise in the area of the dentate line and especially in the tissues immediately above it (Fig. 1). This division of anal tumors has been adopted by the World Health Organization in its publication, 'Histological Typing of Intestinal Tumors' [2].

The rationale for this approach becomes clear when one considers that the epithelium lining the surfaces in the anal region varies significantly at different locations. Cancers in this area assume the characteristics of the cells at the site of origin (Fig. 1). They differ enough in histological appearance, in method of treatment, and in prognosis to justify the division into the two categories.

The management of these cancers is of particular interest for two reasons; first, they are so infrequent that most surgeons are not familiar with their treatment, and second, the management of anal canal cancer, the more common and more lethal type, is changing significantly.

1.1. Anatomy

The anus is the oval aperture at the distal end of the anal canal generally referred to as the anal verge. However, it is often used as in the title of this chapter, to mean the anal region, including the anal canal. The anal canal is described in one of two ways. The surgical version, the longer of the two, is that portion of the tract or channel that is surrounded by the anorectal musculature. The anatomical anal

* The author acknowledges the help of Drs. V.K. Vaitkevicius and B. Considine, Jr. in developing this chemoradiation therapy for anal canal cancer first described in 1974 [45].

J.J. DeCosse and P. Sherlock (eds), Clinical Management of Gastrointestinal Cancer.
© *1984, Martinus Nijhoff Publishers, Boston. ISBN 0-89838-601-2. Printed in The Netherlands.*

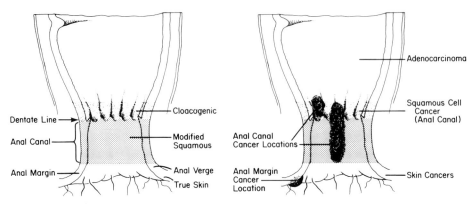

Figure 1. Anal canal lesions shown in the diagram on the right often spread circumferentially, sometimes proximally into the rectum or distally into the perianal skin.

canal extends only from the dentate line to the anal verge. Therefore, the surgical anal canal includes normal rectal epithelium in its proximal third, while the anatomical anal canal, being shorter, does not reach the rectal mucosal level. In this chapter, we will use the anatomical version (Fig. 1).

The dentate line represents the junction between the endodermal and ectodermal layers formed in the embryo when the hindgut meets to join the upward excursion of the skin. This line is identified by a row of anal crypts and their associated epithelial processes called anal papillae. The latter are thought to be remnants of the proctodeal membrane.

The perianal area, as its name implies, is the region surrounding the anal verge. Its outer dimensions are not precisely defined, but it is generally considered to be about 6 cm. in all directions from the anal verge. The skin is arranged in radial folds caused by the action of the underlying muscle. The histological structure of the skin is the same as normal skin elsewhere except that it is slightly more pigmented and it contains an excess of sebaceous and sweat glands plus a growth of hair.

The lining of the anal canal is a mixture of mucocutaneous cells presenting different histologic features at different levels. Beginning at the distal end of the canal, the surface epithelium at the anal verge and outside it is true skin containing glands and hair. Just inside the anal verge, the lining is stratified squamous epithelium without glands and hair. At this point cornification diminishes gradually in a proximal direction until it becomes minimal at the dentate line.

Of particular interest is the fact that the rectal mucosa does not join directly with the modified squamous epithelium of the anal canal at the dentate line as one would expect. Interposed between them is a remnant of embryonic cloaca, specifically the posterior or intestinal part of that structure. The area, called the cloacogenic zone, is only about one cm. in length and has a slightly violaceous appearance (Fig. 1). Here the cells are variable in size and shape, and include transitional cells resembling urinary tract epithelium, stratified cuboidal cells, columnar, and squamous cells. In essence, there is a mixture of these cell types with occasional small islands of normal rectal mucosa from above and stratified squamous epithelium from below. This accounts for the variety of histologic patterns of cancers which arise from this highly variable and unstable area. Though pathologists use terms such as cloacogenic, transitional, basaloid, epidermoid, and squamous cell cancers to describe these lesions, it is best to consider all to be variants of squamous cell cancers. The importance of this will be discussed later.

There is a rich plexus of blood vessels underlying the lining of the anal canal. Superior, middle, and inferior hemorrhoidal arteries and veins contribute to this network. Since the superior hemorrhoidal vein drains into the portal system while the middle and inferior veins drain into the systemic circulation, this is an area of portacaval anastomosis. The systemic venous drainage in the anal canal probably accounts for the occurrence of metastases to the lung from cancers in this location.

There is also a rich lymphatic plexus associated with that of the blood vessels. Lymph drainage, therefore, is upward, lateral and downward. Of special interest is the significant lymph drainage that proceeds laterally and inferiorly to involve the external iliac and the inguinal lymph nodes. The latter are often involved in lesions that have spread downwards from the dentate line and those in the perianal area [3].

2. Anal margin cancer

The *International Histological Classification of Tumors* lists the following types of malignant epithelial tumors of the anal margin [2]:
1. Squamous cell carcinoma
2. Basal cell carcinoma
3. Bowen's disease
4. Paget's disease

Anal margin cancer is not as common as anal canal cancer. Morson [4] analyzed the experience of 157 patients with epithelial cancer of the anal region at St. Mark's Hospital, London during the period 1928–1956. Of these, 38 were anal margin cancer, 103 were anal canal cancer, and in 16 patients the location was not specified. McConnell [5] reviewed 96 patients from the Liverpool Cancer Registry. He found that 41 patients had anal margin cancer while 55 had anal canal cancer. More recently, Hintz, *et al.* [6] suggest that about 25% of tumors are located in the anal margin while 75% occur in the anal canal.

In contrast to adenocarcinoma of the rectum which occurs more often in men, cancer of the anal region has an equal distribution in men and women. However, there is a striking difference in sex incidence between cancer of the anal margin and cancer of the anal canal. Anal margin cancer is more common in males while

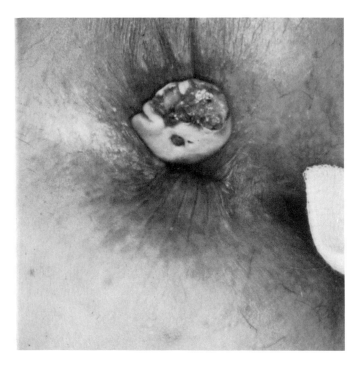

Figure 2. Histologically, the lesion contained a marked degree of keratosis indicating a highly differentiated cancer.

anal canal cancer is more frequent in females. Age incidence is the same in both groups as it is in adenocarcinoma of the rectum [4].

Anal margin cancers are similar to skin cancers in other parts of the body. As such, they do not generally pose a problem in management, and the prognosis is usually good. Therefore, the discussion of the treatment of these tumors is simpler than that of anal canal cancer.

2.1. Squamous cell cancer

This is the most frequent type of malignant tumor of the perianal skin. It is usually a well-differentiated, highly keratinized tumor of relatively small size [7]. The cancers are superficial; they are more often exophatic than ulcerative (Fig. 2). Symptoms are minor; namely the presence of a lump or small ulcer not especially painful or tender. But it does not heal even after several months of local therapy with ointments, baths, etc. Surgical excision is the treatment of choice. The lesion should be removed along with a wide margin of skin around it. In most cases the wound should be left open since it will heal quickly with satisfactory results. Skin

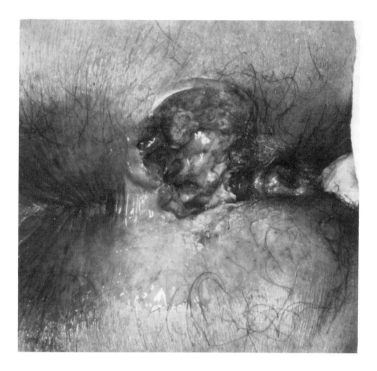

Figure 3. This extensive perineal squamous cell cancer may have originated in the vagina. Today, we would manage this patient with chemoradiation and operation if necessary.

grafts may be applied occasionally when the lesion spreads from outside into the anal canal to a significant degree to help prevent stricture. Recurrence is uncommon, unless the lesion was not completely removed. In this case, surgical excision should be repeated. Inguinal nodes are not involved.

Large, highly invasive ulcerative squamous cancers have been observed in the perineum particularly in women (Fig. 3). These are like cancers that occur in the vagina, and inguinal nodes may be involved [8]. This lesion requires extensive therapy similar to that for invasive cancer of the anal canal described later in this chapter.

2.2. Basal cell cancer

Only ten patients with this lesion of the perianal skin were seen at St. Mark's Hospital in a 25 year period [4]. Similarly, Grodsky [9] in a review of the literature, found that only 50 cases had been reported by 1965. The lesion is similar to 'rodent ulcers' seen on exposed skin, and the average age of patients in 60 years. This lesion should not be confused with basaloid cancer of the anal canal. Symptoms are nonspecific. Any indurated swelling that has been present for months, especially if it is ulcerated, should be suspect as representing a possible low grade cancer. A wide excisional biopsy should be done not only for diagnosis but also for cure.

2.3. Bowen's disease

This is a chronic, intradermal, squamous cell cancer which has a tendency to remain intradermal for years. Clinically, it resembles perianal skin in which chronic pruritus developed. However, the lesion does not respond to routine therapy for uncomplicated perianal dermatitis. This situation suggests the need for biopsy to determine the true nature of the disease process. Microscopically, there is an overgrowth of the superficial layers of the skin, the cells being somewhat disoriented. The characteristic feature, however, is a large atypical cell with a haloed, giant hyperchromatic nucleus. It is thought that intracellular edema causes this haloed effect on the large nuclei. The basal cell layer usually remains intact. Wide local excision is curative. If the margins of the specimen are not free of disease, the edges of the wound should be excised to normal skin. Bowen's disease of the perianal skin is similar to that which occurs in the skin in other parts of the body as reported in the dermatologic literature. There appears to be a correlation between this lesion and the development of a cancer of some other organ at a later date [10].

2.4. Paget's disease

Perianal Paget's disease is an adenocarcinoma of the apocrine sweat glands. It is similar to lesions found elsewhere in the skin in areas where apocrine glands are abundant as they are in the perianal skin. Clinically this disease is similar to chronic perianal dermatitis except that it continues to spread slowly, and it is resistant to therapy for anal pruritus. The diagnosis can only be established by biopsy. The characteristic microscopic feature is a mucus producing 'signet-ring' cell similar to that seen in mucinous adenocarcinoma. Treatment is complete excision of the lesion including a margin of normal skin. If not completely removed, a second, wider excision should be done [11].

This lesion may become a truly invasive carcinoma, penetrating the skin to involve the underlying fat. This occurred in 13 of 38 cases studied by Helwig and Graham [12]. Eleven patients had lymph node metastases, and all of them died of their disease. Patients who are suitable operative risks and have a chance for cure require abdominoperineal resection with wide perineal excision. Inguinal nodes, if involved, should be excised.

2.5. Miscellaneous lesions

Anorectal fistula and cancer are associated only rarely. McAnally and Dockerty estimated that cancer is present in approximately 0.1 percent of all anorectal fistulas [13]. Cancer appears to be associated with fistulas in one of two ways. In the first instance, an adenocarcinoma forms in an anal gland in the area of the dentate line. Eventually, the gland ruptures into the tissues surrounding the anal canal and lower rectum forming a fistula. The patient is unaware of the condition until the fistula forms, causing symptoms which progress until surgery is required. At the time of operation cancer may be suspected because the sinus tract contains a great deal of mucus and the lining has a mucosal appearance. Either the diagnosis is confirmed on frozen section or the pathologist finds it during the routine examination of the operative specimen.

The second situation is quite the reverse. A patient who has had a fistula for many years with minimal symptoms suddenly finds his symptoms worsening. At operation a fistulectomy is done. Generally the surgeon has no reason to suspect malignant degeneration, but the cancer is found in the tissues removed at operation. It is almost always a squamous cell cancer.

In the first type, the cancer causes fistula formation, while in the second, a fistula of long duration degenerates into a malignant phase. It appears that the first type, adenocarcinoma-fistula, is the more common variety [13]. By the time the diagnosis is made, the cancer in both situations has invaded the tissues around the anus, rectum, and even into the buttocks. Occasionally, inguinal lymph nodes are involved [14].

The prognosis in the adenocarcinoma-fistula lesion is generally poor. Abdominoperineal resection with an extensive perineal phase is indicated [15]. An inguinal groin dissection is included as needed. Following recovery from the operation, radiation therapy should be given since perineal recurrences are so common.

The situation is not so lethal with squamous cell carcinoma-fistula lesions. After recovery from fistula surgery, radiation and chemotherapy as outlined below for squamous cell cancer of the anal canal should be given. Abdominoperineal resection may or may not be necessary depending upon circumstances.

Leukoplakia is a clinical term for a dermatitis that has a typical appearance. The tissues are thickened and whitish. It occurs most often in the oral cavity, but is seen occasionally in the modified squamous epithelium in the anal canal, sometimes spreading to the perianal skin. It is thought to be precancerous. However, the few patients we have followed over a period of several years have not developed cancer. We have done local excision only when it is indicated for some associated lesion. Otherwise, operation is not recommended unless the lesion progresses, becoming symptomatic. Even then, local excision is all that is required [16].

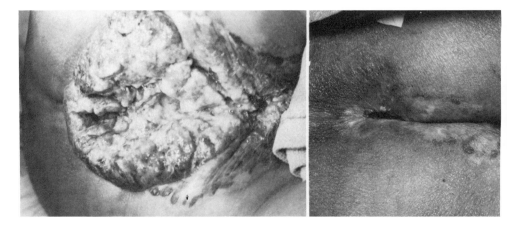

Figure 4. Lesion shown in the left photograph was a mass of recurrent squamous cell cancer and condylomata acuminata. The right photograph shows the patient 3 months after chemoradiation therapy only.

Condylomata acuminata of the perianal area is nearly always a benign disease. However, on rare occasions it is associated with squamous cell cancer. In 1963, Friedberg and Serlin [17] reviewed the association of these two lesions and suggested that giant condylomata, although it does not undergo malignant change, histologically sometimes behaves like carcinoma. More recent articles by Lee, *et al.* [18], and Prasad, *et al.* [19], cite additional case reports, and they advised abdominoperineal resection as the treatment of choice.

We have seen a 32 year old man with a superficial perineal fistula associated with condylomata acuminata. Cancer was not suspected, but after removal of the fistulous tract and condylomata, moderately well differentiated squamous cell cancer was found in the specimen. After the wound healed, the patient was given radiation and chemotherapy according to the regimen described under squamous cell cancer of the anal canal. Abdominoperineal resection was not done and the patient is free of disease 4 years following therapy.

A second patient seen recently had a large mass of perianal condylomata excised in the routine manner. Early squamous cell cancer was found in the specimen, but no further therapy was given. Two years later, the patient returned with a large recurrent mass (Fig. 4) covering the entire perianal area. On biopsy, the tissue contained a mixture of condylomata and squamous cell cancer. The mass was not excised. Instead, the patient was given the radiation-chemotherapy regimen. In three months, the lesion disappeared and there has been no recurrence in 18 months.

On the basis of this brief experience, we advocate the administration of radiation and chemotherapy for condylomata acuminata associated with squamous cell cancer. If the lesion disappears, radical operation may not be required. If the lesion persists, abdominoperineal resection is indicated.

3. Squamous cell cancer of the anal canal

Squamous cell cancer of the anal canal develops in the region of the dentate line. This is the area where in the embryo the skin and the hindgut migrate toward each other but do not quite meet. Interposed between them is the narrow segment of epithelium that is said to be derived from the cloaca. The cells in this narrow segment just above the dentate line vary as has been described in the section on anatomy. Cancers that arise in this tissue also vary in cell type and pathologists label them accordingly. However, the cell type of these tumors is not an important factor in planning therapy [20]. Consequently, it is simpler and less confusing to call these cancers squamous cell cancer of the anal canal.

3.1. Pathology

Most cancers of the anal canal develop from the epithelium of the cloacogenic zone at or just above the dentate line. This epithelium is unstable and there is a mixture of cell types. Histologic features of these cancers also vary. Many tumors consist of several different cell types though usually one predominates. According to Morson [21], these tumors are 'mostly non-keratinizing squamous cell cancers such as those found in the cervix or pharynx'. Cells tend to form mucus rather than keratin.

Among the variety of tumors is one consisting of sheets of small ovoid and spindle shaped cells usually referred to as basaloid. This tumor has no relationship to basal cell cancer of the anal margin. Some anal canal tumors contain small nests of typical squamous epithelium invading from below the dentate line or columnar cells from the rectal mucosa above. These varied patterns of cell types are responsible for the different terms pathologists use to label them. It is important to assess the degree of anaplasia and whether or not there is invasion of vascular, lymphatic, or neural tissues. This information, along with the description of the predominate cell type, although not of importance in planning therapy, is valuable in evaluating prognosis [22].

3.2. Clinical aspects and diagnosis

Unfortunately, early symptoms of anal canal cancer are minimal; usually slight bleeding and discomfort following defecation. Patients assume they have hemorrhoids or a fissure. This leads to self medication and a delay in seeking medical care. As the growth increases in size, the complaints, especially pain, become severe enough to cause the patient to seek medical care. Loss of weight is not common but when present suggests advanced disease. Sometimes patients voluntarily reduce food intake because defecation is so painful. In rare situations, patients will notice a lump in the groin as the first indication of anal canal cancer [22].

The diagnosis is made on examination and biopsy. The long duration of continuous symptoms plus the induration characteristic of cancer suggests the possibility of malignancy and the need for biopsy. The lesion may extend proximally into the rectum or distally to and even outside the anal verge. The cancer is generally ulcerative and the size varies. Some are elongated, elliptical, fissure-like lesions whereas others encircle the anal canal to varying degrees. Advanced cancers may completely encircle it and may extend upward or distally to involve tissues beyond the anal canal. An important point, however, is that all anal canal cancers, whatever their size, involve the area of the dentate line.

In general, adequate appraisal of the location, size and some estimate of the depth of invasion is best done under anesthesia, usually caudal or spinal. Biopsy is done at the same time. If preoperative therapy is a possibility, only a portion of the lesion should be removed for biopsy. Complete removal is unwise because it will not be possible to estimate the effect of the preoperative treatment – hence the decision for further therapy will be more difficult. If the lesion is less than 2 cm., it may be completely excised.

3.3. Staging

The staging of squamous cell cancer of the anal canal is more difficult than that of adenocarcinoma of the rectum. This is due in part to insufficient data because of the low incidence of the disease. A more important reason has to do with the anatomy of the area. The wall of the anal canal is not as clearly delinated into separate compartments as is that of the rectum or colon. The epithelial layer of the anal canal is surrounded by a thick muscle layer consisting of the internal and external sphincter muscles. Degrees of penetration of cancer through it are not as easily categorized as that through the muscle coat of the large bowel. Under these circumstances, the Dukes' Classification is difficult to apply. Since squamous cell cancers may be treated with radiation, the degree of penetration would be unknown in those patients.

Recently, several studies have been reported which show a strong correlation between the size of the primary lesion in squamous cell cancer of the anal canal and prognosis [22–26]. Our experience with 38 patients, described in the section on combined therapy, supports this finding. It appears that patients with lesions that are 6 cm. or more in greatest diameter have a poor prognosis. If the significance of size is confirmed, it suggests that a staging system based on three factors; the size of the cancer, the presence or absence of inguinal lymph node metastases, and the presence or absence of distant metastases, would be both adequate and practical.

3.4. Treatment

In situ squamous cell cancer of the anal canal not suspected clinically but found in tissue removed during hemorrhoidectomy usually does not require additional treatment. Since hemorrhoids are multiple, the specific site from which the cancer cells were removed is unknown. Generally, the *in situ* cancer is completely removed with the hemorrhoids. Nevertheless, patients should be followed closely for at least a year.

Unsuspected cancer has been found in other chronic anorectal conditions in about 2 percent of patients [27]. The most common lesions are fissure, fistula, and condylomata acuminata. The situation in these patients is more complex and management must be individualized. If microscopic cancer is found in a chronic anal fissure, more tissue should be removed to be certain that the excision has been adequate. If cancer is found in tissue removed during fistulectomy or the excision of condylomata acuminata, additional therapy is necessary. This matter is discussed in other sections in this chapter.

Squamous cell cancers of the anal canal that are 2 cm. or less should be excised locally with a fairly wide margin of normal tissue around them. These wounds generally heal well and are best left open because cancer cells on the wound surface are less likely to survive than those in a closed wound. After healing has occurred, the patient should be followed carefully for at least 2 years. If there is recurrence, radical therapy may be indicated.

3.4.1. Surgery

For the past several decades, the accepted treatment for invasive cancer of the anal canal has been radical operation [22, 28, 29, 30]. This consists of abdomino-perineal resection of the rectum with an extensive perineal phase. In women, the rectovaginal septum is often removed. The reported five-year survival rates vary considerably, ranging from less than 30% to more than 60%. The variation seems to be due to differences in sampling. At times authors mix anal margin and anal canal cancers. Naturally, this alters the long-term survival rate. Some authors deal only with cancers of a particular cell type, or report series that have a preponderance of patients with early or advanced disease.

The incidence of local recurrence in anal canal cancer after abdominoperineal resection varies with the stage of the disease, but is higher than in adenocarcinoma of the rectum [31, 32]. The following factors may account for the high local recurrence rate: 1) the anal canal has a profuse network of both blood and lymphatic vessels that may promote early local spread of cancer cells; 2) anatomical constraints around the anal canal prevent the excision of an adequate amount of tissue around the primary lesion; and 3) it is difficult to remove the lateral and downward extensions of the lymphatic vessels and their nodes. Stearns and Quan [20] suggested the addition of pelvic lymph node dissection to the abdomino-perineal resection in selected patients. Although that procedure was of some benefit in reducing recurrence, it also increased morbidity. Therefore, this modification has not been generally adopted.

Nevertheless, radical excision of the rectum continues to be the most widely accepted therapy for invasive squamous cell cancer of the anal canal [33, 34]. For most surgeons, it offers the best long-term results. Thus, the effectiveness of any new therapy must be compared with that of radical surgery. The disadvantages of abdominoperineal resection of the rectum, however, are significant. It results in the loss of bowel function through the establishment of a permanent colostomy, and it frequently causes urinary and sexual dysfunction; especially in males.

3.4.2. Radiation therapy

Squamous cell cancers are generally radiosensitive, so that it is not surprising that radiation has been used in the management of anal cancers for many years. In England, Gordon-Watson in 1935 [35] and later Gabriel in 1941 [1], reported success in controlling these cancers in some patients with interstitial radiation therapy. However, complications were often so severe that this modality was temporarily abandoned.

More recently, improvement in the application of interstitial radiation has restored interest in it. Dalby and Pointon [36] and Papillon [37] advocate its use. Papillon has treated 64 patients with squamous cell cancer of the anal canal with a combination of external beam and interstitial radiation. The five-year survival rate was 68%. Toxic effects were minimized by using a fractioned regimen in which 3000 rads of external beam radiation was given in a 3 week interval followed in 8 weeks by interstitial irradiation. In addition, Puthawala *et al.* [38] have also reported encouraging results in the treatment of extensive anorectal carcinoma by external and interstitial irradiation.

However, at present, radiation therapy for cancer of the rectum and anal canal is most often given as external beam radiation using supervoltage equipment. A number of radiation oncologists maintain that this method of therapy achieves acceptable results [39, 40].

3.4.3. Combined therapy

Recently, *radiation therapy combined with surgery* has become a popular method of treatment for many forms of malignancy, including rectal cancer. Operation is the best way to remove large masses of accessible malignant tissue, while radiation can destroy peripheral extensions of tumor which are not in the surgical field [41]. So it seems logical to combine the two treatment methods. Radiation therapy can be given either before, after, or both before and after operation. Each approach has its advantages. Surgeons generally prefer to use radiation treatment after operation because the extent of disease is known more precisely. This allows the radiation oncologist greater flexibility in treating the patient. Furthermore, operation is not delayed as it is when radiation treatment is given first. However, preoperative radiation also has several advantages. It reduces the size of the primary lesion and may contract its regional extent to a smaller area, making excision more effective. There is also the theoretical possibility that radiation treatment will reduce or prevent the spread of cancer cells during operation.

Chemotherapy, radiation, and surgery in combination may prove to be an even more effective treatment. There is evidence that chemotherapeutic drugs potentiate the effect of radiation. Radiation and 5-FU, for example, appear to interact additively to induce cell killing [42, 43, 44]. This suggests the possibility that smaller, less toxic doses of radiation might be as effective as larger doses if chemotherapy were given at the same time. There is also the possibility that chemotherapy, since it is a systemic modality, might destroy micrometastases. This is, of course, only a theoretical possibility, unsubstantiated as yet. However, it is logical to use both a local and systemic therapeutic approach for the treatment of cancer whenever possible.

In 1974, we published a report on the use of preoperative radiation and chemotherapy followed by abdominoperineal resection in three patients with squamous cell cancer of the anal canal [45]. This brief experience was successful enough to warrant further investigation by others [46, 47, 48], and our series was updated by Buroker, *et al.* [49, 50], and again by Nigro, *et al.* [51]. The following report deals with our experience with the management of squamous cell cancer of the anal canal in a larger number of patients.

Twenty-four women and 14 men ranging in age from 42 to 79 years with biopsy proven squamous cell cancer of the anal canal involving the dentate line are included in this review. All lesions were ulcerated, most were moderately to poorly differentiated, and all but seven were 6 cm or less in greatest diameter (Table 1). Two patients had inguinal metastases, one unilateral and the other had extensive bilateral involvement. There was no evidence of disease in distant organs in any patient, as determined by physical examination, chest x-ray, laboratory studies, radioisotope scans of the liver and bones and CT scans of the head, pelvis and abdomen. All were judged to be candidates for abdomino-perineal resection of the rectum.

The preoperative therapy is summarized in Table 2. Chemotherapy and radia-

Table 1. Squamous cell cancer of the anal canal (38 patients)

Size of lesion	Degree of differentiation	
3 cm – 13	Well	2
4 cm – 11	Moderately	15
5 cm – 3	Poorly	21
6 cm – 4		
7 cm – 2		
8 cm – 5		

tion therapy were begun jointly on day one of the therapy. 5-Fluorouracil was given via a central venous catheter in a dosage of 1000 mg/m^2/24 hr for 4 days as a continuous infusion. This 96-hour infusion was repeated in one month even in the presence of mild bone marrow depression since 5-FU infusions have been shown to be nonmyelosuppressive [52]. Mitomycin C was given as a bolus intravenous injection at a dosage of 15 mg/m^2 on day 1. Radiation therapy was given to 3000 rads (30 Gy), calculated at the central axis mid-plane of the pelvis, at 200 rads (2 Gy) per day, 5 days a week, starting on day one. The parallel-opposing anteroposterior portals included the primary lesion with margin, the true pelvis, and the inguinal lymphatics. Surgery was performed 6 to 8 weeks following completion of the radiation therapy. Leukocyte and platelet counts were obtained weekly until the time of surgery.

All 38 patients were evaluable for the effect of preoperative therapy (Table 3). No tumor was visible or palpable in 33 while in 5, gross cancer was evident but was reduced in size. In these 5 patients the original tumors were large; being more than 6 cm in greatest diameter and nearly all encircling the anal canal.

Sixteen patients had abdominoperineal resection following the preoperative therapy (Table 4). Ten of these patients had no residual cancer in the operative specimen. One patient had only microscopic tumor in the area of the primary lesion while the other 5 had gross tumor. Seven of the 10 patients who had no residual cancer in the operative specimen were treated in the first 3 years of this study. On the basis of these findings, *radical operation was not done routinely after the third year* of the study on patients whose lesion disappeared following the completion of radiation and chemotherapy. Instead, to evaluate the effectiveness of the therapy, these patients were examined under anesthesia and the scar was excised in toto. If the scar involved a significant degree of the circumference of the anal canal, two or three narrow but deep sections were obtained in representative areas.

There was no microscopic tumor found in the excised scar tissue in any of the 20 patients managed in this way. However, one patient was found to have disease only 3 months following the biopsy. The original lesion had spread upward into the rectum in an area not included in the biopsy specimen. An abdominoperineal resection was done. The operative specimen had a small area of residual cancer in

---

Table 2. Preoperative therapy for squamous cell cancer of the anal canal

---

1. External Irradiation.
   300 rads (30 GY) to the primary tumor, pelvic and inguinal nodes. Day 1 to day 21. (200 rads/day).
2. Systemic Chemotherapy.
   A. 5-FU: 1000 mg/m^2/24 hr. as a continuous infusion for 4 days. Start on day 1.
   B. Mitomycin C: 15 mg/m^2 IV bolus on day 1.
   C. 5-FU: repeated day 28 to 31.

---

the primary site with no involvement of the lymph nodes. Two other patients did not have an excisional biopsy. One of these refused to have it done. The other had extensive, bilateral, positive inguinal nodes. Since the primary lesion disappeared, relieving all symptoms, and because the prognosis was poor, radical operation was not judged to be of value.

The long term results in the 30 patients who have survived so far is shown in Table 5. Nine patients, of whom six had abdominoperineal resections and three did not, are apparently free of disease 5 to 10 years after treatment. Of the 21 other patients treated less than 5 years ago, 20 have no evidence of disease. Of these 20 patients, three had radical surgery while 17 did not. One patient who was treated conservatively has extensive metastatic cancer. He is the patient who originally had bilateral inguinal node metastases.

It is worth emphasizing that of the 22 patients who did not have radical surgery, only one was found to have residual disease 3 months after a negative biopsy. Abdominoperineal resection was done and the prognosis appears favorable. Toxicity was not a significant problem in this group of patients, although such effects as stomatitis, loss of hair, mild diarrhea, leukopenia, and thrombocytopenia occurred in about 20% of patients. Great care was taken to identify early manifestations of toxicity such as stomatitis or a drop in the white blood cell

Table 3. Squamous cell cancer of the anal canal (38 patients)

Effect of preoperative therapy		
Anal canal lesion	No gross tumor	33
	Gross tumor present	5*

* Original lesions:

Size	Degree of differentiation	
7 cm	Well	1
8 cm	Moderately well	1
8 cm	Poorly	3

Table 4. Squamous cell cancer of the anal canal. Results after operation

	APR	Excision of scar
No tumor found	10	20
Microscopic tumor only	1	
Gross tumor	5	
Total	16	20

count. If mild degrees of these toxic effects developed, the therapy was interrupted for a few days. All 38 patients completed the treatment regimen without long term toxic effects.

There were eight deaths in the series (Table 6). All these patients had abdominoperineal resections following the chemoradiation therapy. One patient died of an unrelated cause over 4 years after operation. Seven patients died of their disease. Five had distant metastases only, whereas two had both pelvic disease and distant metastases. The initial cancer in all these patients was large; measuring at least 6 cm. in greatest diameter. Five of these cancers did not disappear after preoperative therapy. Interestingly, the lesion disappeared completely in the other two patients, but they died of distant metastases nevertheless.

We have reviewed data recently collected from a questionnaire on an additional 122 patients with squamous cell cancer of the anal canal who received preoperative combined therapy. A few patients received the preoperative regimen outlined in Table 2, but the majority were given larger doses of radiation, usually 4500 to 5000 rads. Several patients had less 5 FU and/or less Mitomycin C. However, all 122 patients received preoperative radiation plus chemotherapy that included 5 FU and Mitomycin C. Although the data is inadequate to draw many conclusions, the study is relevant with regard to the effect of radiation and chemotherapy on the primary lesion.

After radiation and chemotherapy, there was no gross tumor in 113 patients, while some visible tumor remained in nine (Table 7). Abdominoperineal resection was performed in 40 of the 122 patients. No tumor was found in the operative specimen in 27, microscopic tumor only in four, while in nine patients, gross cancer remained (Table 8). Scar tissue was biopsied in another 40 patients whose primary lesions disappeared grossly. There was no tumor in 36 of these patients,

Table 5. Survival data – 38 patients

APR	Excision of scar	No operation
16	20	2

No evidence of disease		
1–10 year	1–7 year	1–3 year
1– 9 year	1–6 year	1–2 year[1]
2– 7 year	1–5 year	
2– 6 year	3–4 year	
1– 3 year[1]	2–3 year	
1– 2 year	5–2 year	
	7–1 year[2]	
8	20	2

[1] Inguinal node positive.

[2] 1 patient, APR 4 months after negative biopsy.

while four had microscopic cancer. Another 42 patients had no operation following combined therapy.

Four patients in the series of 122 had positive inguinal nodes confirmed at biopsy (Table 9). Three of these patients had an abdominoperineal resection with bilateral inguinal node dissection. One died of distant metastases while the other two are apparently free of disease after treatment. The fourth patient had extensive bilateral inguinal node involvement, and since the primary lesion disappeared temporarily, there was no need to operate. The patient later died of liver metastases.

The final results are of interest even though the followup period is less than three years in most patients (Table 10). Of the 40 patients who had radical operation, there were nine deaths due to squamous cell cancer of the anal canal, and one death each from esophageal, breast, and tongue cancer. In the group of 40 who had the scar excised, there were seven local recurrences. The time of recurrence varied from 6 to 24 months. Five of these patients had an abdomi-

Table 6. Squamous cell cancer of the anal canal. Deaths: 8

Metastases	Pelvic	No Cancer
5	2	1
Primary lesion		
2–8 cm	2–8 cm	1–4 cm
2–7 cm		
1–6 cm		

Table 7. Squamous cell cancer of the anal canal. 122 patients[1]

Effect of Preoperative Therapy	
No gross tumor found	113
Gross tumor present	9

[1] Questionnaire survey.

Table 8. Squamous cell cancer of the anal canal. 122 patients[1]

Results after completed therapy

	APR	Excision of scar	No operation
No tumor	27	36	42
Micro tumor only	4	4	0
Gross tumor present	9	0	0
Total	40	40	42

[1] Questionnaire survey.

noperineal resection of the rectum. All are alive without evidence of disease, but again, followup is short. The other two patients were in such poor condition due to extensive local disease that they were given more radiation therapy for palliation. They are still alive with disease. Finally, there were three deaths in the group of 42 patients who had no operation or biopsy of scar. All three died of liver metastases. No other recurrences have been reported in this group thus far.

There was a surprising degree of toxicity from the preoperative radiation and chemotherapy in this group of 122 patients. Fifteen patients required re-hospitalization for severe gastrointestinal signs and symptoms. Three were operated upon. One had an abdominoperineal resection for necrosis of the rectum, one had a colostomy done because of a severe rectal stricture, and the third patient had a sigmoid resection due to perforation. Three other patients died of massive internal hemorrhage from extensive enteritis. Several patients required hyperalimentation and small intestinal intubation.

It would seem that the toxicity from the combined therapy in this group of patients is unacceptable. We believe the potentiating effect of chemotherapy on irradiation is such that when used in combination, the dose of radiation should not exceed 3000 rads. Most of these patients received 4500 to 5000 rads. A second possible cause of toxicity may be improper administration of 5 FU. The daily dose

Table 9. Squamous cell cancer of the anal canal. 122 patients[1]

Inguinal node positive – 4 patients	
APR[2] – 3	No Operation – 1
1 – Died, distant metastases	Died, local and distant metastases
2 – NED	

[1] Questionnaire survey.
[2] Groin dissection with APR.

Table 10. Squamous cell cancer of the anal canal. 122 patients[1]. Results (1–3 years)

APR		Excision of scar		No operation	
40		40		42	
Sq. Cell	9	Alive with disease	2		
Esophageal	1	APR done later	5[2]		
Tongue	1				
Breast	1				
—		—		—	
Deaths	12	Recurrence	7	Deaths	3
NED	28	NED	38	NED	39

[1] Questionnaire survey.
[2] All NED.

suggested in this regimen should be given evenly throughout the 24 hour period. The treatment, both chemotherapy and radiation, should be given by those who are thoroughly familiar with these modalities. Therapy must be interrupted at the first sign of toxicity and resumed only when the patient has recovered.

4. Conclusions

The generally accepted treatment for invasive squamous cell cancer of the anal canal is abdominoperineal resection of the rectum. However, a regimen consisting of 5 FU and Mitomycin C plus external beam irradiation appears to be effective in the management of many patients with this disease. The evidence is derived from a series of 38 patients treated at Wayne State University Affiliated Hospitals plus a series of 122 patients treated by others and reviewed by questionnaire.

Chemoradiation therapy eradicated most primary lesions that were 6 cm. or less in greatest diameter (Fig. 5). Its effect on inguinal lymph node metastasis may be favorable when involvement is modest. However, the evidence for this is still inadequate. Extensive, bilateral involvement of the groin areas is best treated by combined therapy plus additional radiation to the groin. It is only palliative.

It may be true that high dose, external beam irradiation therapy alone administered by newer techniques and equipment can control squamous cell cancer of the anal canal without undue toxicity. The question of whether the addition of chemotherapy to more modest doses of radiation has any advantage over radiation therapy alone can be answered only by a formal randomized study.

Still, we prefer the combined approach because it permits the use of less radiation to obtain the same local effect, and because, on a theoretical basis at least, chemotherapy may act systemically to control micrometastases.

Papillon [53] has recently informed me that since 1976 he has added chemotherapy (5 FU and Mitomycin C) to his method of radiation treatment for patients with squamous cell cancer of the anal canal. He reports better results with the combined therapy.

In conclusion, we advocate chemoradiation therapy with a modest dose of radiation (3000 rads) for all patients with invasive squamous cell cancer of the anal canal. It must be given carefully and monitored closely so that it can be interrupted temporarily at the first sign of toxicity. Such attention to details permits completion of the therapy in most patients without complications. Abdominoperineal resection should be done only in patients whose primary lesion does not disappear.

It is not too farfetched to expect improvement in the systemic part of this therapy through the discovery of better chemotherapeutic drugs and perhaps the addition of new immunological strategies that appear so promising now. Any advance in this area would make abdominoperineal resection, an operation that

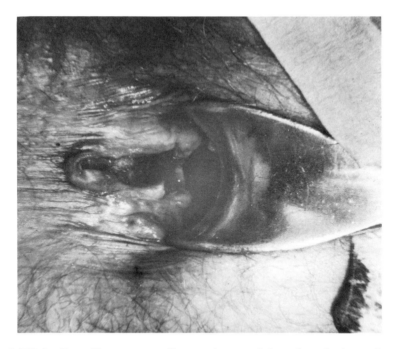

Figure 5. This is a fissure-like squamous cell cancer that extends from above the dentate line to the anus (5¹/₂ cm). Such lesions generally disappear after chemoradiation therapy alone.

results in a permanent colostomy, obsolete. While the first objective of cancer treatment is long term survival, the second is preservation of structure and function. The continued development of combined therapy has an excellant chance to achieve both these objectives in patients with invasive squamous cell cancer of the anal canal.

References

1. Gabriel WB: Squamous-cell carcinoma of the anus and anal canal: analysis of 55 cases. Proc R Soc Med 34: 139–157, 1941.
2. Morson BC: Histological typing of intestinal tumors. In collaboration with LH Sobin: International Histologic Classification of Tumors 15: 62–65, 1976.
3. Rosai J: In: Ackerman's surgical pathology. 6th edition. St. Louis, Mosby, 1981, 559–569.
4. Morson BC: The pathology and results of treatment of cancer of the anal region. Proc R Soc Med 52: 117–118, 1959.
5. McConnell EM: Squamous carcinoma of the anus: a review of 96 cases. Br J Surg 57: 89–92, 1970.
6. Hintz BL, Charyulu KKN, Sudarsanam A: Anal carcinoma: basic concepts and management. J Surg Oncol 10: 141–150, 1978.
7. Morson BC: The pathology and results of treatment of squamous cell carcinoma of the anal canal and margin. Proc R Soc Med 53: 414–420, 1960.
8. Lifshitz S, Savage JE, Yates SJ, Buchsbaum HJ: Primary epidermoid carcinoma of the vulva.

Surg Gynecol Obstet 155: 59–61, 1982.

9. Grodsky L: Rare nonkeratinizing malignancies of anal region. Arch Surg 90: 216–221, 1965.

10. Grodsky L: Bowen's disease of the anal region: squamous cell carcinoma *in situ*. Am J Surg 88: 710–714, 1954.

11. Grodsky L: Extramammary Paget's disease of the perianal region. Dis Colon Rectum 3: 502–510, 1960.

12. Helwig EB, Graham JH: Anogenital (extramammary) Paget's disease. Cancer 16: 387–403, 1963.

13. McAnally AK, Dockerty MB: Carcinoma developing in chronic draining cutaneous sinuses and fistulas. Surg Gynecol Obstet 88: 87–96, 1949.

14. Bretlau P: Carcinoma arising in anal fistula. Acta Chir Scand 133: 496–500, 1967.

15. Kline RJ, Spencer RJ, Harrison JR EG: Carcinoma associated with fistula in ano. Arch Surg 89: 989–994, 1964.

16. Grodsky L: Leukoplakia of the anus. Calif Med 84: 420–423, 1956.

17. Friedberg MJ, Serlin O: Condyloma acuminatum: its association with malignancy. Dis Colon Rectum 6: 352–355, 1963.

18. Lee SH, McGregor DH, Kuziez MN: Malignant transformation of perianal condyloma acuminatum. Dis Colon Rectum 24: 462–467, 1981.

19. Prasad ML, Abcarian H: Malignant potential of perianal condyloma acuminatum. Dis Colon Rectum 23: 191–197, 1980.

20. Stearns Jr MW, Quan SHQ: Epidermoid carcinoma of the ano-rectum. Surg Gynecol Obstet 131: 953–957, 1970.

21. Morson BC, Pang LCS: Pathology of anal cancer. Proc R Soc Med 61: 623–624, 1968.

22. Stearns Jr MW, Urmacker C, Steinberg SS, Woodruff J, Attiyeh F: Cancer of the anal canal. Curr Probl Cancer 4: 4–40, 1980.

23. Dillard BM, Sprat JS, Ackerman LV, Butcher HR: Epidermoid cancer of the anal margin and canal. Arch Surg 86: 772–777, 1963.

24. Richards JC, Beahrs OH, Woolner LB: Squamous cell carcinoma of the anus, anal canal and rectum in 109 patients. Surg Gynecol Obset 114: 475–482, 1962.

25. Kuehn PG, Eisenberg H, Reed JF: Epidermoid carcinoma of the perianal skin and anal canal. Cancer 22: 932–938, 1968.

26. Boman BM, *et al.*: Cancer of the anal canal. The Mayo Clinic experience 1950–1976 (in press).

27. Grodsky L: Unsuspected anal cancer discovered after minor anorectal surgery. Dis Colon Rectum 10: 471–478, 1967.

28. Wolfe HRI, Bussey HJR: Squamous cell carcinoma of the anus. Br J Surg 55: 295–301, 1968.

29. Sawyers JL: Squamous cell cancer of the perianus and anus. Surg Clin North Am 52: 935–941, 1972.

30. Beahrs OH, Wilson SM: Carcinoma of the anus. Ann Surg 184: 422–428, 1976.

31. Sink JD, Kramer SA, Copeland DD, Seigler HF: Cloacogenic carcinoma. Ann Surg 188: 53–59, 1978.

32. Singh R, Nime F, Mittelman A: Malignant epithelial tumors of the anal canal. Cancer 48: 411–415, 1981.

33. Hellman S, DeVita VT, Rosenberg SA: Cancer: principles and practices of oncology. Philadelphia, Lippincott, 1982, 724–731.

34. Goligher JC: Surgery of the anus rectum and colon. 4th ed. London, Balliere Tindall, 1980, 667–677.

35. Gordon-Watson C: The radium treatment of malignant disease of the rectum and anus. Proc R Soc Med 28: 53–59, 1935.

36. Dalby JE, Pointon RS: The treatment of anal carcinoma by interstitial irradiation. Am J Roentgenol 85: 515–520, 1961.

37. Papillon J: Radiation therapy in management of epidermoid carcinoma of the anal region. Dis Colon Rectum 17: 181–187, 1974.

38. Puthawala AA, Sayed AMN, *et al.*: Definitive treatment of extensive anorectal carcinoma by external and interstitial irradiation. Cancer 50: 1746–1750, 1982.

39. Rider WD: Is the Miles operation really necessary for the treatment of rectal cancer. J Can Assoc Radio 26: 167–175, 1975.

40. Kligerman MM: Radiation therapy for rectal carcinoma. Semin Oncol 3: 407–413, 1976.

41. Green JP, Schaupy WC, Cantril ST, School G: Anal carcinoma: current therapeutic concepts. Am J Surg 140: 151–155, 1980.

42. Yuhas JM, Yurconic M, Kligerman MM, *et al.*: Combined use of radioprotective and radiosensitizing drugs in experimental radiotherapy. Radiat Res 70: 433–443, 1977.

43. Lelieveld R, Smink T, VanPutten L: Experimental studies on the combination of radiation and chemotherapy. Int J Rad Onc Bio Physics 4: 37–43, 1978.

44. Looney WB, Hopkins HA, MacLeod MS, *et al.*: Solid tumor models for the assessment of different treatment modalities. XII. Combined chemotherapy-radiotherapy: variation of time interval between time of administration of 5-fluorouracil and radiation and its effect on the control of tumor growth. Cancer 44: 437–445, 1979.

45. Nigro ND, Considine B, Vaitkevicius VK: Combined therapy for cancer of the anal canal. Dis Colon Rectum 17: 354–356, 1974.

46. Newman HK, Quan SHQ: Multi-modality therapy for epidermoid carcinoma of the anus. Cancer 37: 12–19, 1976.

47. Quan SHQ, Magill GB, Leaming RH, Hajdu ST: Multi-disciplinary preoperation approach to the management of epidermoid carcinoma of the anus and anorectum. Dis Colon Rectum 21: 29–31, 1978.

48. Sischy B, Remington J, Hinson EJ, Sobel S, Woll J: Definitive treatment of anal canal carcinoma by means of radiation therapy and chemotherapy. Presented at 63rd annual meeting of American Radium Society, Phoenix, March 4–8, 1981.

49. Buroker T, Nigro ND, Bradley GT, *et al.*: Combined therapy for cancer of the anal canal: a follow-up report. Dis Colon Rectum 20: 677–679, 1977.

50. Buroker T, Nigro ND, Considine B, Vaitkevicius V: Mitomycin C, 5-fluorouracil, and radiation therapy in squamous (epidermoid) cell carcinoma of the anal canal. Mitomycin C. New York, Academic Press, 1979, 183–185.

51. Nigro ND, Vaitkevicius VK, Buroker T, *et al.*: Combined therapy for cancer of the anal canal. Dis Colon Rectum 24: 73–75, 1981.

52. Seifert P, Baker LH, Reed ML, Vaitkevicius VK: Comparison of continuously infused 5-FU with bolus injection in the treatment of colorectal adenocarcinoma. Cancer 36: 123–128, 1975.

53. Papillon J: Personal Communication, December, 1981.

10. Diagnosis and management of gut bleeding in gastrointestinal malignancy

ROBERT C. KURTZ

Introduction

Gastrointestinal bleeding represents one of the most challenging areas in medicine today. This is especially true in the patient with cancer. New techniques and approaches to the diagnosis and management of gastrointestinal bleeding are being rapidly brought into clinical practice. Gut bleeding in the cancer patient often poses special problems, which will be reviewed in this chapter.

1. Upper gastrointestinal bleeding

Upper Gastrointestinal (UGI) bleeding is usually heralded by melanotic stools and either bright-red or 'coffee-ground' emesis. When the bleeding is unusually brisk, bright-red blood or maroon-colored stool may be passed per rectum instead of melena, which may confuse the clinician as to the location of the bleeding site. When red blood is passed from the rectum as a result of an upper gastrointestinal source, hemodynamic instability almost always results.

1.1. Early endoscopy

When confronted with a patient with a presumed UGI hemorrhage, it is most helpful to know the precise cause of the bleeding so that appropriate therapy can be chosen; endoscopy evaluation can be most useful in this regard. Today's modern endoscopes are more flexible, narrower, and have greater tip control than their counterparts of several years ago, and can easily visualize the entire upper gastrointestinal tract through the postbulbar duodenum. In addition to direct visualization of upper gastrointestinal pathology, biopsy material, cytology specimens, photography, and video recording may be obtained during the course of the endoscopic evaluation.

J.J. DeCosse and P. Sherlock (eds), Clinical Management of Gastrointestinal Cancer.
© *1984, Martinus Nijhoff Publishers, Boston. ISBN 0-89838-601-2. Printed in The Netherlands.*

Endoscopic examination in the bleeding patient does not always have to be an emergency procedure, but certainly should be performed before emergency surgery wherever feasible and when the bleeding is not of such magnitude that adequate visualization is impossible. The patient should be hemodynamically stable before any attempt at endoscopy, and blood and clot should be lavaged from the stomach with saline through either a nasogastric tube or Ewald tube to permit adequate endoscopic visualization. If endoscopy is to be performed, it should be done within the first 24 hours of admission. Endoscopy can be expected to identify the site of bleeding in about 90% of patients examined within the first 48 hours. It is important, therefore, to support an aggressive diagnostic approach to the bleeding patient which demonstrates the bleeding source so that rational management decisions may be made from the outset [1, 2].

A differing point of view with regard to early endoscopy has been proposed. In the majority of patients, upper gastrointestinal bleeding will cease regardless of cause [3]. Eastwood and others [4, 5] have suggested that early endoscopic evaluation will not affect the outcome of management of gastrointestinal hemorrhage, particularly in the patient group that stops bleeding. Peterson and co-workers [6] evaluated the role of early endoscopy in a randomized, controlled trial. They randomly assigned 206 patients to routine endoscopy (100 patients) or no routine endoscopy (106 patients). The patients in the two groups were treated similarly with antacids. The 'no-endoscopy' group had endoscopy if bleeding resumed or if upper gastrointestinal x-rays showed a gastric ulcer or suggested neoplasia. The majority of the patients in both groups had peptic ulcer disease as the cause of bleeding, followed by esophageal varices, Mallory-Weiss laceration, gastritis, and gastric cancer. There was no difference in overall mortality or length of hospital stay between the two groups, and there was no difference between the two groups during a 12-month follow-up period. Although they found no benefit from early endoscopy, they also found no harm from it. About 30% of patients in both groups rebled. The more severe the initial hemorrhage, the greater the chance of rebleeding. The authors concluded that making a diagnosis had no influence on patient outcome, which is not surprising as therapy was the same in both groups. They recommended that endoscopy not be used routinely in all patients admitted with upper gastrointestinal bleeding, but should be reserved for those who rebleed or in whom gastric ulcer or tumor are seen on x-ray.

No doubt, if all patients regardless of bleeding site are managed identically, then knowing the diagnosis becomes less important. In addition, there may well be subgroups identified for whom aggressive early endoscopy may prove invaluable, especially if therapy might be different from the standard. Such a patient group would be those bleeding from esophageal varices. Conn [7], in an editorial written in response to this study, feels that physicians should not use 'all or nothing rules' to treat serious conditions. There needs to be room for judgment. This is particularly true as new therapeutic modalities for treating life-threatening gastrointestinal hemorrhage are developed.

Another value of early endoscopy in UGI bleeding is the identification of more than one bleeding site when this occurs. Iglesias and colleagues [8] evaluated 789 patients with UGI bleeding, seen over a 3-year period, who had endoscopy performed within 24 hours of admission. More than one lesion was found in approximately 45 percent of the patients. The most common lesion seen was hemorrhagic gastritis, found in 27.3% of patients.

Early endoscopy will also aid in identifying those patients with a high risk for rebleeding. One such group is the patient who has a 'visible vessel' seen in an ulcer, which is assumed to be the bleeding site. In one study [9], 28 of 317 patients who underwent endoscopy for UGI bleeding were found to have a visible vessel. Surgery was eventually recommended in all 28 patients, because of either recurrent (86%) or uncontrolled (14%) hemorrhage. In contrast, 75% of the remaining patients, whether or not they had ulcer bleeding, had only a single bleeding episode that could be managed conservatively.

It is important to restate that the knowledge gained by early endoscopy in UGI bleeding may prove invaluable for a number of reasons. 1) Subgroups at greater risk for rebleeding can clearly be identified; i.e., those with esophageal varices and where an ulcer contains a visible vessel. 2) Bleeding may be originating from more than one UGI source. 3) Therapy for various bleeding lesions is expanding and it is important to identify the bleeding site if laser or electrocoagulation, for example, are to be used. 4) Present-day endoscopic instruments are thin, easily swallowed, and yield an accurate and safe picture of the bleeding site in the vast majority of patients.

1.2. Major causes of upper gastrointestinal bleeding

1.2.1. Gastritis and stress erosions

Patients with cancer may have upper gastrointestinal bleeding related to the cancer as a result of cancer treatment or as a complication of therapy. Klein and co-workers [10], in a retrospective study at Memorial Sloan-Kettering Cancer Center (MSKCC), reviewed 49 patients with UGI bleeding severe enough to produce hematemesis, a fall in blood pressure, or a 5% drop in hematocrit. Of this group, 16 (32%) were found to have acute mucosal erosions (stress ulcers) as the cause for their bleeding. These ulcerations were quite superficial and extended down to but not through the muscularis mucosa. Endoscopy was the best way to accurately identify these lesions, as they will not be seen on barium x-rays. In every patient an identifiable contributing factor was found to cause the stress ulcer bleeding. These factors included steroids, sepsis, renal or hepatic failure, and surgery. The mortality rate for these patients approached 100%. It is interesting to note that as stress ulcer and gastritis bleeding was the most common cause of UGI bleeding in these oncology patients, it is also the most common cause of UGI bleeding in patients without cancer.

A second study from MSKCC [11], applying endoscopy, prospectively evaluated 65 patients with cancer and UGI bleeding. The majority (40%) of patients again were found to be bleeding from hemorrhagic gastritis. These patients could be further divided into two groups: those in whom exogenous agents such as steroids, alcohol, or aspirin were implicated in the development of the hemorrhagic gastritis; and, those in whom the endogenous stress of sepsis, renal or hepatic failure could be implicated as an etiologic factor of the bleeding. Those patients with endogenous stress frequently bled massively, requiring four times as many blood transfusions, and the bleeding lasted twice as long as the group with gastric irritants only.

Chait and colleagues [12] reviewed the anatomic distribution of gastric stress erosions, as seen in patients with cancer and bleeding, associated with physiological stress, exogenous gastric irritants, or both. The percentage of patients receiving chemotherapy was the same in each of the three groups. Eighty-seven patients formed the basis for this study, and 82 (95%) had cancer at the time of the bleeding episode. The most common cancers were breast, lymphoma, leukemia, colorectal, and bladder cancer. Fifteen patients (17%) had a past history of peptic ulcer disease, and these patients were distributed approximately equally among the three groups.

In the group with physiological stress, 60% of patients had erosions in the proximal stomach, 13% had distal lesions, and 27% had generalized erosions. This proximal distribution of erosions was even more dramatic (74%) in the physiologic stress group without concomitant gastric irritants. In the patients with gastric irritants alone, the distribution of erosions differed significantly ($p<0.01$) from either group of stress patients. The distribution was distal in 54%, proximal in 33%, and generalized in 13%. In none of the patients studied did the gastritis appear to be directly related to the underlying cancer.

Patients who had gastritis due to exogenous gastric irritants alone usually had a mild course and improved rapidly when the medication was withdrawn. All the patients in this group survived. The most commonly associated cancer in this group of patients was breast cancer; whereas, lymphoma and leukemia were the most commonly associated malignant diseases in patients with endogenous stress erosions.

The mechanism by which stress causes gastric ulcerations is still somewhat controversial. Reduction in mucosal blood flow has been demonstrated to cause acute stress ulceration in rabbits [13]. Menguy and co-workers have shown a significant decrease in gastric mucosal ATP-ase, which is more marked in the fundus and body of the stomach than in the antrum [14, 15]. The gastric mucosa will develop ulcerations in this setting in the presence of a critical intraluminal acid concentration, and ulceration may be further promoted by bile acids [16, 17]. Presumably, acid-back diffusion through the altered gastric mucosal barrier is the event that leads directly to the development of the gastric erosions [18]. These mechanisms are no doubt compounded in the cancer patient who is receiving cytotoxic chemotherapy, particularly those drugs that alter DNA synthesis. Experimental evidence suggests that altered DNA synthesis may also be an important mechanism in the pathogenesis of stress ulcerations in the mouse [19].

1.2.2. Peptic ulcers

Peptic ulcer disease is common in the United States. Estimates suggest that approximately 10% of the adult population will be expected to develop peptic ulcer at some time. It would, therefore, be expected that bleeding from peptic ulcer disease would be seen frequently in a population of patients with malignant disease.

In the MSKCC prospective study [11], 18 patients (22%) bled from benign peptic ulcer disease. These ulcers occurred with less than one half the frequency of the acute gastric erosions. All of the ulcers showed histologic evidence of chronicity with edematous reactive margins or fibrosis. The ulcers were approximately equally divided between stomach and duodenum. A marginal ulceration was seen in a patient who had had a subtotal gastric resection with Billroth II anastomosis for duodenal ulcer disease and who was later found to have the Zollinger-Ellison syndrome. In the duodenum, multiple small erosions were frequently seen in association with a deformed bulb, larger ulceration, or both.

The overall incidence of peptic ulcer disease and related complications of hemorrhage and perforation are declining. Brown and colleagues [20] noted an overall decrease of 26% in hospitalizations in England, Wales, and Scotland, for both duodenal (16%) and gastric ulcer (41%) over the 14-year period from 1958 to 1972. Elashoff and Grossman [21] noted similar data in the United States, where admissions for peptic ulcer disease to short-term, nonfederal hospitals during the 9-year period, 1970–1978, declined by 26% from an estimated 463,463 in 1970 to 341,743 in 1978. The decline was mainly for duodenal ulcer disease. Hospital admissions for gastric ulcer in the United States have remained relatively constant. Of particular importance over this 9-year period was a decline of 37% in ulcer patients with hemorrhage. There has also been a decline in the death rate from peptic ulcer disease due to hemorrhage and perforation, an increase in age in the peptic ulcer patient, and a steady fall in the male/female ratio to 1.2:1. The authors suggested that endoscopy may have made the diagnostic criteria for peptic ulcer disease much more stringent, that multiple admissions for the same patient may have declined, that uncomplicated duodenal ulcers may be admitted to a hospital less frequently, and that better medical and surgical management for bleeding and perforation may be responsible for the reduced death rates.

Analgesics have been implicated as a major etiologic factor in the development of chronic peptic ulcer disease and bleeding. In one nonendoscopy study [22] of aspirin use in 24 Boston hospitals, done in 1972, a possible causal relationship was found between regular 'heavy' aspirin intake and both benign gastric ulcer and major upper gastrointestinal hemorrhage. No evidence was found associating aspirin use and uncomplicated duodenal ulcer.

An Australian study [23] compared the patterns of analgesic ingestion in patients with gastric and duodenal ulcer disease with age and sex matched controls. A strong positive association was found between heavy analgesic use and chronic gastric ulcer disease. This association was most marked in women and was approximately equivalent for drugs containing either aspirin or acetaminophen. The authors found no association between chronic duodenal ulcer disease and analgesic ingestion. Aspirin and other drugs can account for the development of gastritis, and chronic gastric ulcer disease may also be related to the use of analgesic agents. These drugs are frequently part of the pain management program in patients with cancer.

On rare occasion peptic ulcerations and gastrointestinal hemorrhage may be related to non-B islet cell tumors of the pancreas that produce gastrin and massive gastric hypersecretion of acid (Zollinger-Ellison syndrome). Upper gastrointestinal tract bleeding and perforation occur frequently in these patients [24]. Serum gastrin levels may approach 1,000 pg/ml or more, and when an analysis of gastric acid output is obtained, the basal to maximal acid output ratio approximates 1:1. Ulceration may occur throughout the upper gastrointestinal tract but is most common in the duodenal bulb. When confronted with a patient with severe peptic ulcer disease and high serum gastrin levels, the diagnosis of the Zollinger-Ellison syndrome can be confirmed by either intravenous calcium or secretin-stimulated release of gastrin from the gastrinoma [25]. Treatment of patients with this syndrome is directed toward reducing gastric acid production instituting either high-dose H_2-receptor antagonists, such as cimetidine or ranitidine, or surgery. The operative procedure of choice is total gastrectomy. In one large series of patients with documented metastatic gastrinoma treated by total gastrectomy, 42% were alive at ten years compared to only 18% alive at ten years when a lesser operative procedure was performed [26].

1.2.3. Tumor as a cause for bleeding

Cancer involving the proximal gastrointestinal tract may bleed, but the frequency of cancer is less than either hemorrhagic gastritis or peptic ulcer disease. In the MSKCC study [11], 18 patients had tumor seen endoscopically in the stomach, but in only ten patients was the tumor felt to be the direct source of the bleeding. The remaining eight patients had hemorrhagic gastritis in five, esophagitis in two, and duodenal ulcer in one identified as the cause of bleeding. Four patients with primary adenocarcinoma of the stomach were in this study. In three, bleeding was coming from the cancer; in the fourth, esophagitis was the cause. There was, in addition, one patient with an ulcerated leiomyoma that bled. Metastatic tumor involving the stomach was less likely to represent the bleeding source than primary gastric cancer, with only two of nine patients with bleeding metastatic tumors (one breast carcinoma and one malignant melanoma). Lymphoma, however, when it involved the stomach, was likely to bleed, as all four of the patients seen with gastric lymphoma were bleeding from this tumor.

In general, carcinoma of the stomach does not present with massive upper gastrointestinal bleeding. More commonly, the bleeding is chronic. Stools may or may not be grossly melanotic, but they are often occult blood-positive. Significant bleeding has been reported in patients with primary gastric cancer and associated coagulopathy such as disseminated intravascular coagulation [27]. Green and colleagues [28] compared 28 patients with early gastric cancer with 130 patients with advanced disease. They found that the patients with early gastric cancer were more likely to have a history of chronic peptic ulcer disease, and presented more frequently with hematemesis and melena than their counterparts with advanced gastric cancer.

Medications may increase the risk of gastrointestinal metastasis and bleeding. Hartmann and Sherlock [29] described the phenomenon of adrenal steroids potentiating the likelihood of metastatic breast cancer spreading to the stomach or duodenum. They reviewed 204 patients who died of mestastatic breast cancer. Twenty-six had gastroduodenal metastases, of whom 24 had been receiving adrenal steroids. In the 68 patients who had not been on steroids, only two had gastroduodenal metastases. Ulceration of the metastases in the stomach and duodenum was more likely to occur in the steroid-treated group with concomitant massive hemorrhage.

Duodenal tumors are a rare cause of UGI hemorrhage. In a recent study [30], the incidence of bleeding from primary and metastatic tumors of the duodenum was less than 1% (8 of 859). Three of these eight patients had a primary duodenal neoplasm, two had metastatic involvement, and three had invasion of the duodenum by pancreatic cancer.

1.2.4. Portal hypertension and variceal bleeding

Portal hypertension and esophageal varices occur in patients with cancer, both due to chronic liver disease secondary to viral infections and alcohol, as well as tumor replacement of the liver. In patients with cancer, esophageal or gastric varices account for gastrointestinal hemorrhage only rarely but should still be considered as a diagnostic possibility, particularly if liver metastases are massive. Luna and colleagues [31] evaluated 46 consecutive patients with extensive hepatic involvement by tumor and found five patients with esophageal varices.

A retrospective MSKCC study [32] reviewed 20 years of patients' records and identified 72 patients who met radiologic, endoscopic, or postmortem criteria for esophageal varices. In all, 72 patients were identified with esophageal varices. Of these, 38% were secondary to alcoholic cirrhosis, and 12.5% related to post-necrotic cirrhosis. The remaining 52 patients were felt to have portal hypertension and varices from hepatic replacement by tumor. About one half of these (25 patients) had postmortem documentation. In 17 patients, metastatic tumor deposits were believed to be the cause of the portal hypertension. Four patients had portal vein obstruction by the cancer, and four had both metastatic cancer in the liver coupled with cirrhosis. Sixty-five % of the patients bled from their esophageal varices, and 47% developed hepatic coma during the course of their illness.

Portal or splenic venous obstruction can lead to the development of esophageal varices. Three of the four patients with portal vein obstruction had hepatocellular carcinoma. Albacete, *et al.* [33] found 8 of 25 patients (32%) with hepatoma to have portal vein obstruction. Pancreatic cancer can also cause portal or splenic vein obstruction with subsequent esophageal varices [34].

Hepatic veno-occlusive disease, when chronic, can lead to portal hypertension and esophageal varices. The entity of veno-occlusive disease is being described as a complication of allogenic bone marrow transplantation, performed as treatment for leukemia and complicated by graft versus host disease [35]. Varices have not been described in this complication. Most of these patients died of hepatic failure and did not develop chronic hepatic disease, although one patient in this series died with gastrointestinal bleeding, azotemia, coagulation abnormalities, and shock.

1.2.5. Esophagitis

Esophagitis, caused by acid reflux through an incompetent lower esophageal sphincter, rarely causes massive UGI hemorrhage but may represent a source of chronic blood loss. This problem may be further compounded by drugs that have an anticholinergic effect on the lower esophageal sphincter; the use of prolonged nasogastric intubation in the supine patient; operative procedures that remove the lower esophageal sphincter, such as an esophagogastrectomy for cardio-esophageal cancer; and, the use of prosthetic endoluminal tubes, such as a Celestin tube to maintain esophageal patency as palliation for esophageal cancer. Bile reflux in patients who have had major gastric resections may also cause both severe inflammation in the gastric remnant and a bleeding esophagitis.

There are infectious agents that will also cause severe esophagitis, particularly in the immunocompromised patient. Perhaps the best-known of the infectious forms of esophagitis is esophageal candidiasis. In a study done at MSKCC, Eras, Goldstein, and Sherlock [36] reviewed over 2,500 autopsy protocols and found 109 patients who had evidence of gastrointestinal involvement with fungus. They divided their patients into those who had leukemia or lymphoma and those with solid tumors. There were 76 patients with fungal infection and either lymphoma or leukemia, whereas there were only 33 patients in the solid tumor group. The esophagus and stomach were the most frequently involved single sites, and the esophagus was involved as well in all but six patients with multiple sites of involvement. Gastrointestinal bleeding, as a result of fungal involvement of the esophagus occurred in 20 of 70 patients and represented the most common symptom of fungal esophagitis. In one patient, a fungal ulceration eroded into a major blood vessel.

The diagnosis of Candida esophagitis should be considered when an immuno-suppressed patient complains of dysphagia or odynophagia, with or without upper gastrointestinal bleeding. The presence of characteristic lesions of thrush in the mouth or posterior pharynx may be helpful. The characteristic findings on barium esophagram include a shaggy appearance of the distal esophagus and filling defects or poor coating of the mucosa by the barium. Fluoroscopy or cine radiography studies may show hypomotility. A barium esophagram will miss some patients with fungal esophagitis, and endoscopy should be considered if the diagnosis is unclear. The endoscopic appearance is characteristic, and biopsy and brush cytology smears will usually confirm the presence of Candida.

Candida agglutinin titers may also be helpful in the diagnosis of Candida esophagitis, since titers are frequently elevated above 1:160 [37]. In general, studies of immunologic function in patients with Candida esophagitis have shown normal humoral immunity with defects in the cell-mediated immune system. Control of the esophagitis usually parallels the response of the underlying lymphoma or leukemia to therapy. In addition, oral nystatin suspension may be used, but often 'low-dose' amphotericin B is required to treat the infection.

Viral infections of the esophagus, particularly herpes simplex virus, may occur concomitantly with a Candida infection. This is often a preterminal event in a severely immunocompromised patient. The symptoms of herpes esophagitis can be indistinguishable from those of Candida infection and include dysphagia, odynophagia, and ulcerations with serious bleeding [38]. In a series at MSKCC [39], 25 patients with herpetic esophagitis were reported where the esophagus was the only organ in which herpes viral inclusions were noted. Almost all of the patients studied had either lymphoma or leukemia. Esophagoscopy can aid in identifying herpetic ulcerations, and confirmation may be made by brush cytology or biopsy, particularly of the mucosa adjacent to the ulcerations where typical herpes inclusions are found [40]. Complement-fixing antibodies may also be useful. Therapy for herpes virus infections is still experimental with drugs, such as arabinosyl ademine (ARA-A), 2'fluoro-5-iodo-arabinosylcytosine (FIAC), or interferon.

1.2.6. Mallory-Weiss syndrome

In 1929, Mallory and Weiss [41] described the autopsy findings in four patients who died from massive gastrointestinal hemorrhage due to lacerations of the gastric mucosa near the cardioesophageal junction. These lacerations were felt to be secondary to the rapidly rising, high intragastric pressures associated with hiatus hernia, retching, or vomiting, and the use of alcohol, aspirin, or both. The lacerations were most commonly in the stomach and were associated with other gastric lesions, which could have been the reason for retching in 83% of instances. Blood loss was often substantial, but medical management was successful in all but five patients (8.5%).

In patients who continue to bleed or who rebleed, angiotherapy may be attempted preoperatively. Fifteen such patients were treated with intraarterial vasopressin or arterial embolization. Permanent hemostasis was achieved in the majority of patients so treated [43]. Chemotherapy and radiation therapy will often cause nausea, vomiting, and retching. No doubt Mallory-Weiss tears of the gastric and esophageal mucosa will be seen more frequently in the oncologic population as drug therapy becomes more aggressive.

1.3. Prevention and drug treatment of upper gastrointestinal hemorrhage

1.3.1. Growth hormone

As gastric stress erosions and hemorrhagic gastritis represent the most important source of UGI bleeding in the cancer patient, a number of pharmacologic agents have been studied in attempts to halt or prevent this type of life-threatening hemorrhage. Bovine growth hormone was shown to have a beneficial effect on prevention and healing of restraint-induced gastric ulcerations in rats [44]. Eight patients at MSKCC, with cancer and massive hemorrhage from stress ulcers, were treated with human growth hormone [45]. Bleeding stopped in six. The two patients in whom bleeding was not controlled died. The authors speculated that the deleterious effect of stress on gastric mucosal nucleic acid, protein synthesis, and cell proliferation could be counteracted by the beneficial stimulating effect of growth hormone.

1.3.2. Antacids and cimetidine

Other pharmacological approaches to upper gastrointestinal bleeding have been directed to reduction or neutralization of gastric acid applying H_2-receptor antagonists such as cimetidine and ranitidine, antacids, and prostaglandins. Simonian and Curtis [46] administered large quantities of antacids to completely neutralize gastric acid in patients with active bleeding from stress ulcerations. They advocate starting with 60 ml of antacid by nasogastric tube, to be followed by 30 ml every 15 minutes until the total hourly dose necessary to maintain intragastric pH at 7 or higher was determined. This was as much as 180 ml of antacid per hour, which was given by tube after the contents of the stomach were aspirated. The hourly dose of antacids was continued for 24 hours and then decreased to every 2 to 4 hours if the bleeding stopped. Applying this technique, the authors successfully stopped the bleeding in 44 of 49 patients (89%). This study was uncontrolled, and it is quite possible that the success rate might have been achievable without high-dose antacids. Additionally, such large volumes of antacids might create problems with aspiration in critically ill patients.

H_2-receptor antagonists, such as cimetidine, have been used to stop hemorrhage from upper gastrointestinal sources, such as gastric stress erosions and gastric and duodenal ulcers. Cimetidine and related compounds, such as metiamide and ranitidine, act as a specific competitive blocking agent of histamine on the gastric parietal cell, and substantial reduction in both basal and stimulated gastric acid secretion is produced. MacDonald and associates [47], in an uncontrolled prospective study, treated 11 patients with documented bleeding from hemorrhagic gastritis. In nine patients, the bleeding was controlled.

In another study, nonrandomized and retrospective, 13 patients bleeding from hemorrhagic gastritis were treated with varying doses of cimetidine [48]. The majority received 300 mg of cimetidine intravenously every 6 hours. After the bleeding stopped, they received 300 mg every 8 hours until they died or were discharged. Twelve of the thirteen patients stopped bleeding. Three of the twelve rebled, of whom two required surgery to control the hemorrhage. Nine of the 13 patients eventually died, but only one died of hemorrhage. The authors concluded that cimetidine is a safe and effective way to halt stress ulcer bleeding.

In a controlled trial, Pichard, et al. [49] used cimetidine to treat patients with bleeding gastric and duodenal ulcers. Rebleeding occurred in 8 out of 17 patients treated with cimetidine and in 8 out of 22 patients treated with placebo. Hoare and colleagues [50], in a controlled, prospective trial in 66 patients, found mixed results. They found no effect on the rebleeding rate in patients with duodenal ulcers, but there did appear to be some advantage to cimetidine in the patients bleeding from gastric ulcer disease. In another randomized, controlled study, Kayasseh, et al. [51] compare somatostatin and cimetidine in the treatment of severe, persistent bleeding from peptic ulceration. They treated 20 patients, each receiving either cimetidine or somatostatin. In seven of the ten pairs of patients, somatostatin was more effective; in 2 pairs, both drugs were ineffective; and in 1 pair, cimetidine appeared more beneficial.

It would appear from the above studies that there is still a great deal of debate as to whether or not antacids and H_2-receptor blocking agents will halt the bleeding found in patients with peptic ulcer disease and hemorrhagic gastritis.

The prevention of stress ulcer or hemorrhagic gastritis bleeding is another area where trials of these drugs, alone and in combination, have been ongoing. In 1977, MacDougall, Baley, and Williams [52], in a controlled, prospective study, treated 75 patients with fulminant hepatic failure with antacids or cimetidine (or metiamide). Only 1 of 26 patients in the cimetidine group bled, whereas 13 patients of 24 (54%) in the control group bled. The results were highly significant (p<0.001). Of note, cimetidine was infused continuously in this study, and intragastric pH was maintained at 5 or higher.

Hastings and colleagues [53], in Boston, studied the effectiveness of antacids in a controlled, randomized trial of 100 patients admitted to the Respiratory-Surgical Intensive Care Unit of the Beth Israel Hospital over a 5-year period. They used an initial dose of 30 ml of antacid and checked the pH of the gastric contents on an hourly basis. They instilled 30 ml of antacid hourly if the pH was 3.5 or higher and 60 ml if the pH was less than 3.5. Fifty-one patients were randomized to receive the antacid therapy, and 49 were in the control group. Only two patients developed upper gastrointestinal bleeding on antacids (3.9%), whereas 12 patients (24.5%) in the control group bled. The difference was statistically significant (p <0.005). They also showed that as the number of risk factors for hemorrhagic gastritis increased, the chance of bleeding also increased. Among those patients in whom four or more risk factors were present (respiratory failure, sepsis, peritonitis, jaundice, renal failure, or hypotension), the frequency of bleeding was 40% without antacids versus 10.5% with antacids (p<0.05).

An uncontrolled, retrospective study from Minnesota [54] examined the use of Vivonex, an elemental standard diet, in conjunction with antacids in preventing stress ulcerations (Curling's ulcers) in burn patients. They studied 106 patients who survived longer than 8 days. Only three patients developed clinically evident Curling's ulcer, but 30% developed 2, 3, or 4 plus guaiac-positive nasogastric aspirates. The authors concluded that 'intense' antacid therapy protected against clinically evident Curling's ulcer.

Jones and colleagues [55] used cimetidine prospectively and evaluated 35 consecutive patients who had renal transplantation. Their starting dose was 200 mg intravenously every 12 hours. The dose was tailored to renal function and was given orally when appropriate. These patients did not receive antacids routinely. All patients were receiving Prednisone and azathioprine. This group was compared to a retrospective control group. After eliminating several postoperative deaths, 30 patients were followed for 4 months post-surgery. None of the 30 patients who were treated with cimetidine bled, whereas 6 of 33 in the retrospective control group bled. The authors concluded that the prophylactic use of cimetidine in this population was worthwhile.

Another controlled, prospective study, reported in 1980, evaluated cimetidine prophylaxis for stress ulcer bleeding in patients with severe head trauma [56]. Twenty-six patients were randomized into the cimetidine group and 24 in the control group. All patients received steroids and anticonvulsant therapy. The mean volume of secretion and titratable gastric acid increased in the control group on the third and sixth day after injury. Values for both of these were reduced in the cimetidine group. The gastric pH was 3.5 or higher in 65% of the cimetidine group, compared with 18% in the control group. Five of the 26 patients (19%) in the cimetidine group had gastrointestinal bleeding. Eighteen of the 24 control patients (75%) had bleeding, and in eight the bleeding episode was significant ranging from 2 to 24 units of blood. Endoscopy was performed in 14 of the 26 patients treated with cimetidine. Five had gastritis, two had gastroesophageal junction ulceration, and one had a prepyloric antral ulcer. Eleven of the 24 control patients underwent endoscopy. Six had gastritis, one had duodenitis, and one had a deep ulcer which eventually perforated. Cimetidine prophylaxis did not appear to reduce the development of mucosal lesions, but significantly reduced the risk of bleeding from these lesions.

At this point it would appear that either antacids or cimetidine are effective in lowering gastric acid secretion and preventing bleeding in the critically-ill patient. Is there an advantage of one drug over the other? Priebe and colleagues [57] addressed this question, updating data reported by Hastings [53] two years earlier. They again used the patients admitted to the Respiratory-Surgical Intensive Care Unit at Beth Israel Hospital in Boston. They randomized 75 patients to either antacids (37 patients) or cimetidine (38 patients), and there was no difference between the characteristics of either group. In the cimetidine group, failure to achieve a pH of 3.5 or greater on one or more occasion occurred in 18 patients who were started on this drug at a dose of 300 mg every 6 hours and in nine given 300 mg every 4 hours. Seven of eight patients who required 400 mg of cimetidine every 4 hours had a pH less than 3.5 on one or more determinations, even at this higher dosage. In contrast, failure to achieve an intragastric pH at 3.5 or more occurred in nine patients started on 30 ml of antacid hourly, in 6 on 60 ml, and 1 started on 120 ml. However, when all of the pH measurements were tabulated, the gastric pH was less than 3.5 in only 1.7 percent. The results of this study showed that seven of the 38 cimetidine-treated patients bled, whereas none of the antacid-treated patients had bleeding ($p < 0.01$). The authors concluded that cimetidine was less effective than antacids and speculated that the active secretory state of the gastric mucosa is what protects it from injury. Thus 'turning off' the secretory capacity of the gastric mucosa with cimetidine would be a less effective way to reduce the risk of stress ulcer bleeding than simply neutralizing the acid after it has been produced. Perhaps this is related to the buffering effect of the bicarbonate produced during active mucosal acid secretion and its presence in the mucosa.

A similar study done in Seattle [58], showed that antacids offered a consistent effect against gastric acidity and were 100% effective in maintaining a pH of 4 or greater. Cimetidine, in the standard dose of 300 mg 4 times daily, was effective in only 47% of patients and at maximal dose in only 74% of patients. It would, therefore, appear that antacids given orally or by nasogastric tube hourly to keep the gastric pH at 3.5 to 4 or higher is the method of choice to prevent stress-induced upper gastrointestinal bleeding. Care must be taken, however, that complications secondary to the antacid therapy do not occur. Antacids can cause hypermagnesemia in patients with renal failure; if there is sufficient volume in the stomach, aspiration may occur, and, antacids in large quantities have been associated with diarrhea which if severe enough may create problems in an intensive care unit setting.

1.3.3. Prostaglandins

Prostaglandins have been shown to protect the gastric mucosa against several forms of experimental injury [59]. Robert and colleagues [60] have shown that small intragastric amounts of prostaglandin, instilled about one minute before such noxious agents as absolute ethanol, boiling water, strong acid, and alkali, can protect the gastric mucosa. Prostaglandins can inhibit acid production, but the mechanism of cytoprotection is probably different from that of acid inhibition. The cytoprotective dose may be too small to inhibit acid secretion. These compounds would seem to be ideal to use both in the therapy of active stress ulcer bleeding, as well as in stress ulcer prophylaxis. Such studies in humans are presently underway and until such time as the effectiveness and safety of prostaglandin in these situations has been established the use of these compounds will remain experimental.

1.3.4. Vasopressin (Pitressin)

Vasopressin has been used for control of both variceal and nonvariceal upper gastrointestinal bleeding. After selective superior mesenteric artery catheterization, Baum and Nusbaum [61] reported the successful control of upper gastrointestinal hemorrhage when vasopressin was infused intraarterially. Athanasoulis and co-workers [62] performed angiography in 50 patients with gastric mucosal hemorrhage. The diagnosis was based on endoscopic findings in 10 patients, angiography in 28 patients, both procedures in 10, and surgery in 2 patients. In 37 patients, vasopressin was infused selectively into the bleeding artery, and the hemorrhage was controlled both clinically and angiographically in 31 (84%). Only two of these patients developed rebleeding. Four of the six patients who could not be controlled had surgery. In the remaining 13 patients, infusion with vasopressin could not be performed, due either to technical reasons or to other associated conditions. Ten of these 13 patients had surgery. This group included 27 patients with true stress-induced gastric erosions, as well as ulcerations associated with anti-inflammatory drugs and ethanol. There were two patients who had Mallory-Weiss tears. There were no major complications of the vasopressin therapy that necessitated cessation of the infusion. In four patients, the infusion had a definite antidiuretic hormone effect.

It is assumed that vasopressin infusion into the left gastric artery reduces blood flow to the stomach and causes cessation of the gastric mucosal hemorrhage. Complications of infusional therapy with vasopressin can occur and generally are either cardiac or vascular in nature.

Conn and co-workers [63], in New Haven, evaluated intraarterial vasopressin in a prospective controlled trial. They treated a total of 60 episodes of upper gastrointestinal hemorrhage. Thirty-eight patients had conventional management, and vasopressin was administered in 28 patients. The majority of patients in both groups had either documented or suspected variceal bleeding. The vasopressin group was successfully managed in 20 instances (71%), whereas conventional therapy was successful in 9 (28%). The difference was statistically significant (p <0.001). Transfusion requirements were significantly lower in the vasopressin group. The response to therapy with vasopressin, however, did not influence the overall survival.

Another controlled study from New Haven [64] compared the use of continuous intraarterial infusions of vasopressin with the same drug administered intravenously in treating patients with hemorrhage from esophageal varices. Twenty-two patients were randomized. The intraarterial vasopressin group was started at $0.1\,\mu$/minute and increased, as necessary, up to $0.5\,\mu$/minute. Intravenous vasopressin was begun at 0.5 μ/minute and increased in steps up to a maximum dose of 1.5 μ/minute. Hemorrhage was controlled in 50% of bleeding episodes in both groups. Mortality for the intravenous-treated group was 70%, and mortality in the group given intraarterial vasopressin was 75%. Serious complications occurred in three patients in each group and were either cardiovascular, pulmonary, or infectious. Since the effectiveness and complication rates of both routes of administration of vasopressin are similar, the authors recommended use of the intravenous method. It is much easier and can be used early in the management as a brief therapeutic trial.

Recently a placebo-controlled trial of intravenous vasopressin was reported [65]. In this study 60 patients were randomized to either 40 μ/hour of intravenous vasopressin or placebo. Six hours after the beginning of the infusion, 13 patients in the vasopressin group and 11 in the placebo group had stopped bleeding. By 24 hours, 17 in the vasopressin group and 14 in the placebo group had stopped bleeding. There was little difference in the two groups as far as number of units of blood transfused, number of patients needing surgery, or the number of deaths. Even when analysis of the two groups was restricted to variceal bleeding, no difference was noted. The authors concluded that continuous intravenous infusion of vasopressin does not help to control bleeding or change the clinical outcome.

1.3.5. Embolic therapy

Embolizing the artery supplying the bleeding point may be considered for bleeding ulcers or tumors in the patient who is a poor surgical risk. This can be performed by injecting small bits of Gelfoam or autologous clot intraarterially through the angiography catheter at the time of the arteriogram. This procedure carries with it the risk of infarction of the tissue in the distribution of the artery embolized, and it requires considerable expertise. Embolic occlusions might be an alternative therapeutic method to intraarterial drug infusion for controlling bleeding from lesions, such as Mallory-Weiss mucosal tear, hemorrhagic gastritis, or tumor.

1.4. Endoscopic methods of controlling bleeding

A variety of new techniques have been developed for the control of upper gastrointestinal hemorrhage utilizing fiberoptic endoscopy. These techniques include laser photocoagulation, topical sprays, electrocoagulation, thermal probes, and topical injections. Perhaps the most difficult part of the endoscopic management of upper gastrointestinal bleeding is visualizing the bleeding site. This will often require careful saline lavage until a discrete bleeding point is identified, and a continuous saline or CO_2 jet spray to keep the bleeding point clear.

1.4.1. Laser photocoagulation

The word LASER is an acronym for *L*ight *A*mplification by *S*timulated *E*mission of *R*adiation. The energy of the monochromatic light emitted by the laser can be directed by way of a fiberoptic probe through an endoscope toward a discrete bleeding point. This energy, measured in watts, will be absorbed by blood and tissue and cause coagulation of protein. There are two types of laser currently being studied for endoscopic use; the neodymium-yttrium-aluminium-garnet (Nd:YAG) laser, and the argon laser.

The argon laser has a shorter wavelength and emits a blue-green light, which is readily absorbed by red-colored tissues such as blood. It is usually used with a coaxial jet of CO_2 gas which aids in keeping the target free of fresh blood so that all of the argon laser's energy can be directed to the bleeding vessel.

The Nd:YAG laser has a longer wavelength, but its energy is also readily absorbed on red surfaces. It will penetrate tissue substantially deeper than the argon laser and has a much greater power output. Both the argon laser and the Nd:YAG laser can be used efficiently and safely to stop ulcer bleeding in experimental animals. There have been uncontrolled studies that purport to demonstrate the usefulness of the laser in stopping gastrointestinal hemorrhage in man, as well [66, 67]. Controlled studies have also been done. The most recent one, from Leuven, Belgium [68], studied 152 patients. The first 23 patients were studied in an uncontrolled fashion. Where arterial spurting was encountered, bleeding could be stopped by Nd:YAG laser therapy in 87%. However, there was a high rate of recurrent bleeding (55%), and 61% of this group required surgery.

The next group of 129 patients were randomized to either receive Nd:YAG laser treatment or conservative management. In 86 patients in the control study, the Nd:YAG laser was significantly better ($p < 0.001$) in stopping bleeding of the nonspurting variety than conservative measures. The rate of bleeding and the need for eventual surgery was not statistically different between the laser and the control groups. In 43 patients with 'stigmata of recent hemorrhage', either fresh clot or visible vessel, there was no statistical benefit from laser therapy, and mortality rates were not influenced in any of the groups. The majority of bleeding sites in all groups were gastric and duodenal ulcers or erosions followed by Mallory-Weiss tears. Only one patient in the control group was bleeding from a stomach cancer.

Vallon and colleagues [69] applied the argon laser and evaluated 28 spurting lesions with concurrent controls. Although their data suggest that the argon laser is effective in stopping such bleeding, statistical significance was not reached. They also studied 78 patients in whom the bleeding had ceased. Again there was no statistical significance between the control or treatment groups; rebleeding rates were similar for both groups.

It would appear from these two studies that laser therapy is safe and reasonably effective in stopping the bleeding from 'spurting' peptic ulcer, but the need for surgery and overall mortality is not substantially changed. To date, laser treatment is still experimental and should only be used in the setting of clinical trials. As additional data is forthcoming, it is hoped that the precise benefits and indications for laser therapy will be defined.

1.4.2. Electrocoagulation

Because of the relatively inexpensive and readily available equipment, physicians have had a much wider clinical experience with electrocoagulation than with laser therapy. Electrosurgery is used endoscopically for polypectomy and papillotomy where coagulation currents and mixed cutting and coagulation wave forms are used. Either monopolar or bipolar electrodes may be passed through the biopsy channels in the fiberoptic endoscope and appropriate current applied to the observed bleeding site. The bipolar electrode has the potential for less tissue injury than the monopolar electrode. In a review, Papp [70] noted that endoscopic electrocoagulation was successful in 98 percent of his patients so treated. Unfortunately, these studies have been for the most part uncontrolled.

Papp [71] recently published a controlled study of electrocoagulation instituted whenever a visible vessel was seen in an ulcer at the time of diagnostic endoscopy. Between 1977 and 1979, 103 patients with ulcer disease were seen of whom 32 were found to have a visible vessel. Sixteen patients each were randomized to the control or electrocoagulation group. The 16 patients in the control group received cimetidine and antacids. Thirteen patients (81%) in this group rebled. Nine went to surgery, four required eventual electrocoagulation, and one patient in the control group died. The electrocoagulation group fared much better in that only one out of the 16 rebled (6%) and required surgery. There were no deaths nor were there any complications of the electrocoagulation. Follow-up endoscopy, done 8 weeks after the electrocoagulation, showed complete ulcer healing in all patients. The length of hospital stay and cost of hospitalization were reduced in the electrocoagulation group. Papp recommended that monopolar electrocoagulation should be an availabe tool to the endoscopist who manages patients with upper gastrointestinal bleeding.

Complications, such as perforation, do occur with the monopolar electrode. Additional studies enrolling larger numbers of patients will be necessary to fully define the role of electrocoagulation in gastrointestinal bleeding.

1.4.3. Endoscopic sclerosis of varices

A rebirth of interest in endoscopic sclerotherapy for esophageal varices is occurring. The original idea dates back to 1939 [72]. The flexible fiberoptic endoscope is now applied, and several different sclerosing agents have been tried. Perhaps the largest experience has been with sodium morrhuate and ethanolamine. Virtually all of the sucessful reports on the use of sclerotherapy have been uncontrolled studies. In 1980, a prospective trial was published [73]. In this study, 64 patients were randomized to medical management [28] versus sclerotherapy [36]. The patients were evenly distributed in terms of the Child's classification. A flexible esophageal sheath was used together with the fiberoptic endoscope so that the varix to be injected could be isolated and protrude into the lumen. Ethanolamine was the sclerosing agent used. Rebleeding occurred in 12 (33%) of the sclerotherapy group and 19 (68%) of the control group. The risk of bleeding per patient-month of follow-up decreased more than threefold in the sclerotherapy group, and the number of patients rebleeding at 2, 6, and 12 months was reduced significantly ($p<0.05$). The 12-month survival was also statistically significant for the sclerotherapy group (46% versus 6%) ($p<0.02$).

A second report from the same group was published in 1982 [74]. They added an additional 43 patients to the study and extended the follow-up for the original group of patients to 4 years. Again, the control and treatment group were similarly composed. In the sclerotherapy group, 22 (43%) had further episodes of bleeding with follow-up of up to 44 months (mean 14.4 months). When rebleeding occurred, it was almost always before complete obliteration of the varices was achieved. Of the 42 patients who lived long enough to have complete obliteration of their varices, episodes of rebleeding occurred in only four. In the control group rebleeding occurred in 42 of the 56 patients (75%), a significantly higher percentage ($p<0.01$). Survival data showed that 75% of the sclerotherapy group were alive at one year compared to 58% in the control group. This difference too was significant. A total of 240 courses of injections were given during the trial, and 21 patients had complications consisting of esophageal ulcerations (15 patients) and strictures (9 patients). Two patients developed perforation of the esophagus.

As Graham and Smith [75] pointed out in a review of 85 consecutive variceal bleeders, substantially better long-term survival must result from improved survival during the early period after the bleeding episode. It is quite possible that sclerotherapy may just do that. Virtually all of the studies on various modalities of treating bleeding esophageal varices are based on cirrhotic patients. Because the incidence of bleeding esophageal varices secondary to metastatic or primary liver cancer is minute by comparison, one can only extrapolate the usefulness of sclerotherapy to the cancer population. It would, however, seem to represent an inexpensive and safe way to control variceal hemorrhage in this group of patients.

2. Small intestinal bleeding

As with upper gastrointestinal bleeding, hemorrhage from a source distal to the ligament of Treitz may be a direct result of malignancy, may be related to therapy for malignancy, or totally unrelated to the underlying cancer. Small intestinal bleeding is much less common that UGI bleeding, and is also much more difficult to identify.

2.1. Causes

Briley and colleagues [76] studied 305 patients with gastrointestinal hemorrhage. The vast majority (259) were bleeding from an upper gastrointestinal source. Only 2 of the 259 were shown on angiography to be bleeding from a small intestinal source. Of the 46 patients who presented with an acute lower gastro-intestinal bleed, 14 (30.4%) had an angiographically demonstrated bleeding site in the small bowel. The sources of small bowel bleeding were primary tumor (3), vascular malformation (3), aorto-enteric fistula (2), trauma (2), metastatic tumor (1), ulcer (2), enteritis (1), tuberculous ileitis (1), and sarcoidosis (1). The authors were somewhat surprised that, in an angiographic study, approximately 30% of patients with presumed large bowel bleeding were in reality bleeding from a small intestinal site.

2.1.1. Primary tumors of the small bowel

Adenocarcinoma of the small bowel is a distinctly uncommon form of cancer. In a recent review, 338 patients with adenocarcinoma of the small bowel were found in the Connecticut Tumor Registry over a 33-year period (1935–1978), or about 10 patients per year [77]. The presenting symptoms were usually related to intestinal obstruction, but anemia from either gross or occult blood loss occurred in over 70% of patients in a New York series [78]. Perhaps even more important, 17 of the 43 patients analyzed had 'unexplained' gastrointestinal bleeding. Primary lymphoma of the small intestine may present with occult fecal blood loss or may present with profound anemia due to malabsorption of iron, folate, or Vitamin B_{12}. Leiomyoma and leiomyosarcoma of the small bowel may develop central ulcerations and bleed in a similar fashion to their counterparts in the stomach. This point was also emphasized by Darling and Welch [79]. One common error in diagnosing small intestinal tumors is that a barium upper gastrointestinal series may be ordered with films following the barium column, stopping just distal to the ligament of Treitz, missing the more distal small bowel tumor. The sensitivity of the barium meal in detecting small intestinal tumors will vary with the ability and interest of the radiologist performing the study.

Carcinoid tumors of the small bowel are perhaps the most common small bowel tumor found at autopsy. They rarely cause symptoms and rarely bleed. A recent report [80] described a 55-year-old man who had numerous massive bleeding episodes due to multiple small ileal carcinoid tumors. Extensive endoscopic and radiologic preoperative studies failed to identify the bleeding source in this patient.

2.1.2. Metastatic small bowel tumors

The small bowel is the site of metastatic implants far more frequently than the stomach and colon. This may relate to its greater surface area. As with primary small bowel tumors, they present with either obstruction, bleeding, or both.

Melanoma is the most common tumor to spread to the small bowel [81]. Often, no primary lesion can be identified, or the melanoma may have been removed surgically many years before [82]. Melanoma metastases to the small bowel are frequently multiple. Barium x-rays will show characteristic intraluminal polypoid masses, occasionally with a central ulceration, producing a 'bulls-eye' or 'target' appearance [83]. Breast cancer will also commonly spread to the small bowel, and as with gastric metastasis from breast cancer, this appears to occur more commonly in women who have been treated with adrenal steroids [29]. Tumors that spread to retroperitoneal lymph nodes, such as germ-cell tumors of the testis, can involve the small bowel, and as with other types of metastatic tumors, these tumors can cause obstruction and bleeding, if the mucosa is involved [84].

2.1.3. Cancer therapy

Cancer treatment may also be responsible for small intestinal bleeding. The mucosa of the small intestine is quite radiosensitive, and abdominal radiation much above 4,500 to 5,000 rads may cause significant damage. Early symptoms of radiation bowel damage may include nausea and vomiting, but often diarrhea or constipation may also occur. Bleeding may occur either early or late, and rarely be massive [85]. Malabsorption may also occur, as well as enteric fistula, and anemia in patients with longstanding radiation enteritis may be related to this feature.

2.2. Diagnosis of occult small bowel bleeding

Barium small intestinal x-rays, as well as small bowel enema are important initial diagnostic steps in detecting small intestinal bleeding lesions. However, they are not always accurate. When there is continuous occult gastrointestinal bleeding and a small intestinal source is suspected, a tube aspiration test may be performed. A narrow, long tube with a mercury-weighted tip and aspiration holes is swallowed. As the tube progresses through the small bowel, material is periodically aspirated and tested for occult blood. When blood is detected, barium is swallowed, and careful spot films of the small intestine are obtained near the tip of the tube. An alternate test is the string test. A weighted string is swallowed and allowed to pass the length of the small bowel. It is then retrieved and tested chemically for blood. When bleeding is more active and acute, angiography will often identify the small bowel source [76]. Radionuclide scanning is also becoming more widely applied, primarily for lower gastrointestinal hemorrhage.

3. Large intestinal bleeding

Bright-red rectal bleeding may pose a difficult management problem. Misinterpretation of rectal bleeding by the physician can lead to the diagnosis of unimportant sources of bleeding, such as hemorrhoids or fissures, while a major, more proximal, lesion such as a cancer may be overlooked. Patients tend to underestimate the seriousness of rectal bleeding, particularly if they have had multiple episodes over many months or years, which may have been attributed to hemorrhoids, perhaps due to incomplete evaluation.

Most patients presenting with rectal bleeding can be placed into one of two groups, dependent on the severity of the bleeding episode. The most common group is that of submassive hemorrhage, which theoretically can range from an occasional drop or two of blood on the toilet tissue to substantial rectal bleeding, requiring hospitalization for observation and perhaps blood transfusion. The amount of bleeding is less than 1,500 ml in 24 hours, and the patients are generally hemodynamically stable.

The second, less common type of bleeding is massive hemorrhage. Here bleeding is more than the arbitrary 1,500 ml in 24 hours, and the patient is often hemodynamically unstable. These patients will require immediate medical attention directed to volume replacement with blood products and then diagnostic procedures. The importance of categorizing the bleeding patient is primarily for the selection and sequencing of the most appropriate diagnostic studies.

3.1. Major causes of large bowel hemorrhage

3.1.1. Colonic diverticulosis
Colonic diverticulosis is a common cause of submassive colonic bleeding and the most common cause of massive colonic bleeding, accounting for approximately 70% of these episodes [86]. Diverticulosis is a common finding in asymptomatic older patients in our society. The incidence of bleeding from diverticulosis ranges from 10% to 30%, with massive hemorrhage occurring in about 5% [87]. It is indeed fortunate that in 95% of patients diverticular bleeding stops spontaneously.

The pathogenesis of diverticular bleeding is not well understood, Meyers and colleagues [88], using arteriographic and microangiographic techniques, localized the site of bleeding in eight of ten patients studied. Serial histological sections identified consistent changes, which included absence of diverticulitis and asymmetric rupture and intimal thickening of the vas rectum near the bleeding point. These findings suggested that trauma to the diverticulum predisposed to rupture and bleeding. Evaluation of bleeding due to diverticulosis will depend on the rapidity and amount of blood loss, and is discussed in the sections on submassive and massive bleeding.

3.1.2. Large bowel cancer and polyps
Cancer of the large bowel, particularly in the rectum and left colon, will cause

rectal bleeding. The bleeding is almost always submassive. Cancers involving the right colon are more likely to produce melanotic stools or occult bleeding with gradual development of iron deficiency anemia. Colonic polyps may also present with bright-red rectal bleeding or occult blood loss (which can be determined by fecal occult blood testing). As with colon cancer, presentation is often dependent on size and location in the colon. Evaluation of such bleeding should involve sigmoidoscopy, air-contrast barium enema, and colonoscopy. Angiography is rarely needed. Bleeding should not automatically be attributed to the presence of hemorrhoids or diverticulosis, because up to 50% of these patients may have concomitant colon polyps or cancer.

Attempts have been made to quantitate fecal blood loss in the presence of colonic polyps. In a recent study [89], Cr^{51}-labeled red blood cells were injected intravenously in 44 patients with colonic polyps, and in 11 control patients the quantitative fecal blood loss was compared with a stool Hemoccult test. A total of 642 stool specimens were analyzed. The mean daily fecal blood loss in 34 patients with adenomatous polyps of the descending and rectosigmoid colon was 1.36 ± 0.14 ml/day. In ten patients with polyps in the ascending or transverse colon it was slightly less at 1.28 ml ± 0.13 ml/day. The 11 control patients' mean fecal blood loss was 0.62 ± 0.07 ml blood/day. The control group had negative Hemoccult slide tests. In patients with sigmoid and descending colon polyps with stool containing 2.0 to 3.99 ml blood/day, the Hemoccult test was positive in 86 percent. In the whole group of patients with descending colon or rectosigmoid polyps, the Hemoccult test was positive in 54%. The Hemoccult test was positive in only 17% of patients with right colon or transverse colon polyps. When patients with transverse or right colon lesions were separated into those with stool containing 2.0 to 3.99 ml blood/24 hours, the Hemoccult test was positive in 26%.

3.1.3. Angiodysplasia

Angiodysplasia is now being diagnosed more frequently than it used to be in patients with lower gastrointestinal hemorrhage. The characteristic lesions are frequently found in the right colon or distal small bowel. They are not seen on barium enema and also may be missed on colonoscopy, although more and more endoscopists can now identify angiodysplasia during colonoscopy. Surgeons may have a difficult time finding the lesion at laparotomy and where angiodysplasia is suspected, injection of the surgical specimen's vasculature in the operating room with a silicone rubber compound will help the pathologist identify the abnormality. To date, angiography is the best way to make the diagnosis.

The patient with hemorrhage from an angiodysplastic lesion is usually elderly, although such bleeding has occurred in patients as young as 30. There may be an association with valvular heart disease, particularly aortic stenosis. Angiodysplastic lesions may be found throughout the gastrointestinal tract. Weaver and colleagues [90] have suggested that there is a spectrum of vascular abnormalities, from inherited telangiectasia, such as seen in the Osler-Weber-Rendu syndrome, to the acquired angiodysplasia associated with aortic stenosis.

Hemorrhage from angiodysplasia may be intermittent and of a chronic nature, with iron deficiency anemia as a major problem. Baum and colleagues [91], however, found that one half of their patients presented with massive hemorrhage. The diagnosis may best be made by angiography at the time of massive hemorrhage. There are typical radiographic findings of angiodysplasia, which include a thick-walled veinule and early drainage from the veinule. If these findings are present and there is extravasation of contrast material into the bowel lumen, one can be confident that the bleeding point is identified. Demonstration of angiodysplasia by arteriography does not necessarily mean that this is the bleeding site; contrast extravasation must also be seen. In one study, 53% of a group of elderly patients with no history of gastrointestinal bleeding showed submucosal evidence of angiodysplasia, and 27% also had frank mucosal abnormality [92]. These findings suggest that angiodysplasia is a common degenerative lesion and is present in a significant number of people over 60 years of age, with or without rectal bleeding.

3.1.4. *Upper gastrointestinal bleeding*
Massive upper gastrointestinal hemorrhage from any source may present with bright-red rectal bleeding. Usually this occurs in a life-threatening bleeding episode, and may initially be difficult to distinguish from a massive lower gastrointestinal hemorrhage. Nasogastric intubation with aspiration of gastric contents has been advocated in all patients with lower gastrointestinal hemorrhage, but patients with duodenal ulcer bleeding may be missed. Therefore, upper gastrointestinal endoscopy should be performed early in patients with massive rectal hemorrhage. If the nasogastric aspirate is negative for blood, such endoscopy should specifically include the duodenal bulb and duodenal sweep. If arteriography proves necessary to confirm the bleeding site, celiac axis study need not be done if endoscopy has eliminated the upper gastrointestinal tract as a source for the massive hemorrhage.

3.1.5. *Inflammatory bowel disease*
Rectal bleeding may be minimal and associated with mild abdominal cramping and diarrhea, or the patient may present with fulminant diarrhea and massive colonic hemorrhage. Crohn's disease will often produce diarrhea, but it is usually nonbloody. Yet, anemia may be present due to chronic occult blood loss. If the disease involves the rectosigmoid area of the colon, some patients will have bloody stools.

3.1.6. *Antibiotic-induced colitis*
Many antibiotics can cause pseudomembranous colitis. Usually the disease occurs on the left side, and the associated diarrhea contains only small amounts of blood. However, the bleeding may also be substantial in some patients. On

sigmoidoscopy, the typical appearance of the pseudomembrane is diagnostic, and tissue obtained by scope can be cultured for C. difficile and an assay for clostridia toxin can be performed. Interestingly, this disease may also occur more proximally in the colon, where it may be missed by sigmoidoscopy. One report describes eight patients with acute right-sided hemorrhagic colitis related to Ampicillin use. Diagnosis was made by early colonoscopy [93]. The lesions started in the descending colon or even more proximally in all of the patients. Some patients with antibiotic-associated colitis may benefit from oral vancomycin therapy.

3.1.7. Typhlitis

Typhlitis, or inflammation of the cecum and surrounding tissues, is seen in approximately 10% of leukemic patients at postmortem examination, although the antemortem diagnosis is made much less frequently [94]. The majority of patients with typhlitis die from gastrointestinal bleeding and sepsis. Symptoms are often vague, but frequently pain is localized to the right lower quadrant. Fever and diarrhea are usually present, and sepsis is seen in 75% of patients. Plain films of the abdomen may show a lack of bowel gas in the right lower quadrant [95]. A cautiously performed barium enema can show cecal distortion. Colonoscopy can also be helpful in the diagnosis, but care must be taken in the leukemic patient with severe thrombocytopenia and leukopenia. Surgery, in general, should be avoided. In those few long-term survivors where right hemicolectomy was performed, remission of the leukemia occcurred soon after the surgery [96].

3.2. Diagnostic approach to large bowel hemorrhage

3.2.1. Submassive bleeding

Following digital rectal examination and sigmoidoscopy, air-contrast barium enema is frequently obtained. The barium enema is an important diagnostic tool, but care must be taken to insure a good, carefully done air-contrast study. The standard barium enema without air contrast will miss a number of polypoid lesions and probably should not be done in the evaluation of a patient with rectal bleeding. One can never be sure that a lesion identified on barium enema is, in fact, the bleeding lesion. Diverticulosis, for example, might be expected to be seen in up to 30% of all barium enemas performed in individuals over 60 years of age, whether or not they are bleeding. Angiodysplasia will not be diagnosed by barium enema, and polyps and small colon cancers may be missed.

Colonoscopy can be expected to identify lesions that barium enema does not, such as small polyps and angiodysplasia. The endoscopist may be able to identify the source of mild to moderate colonic bleeding by actually seeing the lesion while it is bleeding. Where diverticulosis is the cause of bleeding, blood clot may be found in the opening of the diverticulum. Colonoscopy should be performed by an experienced endoscopist. Often the preparation of the colon is not ideal, and this can add to the difficulty of performing the procedure and interpreting the findings.

Knutson and Max [97] studied 168 patients referred for colonoscopy because of rectal bleeding unexplained by both rigid proctosigmoidoscopy and barium enema. The cecum was visualized in 109 of 134 attempts (81%), and they identified 46 unsuspected lesions in 39 patients. The majority of these lesions were benign adenomas, but 3 *in situ* and 7 invasive cancers were detected, as also were 5 angiodysplastic lesions. It is difficult to know whether or not these lesions were responsible for the rectal bleeding in all cases, but certainly an impressive number of clinically important lesions were identified. Tedesco and colleagues [98] reported on 258 patients with rectal bleeding. Their patients also had a negative proctosigmoidoscopy and a barium enema that was negative or showed only diverticula, yet significant lesions were identified by colonoscopy in 41.5%. Twenty-nine patients (11.2%) had cancer, and 17 patients (6.6%) had cecal angiodysplasia.

If after colonoscopy no diagnosis is obvious, either angiography or radionuclide scanning should be done. Radionuclide scanning is gaining in popularity as a diagnostic tool in the patient with large bowel bleeding. One technique is to label red blood cells in vitro with technetium Tc99m. Bunker, *et al.* [99] studied 16 patients by this technique, in which 11 had active bleeding. Ten of the 11 patients had positive scans. This procedure directed appropriate additional diagnostic studies or surgery to the correct location, which was the ascending colon (1), rectosigmoid (4), transverse colon (1), and duodenum (1). In three patients, bleeding ceased before the exact location could be confirmed by other studies. Five patients with minimal evidence of active bleeding at the time of the study had negative scans. None of these patients required more than one unit of blood over a 24-hour period. One of these patients was later found to have a rectosigmoid colon cancer.

Because the red blood cells are labeled, serial abdominal imaging may be performed for 24 hours or more so that slow or intermittent bleeding should be identified by this technique. Additionally, labeling the red blood cells minimizes the amount of label that enters the gastric juice, a frequent cause of false-positive results.

More recently, Markisz and co-workers [100] reported their results with 99mTc-labeled, in vitro-labeled red cells. They studied 39 patients. Seventeen (44%) had a scan that showed active bleeding. In eight of this group (47%), the scan became positive 6 hours or more after injection. In 11 patients, the bleeding site was further confirmed by angiography, surgery, or colonoscopy. The scan was correct in 10 of these 11 patients (91%).

Several interesting points came out of this study. Deaths occurred only in the scan-positive patients, and no deaths occurred in the scan-negative patients. Also, no patient with a negative scan had a positive angiogram.

If there is still no diagnosis after colonoscopy and radionuclide scanning, angiography might then be considered. The lesion one hopes to find in this setting would be a right colon or ileal angiodysplasia. If such a lesion is identified, elective surgery may be considered. Another approach would be to wait until rebleeding occurs and repeat the angiogram at that time, with the hope of identifying extravasation of contrast into the bowel lumen in the area of the lesion. There are advocates of both approaches.

3.2.2. Massive bleeding

After ruling out a rectal cause for hemorrhage with digital rectal exam and proctosigmoidoscopy, gastroscopy should be performed to identify or eliminate an upper gastrointestinal source for the bleeding. With a negative upper gastrointestinal endoscopy, radionuclide scanning or angiography should be performed. In order to demonstrate extravasation of contrast into the bowel lumen on angiogram, the bleeding should be brisk, that is between 1 and 2 ml per minute. Casarella and colleagues [101] studied 60 consecutive patients, with massive rectal hemorrhage, utilizing angiography. The bleeding lesion was demonstrated in 40 of the 60 patients. Twenty-four patients had either bleeding diverticula or angiodysplasia; three had colon cancer. Interestingly, in those patients bleeding from diverticula, all of the bleeding points but one occurred proximal to the splenic flexure even though most of the diverticula were in the left colon. Another interesting finding was that 11 of the 40 patients had bleeding sites that were proximal to the large bowel. The majority of those patients not diagnosed by angiography were believed to be bleeding from either diverticulosis or peptic ulcer. Subsequent barium enemas revealed nothing other than colonic diverticula.

As with some forms of upper gastrointestinal hemorrhage, treatment of massive hemorrhage can also be initiated with angiography. Vasopressin and other vasoconstrictive substances can be infused directly through the angiography catheter, often with dramatic temporary results.

If angiography does not demonstrate a bleeding site, colonoscopy can be attempted. However, this is a most difficult procedure in the presence of active massive colonic hemorrhage. Even an instrument with a large aspiration channel will frequently become clogged with aspirated blood clot. If colonoscopy cannot be successfully and safely performed, the procedure should be terminated. Fortunately, the vast majority of acute massive hemorrhages will stop spontaneously, allowing repeat colonoscopy in 24 to 48 hours, when conditions are more satisfactory. If the bleeding does not stop, some have advocated barium enemas as a possible therapeutic as well as diagnostic tool. One author [102] suggests that the barium may help stop diverticular bleeding. However, this is based on an uncontrolled study; and if the bleeding does not stop, one is then faced with operating on a patient with a barium-filled colon.

In the uncommon patient in whom no bleeding site can be demonstrated and massive bleeding persists, emergency subtotal colectomy with ileorectal ana-stomosis should be the surgical procedure of choice. 'Blind' resection of either the right or left colon is fraught with difficulty, including continued or recurrent postoperative bleeding. Multiple intraoperative colotomies looking for the bleeding site can lead to fecal peritoneal contamination and sepsis. Another approach in undiagnosed massive hemorrhage involves intraoperative colonoscopy. The surgeon, with the abdomen open, can guide the colonoscope to the right colon. If this is successful and the bleeding site identified, a segmental resection can be performed. This procedure usually produces good results and has a low mortality rate [103].

4. Conclusions

It is important to maintain a perspective in the diagnosing and management of gastrointestinal hemorrhage in patients with cancer. Clinical judgment should prevail over any algorithm. The clinician must take the patient's underlying malignancy into consideration. The patient with far-advanced cancer with liver metastases and bleeding from esophageal varices will be managed differently from the patient with a gastrointestinal lymphoma in remission bleeding from peptic ulcer disease. As the array of diagnostic and therapeutic tools continues to increase in number, the options available to the clinician will also increase to the benefit of the patient.

References

1. Palmer ED: Diagnosis of upper gastrointestinal hemorrhage, Charles C. Thomas Publisher, Springfield, Mass, 1961.
2. Palmer ED: The vigorous diagnostic approach to upper gastrointestinal tract hemorrhage: a 20-year prospective study of 1400 patients. JAMA 207: 1477–80, 1969.
3. Schiller KFR, Truelove SC, Williams DG: Haematemesis and melena, with special reference to factors influencing outcome. Br Med J 2: 7–14, 1970.
4. Eastwood GL: Does early endoscopy benefit the patient with active upper gastrointestinal bleeding? Gastroenterology 72: 737–9, 1977.
5. Winans CS: Emergency upper gastrointestinal endoscopy: does haste make waste? Am J Dig Dis 22: 536–40, 1977.
6. Peterson WL, Barnett CC, Smith HJ, Allen MH, Corbett DB: Routine early endoscopy in upper gastrointestinal tract bleeding. N Engl J Med 304: 925–9, 1981.
7. Conn HO: To scope or not to scope (Editorial). N Engl J Med 304: 967–9, 1981.
8. Iglesias MC, Dourdourekas D, Adomavicius J, Villa F, Shobassy N, Steigmann F: Prompt endoscopic diagnosis of upper gastrointestinal hemorrhage: its value for specific diagnosis and management. Ann Surg 189: 90–5, 1979.
9. Griffiths WJ, Neumann DA, Welsh JD: The visible vessel as an indicator of uncontrolled or recurrent gastrointestinal hemorrhage. N Engl J Med 300: 1411–3, 1979.
10. Klein MS, Ennis F, Sherlock P, Winawer SJ: Stress erosions: a major cause of gastrointestinal

hemorrhage in patients with malignant disease. Am J Dig Dis 18: 167–71, 1973.

11. Lightdale CJ, Kurtz RC, Sherlock P, Winawer SJ: Aggressive endoscopy in critically ill patients with upper gastrointestinal bleeding and cancer. Gastrointest Endosc 20: 152–3, 1974.

12. Chait MM, Turnbull AD, Winawer SJ: The anatomic distribution of gastric erosions from stress and gastric irritants in patients with cancer. Gastrointest Endosc 24: 233–5, 1978.

13. Harjola PT and Sivula A: Gastric ulceration following experimentally induced hypoxia and hemorrhagic shock: in vivo study of pathogenesis in rabbits. Ann Surg 163: 21–8, 1966.

14. Menguy R, Deshaillets L, Masters R: Mechanism of stress ulcer: influence of hypovolemic shock on energy metabolism in the gastric mucosa. Gastroenterology 66: 46–55, 1974.

15. Menguy R, Masters YF: Mechanisms of stress ulcer IV. Influence of fasting on the tolerance of gastric mucosal energy metabolism to ischemia and on the incidence of stress ulceration. Gastroenterology 66: 1177–86, 1974.

16. Mersereau W, Hinchey EJ: Effect of gastric acidity on gastric ulceration induced by hemorrhage in the rat, utilizing a gastric chamber technique. Gastroenterology 64: 1130–5, 1973.

17. Ritchie WP Jr: Acute gastric mucosal damage induced by bile salts, acid, and ischemia. Gastroenterology 68: 699–707, 1975.

18. Davenport HW: Back-diffusion of acid through the gastric mucosa and its physiological consequences. In: Progress in Gastroenterology, Vol II, Jerzy-Glass G (ed), Grue and Stratton (1970), p 42–56.

19. Kim YS, Kerr R, Lipkin M: Cell proliferation during the development of stress erosions in the mouse stomach. Nature 214: 1180–1, 1967.

20. Brown RC, Langman MJS, Lambert PM: Hospital admissions for peptic ulcer during 1958–1972. Br Med J 1: 35–7, 1976.

21. Elashoff JD, Grossman MI: Trends in hospital admissions and death rates for peptic ulcer in the United States from 1970–1978. Gastroenterology 78: 280–5, 1980.

22. Levy M: Aspirin use in patients with major upper gastrointestinal bleeding and peptic ulcer disease. N Engl J Med 290: 1158–62, 1974.

23. Piper DW, McIntosh JH, Ariotti DE, Fenton BH, Maclennan R: Analgesic ingestion and chronic peptic ulcer. Gastroenterology 80: 427–32, 1981.

24. Way L, Goldman L, Dunphy JE: Zollinger-Ellison syndrome: an analysis of twenty-five cases. Am J Surg 116: 293–303, 1968.

25. Kolts BE, Herbst CA, McGuigan JE: Calcium and secretin-stimulated gastrin release in the Zollinger-Ellison syndrome. Ann Int Med 81: 758–62, 1974.

26. Fox PS, Hofmann JW, DeCosse JJ, Wilson SD: The influence of total gastrectomy on survival in malignant Zollinger-Ellison tumors. Ann Surg 180: 558–66, 1974.

27. Fung WB, Barr A: Fulminant disseminated intravascular coagulation in advanced gastric cancer. Am J Gastroenterol 171: 210–2, 1979.

28. Green PHR, O'Toole KM, Weinberg LM, Goldfarb JP: Early gastric cancer. Gastroenterology 81: 247–56, 1981.

29. Hartmann WH, Sherlock P: Gastroduodenal metastases from carcinoma of the breast: an adrenal steroid-induced phenomenon. Cancer 14: 426–31, 1961.

30. Sharon P, Stalnikovicz R, Rachmilewitz D: Endoscopic diagnosis of duodenal neoplasms causing upper gastrointestinal bleeding. J Clin Gastroenterol 4: 35–8, 1982.

31. Luna A, Meister P, Szanto PB: Esophageal varices in the absence of cirrhosis. Am J Clin Pathol 49: 710–7, 1968.

32. Kurtz RC, Sherlock P, Winawer SJ: Esophageal varices: development secondary to primary and metastatic liver tumors. Arch Int Med 134: 50–1, 1974.

33. Albacete RA, Matthews MJ, Saini N: Portal vein thrombosis in malignant hepatoma. Ann Int Med 67: 337–48, 1967.

34. Duff GL: The clinical and pathological features of carcinoma of the body and tail of the pancreas. Bull Johns Hopkins Hosp 65: 69–100, 1939.

35. Berk PD, Popper H, Krueger RF, Decter J, Herzig G, Graw RG: Veno-occlusive disease of the liver after allogenic bone marrow transplantation. Ann Int Med 90: 158–64, 1979.
36. Eras P, Goldstein MJ, Sherlock P: Candida infection of the gastrointestinal tract. Medicine 51: 367–79, 1972.
37. Kodsi BE, Wickremesinghe PC, Kozinn PJ, Kadirawelpillai I, Goldberg PK: Candida esophagitis. A prospective study of 22 cases. Gastroenterology 71: 715–9, 1976.
38. Fishbein PG, Tuthill R, Kressel H, Friedman H, Snape WJ Jr: Herpes simplex esophagitis: a cause of upper gastrointestinal bleeding. Dig Dis Sci 24: 540–4, 1979.
39. Rosen P, Hajdu SI: Visceral herpes virus infections in patients with cancer. Am J Clin Path 56: 459–65, 1971.
40. Lightdale CJ, Wolf DJ, Marcucci RA, Salyer WR: Herpetic esophagitis in patients with cancer: antemortem diagnosis by brush cytology. Cancer 39: 223–6, 1977.
41. Mallory GK, Weiss S: Hemorrhages from lacerations of the cardiac orifice of the stomach due to vomiting. Am J Med Sci 178: 506–15, 1929.
42. Knauer CM: Mallory-Weiss syndrome. Gastroenterology 71: 5–8, 1976.
43. Fisher RG, Schwartz JT, Graham DY: Angiotherapy with Mallory-Weiss tear. Am J Roent 134: 679–84, 1980.
44. Vanamee P, Winawer SJ, Sherlock P, Sonenberg M, Lipkin M: Decreased incidence of restraint-stress induced gastric erosions in rats treated with bovine growth hormones. Proc Soc Exp Biol Med 135: 259–62, 1970.
45. Winawer SJ, Sherlock P, Sonenberg M, Vanamee P: Beneficial effect of human growth hormone on stress ulcers. Arch Int Med 135: 569–72, 1975.
46. Simonian SJ, Curtis LE: Treatment of hemorrhagic gastritis by antacid. Ann Surg 184: 429–34, 1976.
47. MacDonald AS, Steele BJ, Bottomley MG: Treatment of stressinduced upper gastrointestinal haemorrhage with metiamide. Lancet 1: 68–70, 1976.
48. Dunn DH, Fischer RC, Silvis SE, Onstad GR, Howard RJ, Delaney JP: The treatment of hemorrhagic gastritis with cimetidine. Surg Gynecol Obstet 147: 737–9, 1978.
49. Pickard RG, Sanderson I, South M, Kirkham JS, Northfield TC: Controlled trial of cimetidine in acute upper gastrointestinal bleeding. Br Med J 1: 661–2, 1979.
50. Hoare AM, Bradley GVH, Hawkins CF, Kang JY, Dykes PW: Cimetidine in bleeding peptic ulcer. Lancet 2: 671–3, 1979.
51. Kayasseh L, Gyr K, Keller U, Stalder GA, Wall M: Somatostatin and cimetidine in peptic ulcer hemorrhage. Lancet 1: 844–6, 1980.
52. MacDougall BRD, Bailey RJ, Williams R: H_2-receptor antagonists and antacids in the prevention of acute gastrointestinal hemorrhage in fulminant hepatic failure: two controlled trials. Lancet 1: 617–9, 1977.
53. Hastings PR, Skillmann JJ, Bushnell LS, Silen W: Antacid titration in the prevention of acute gastrointestinal bleeding. A controlled, randomized trial in 100 critically ill patients. N Engl J Med 298: 1041–5, 1978.
54. Solem LD, Strate RG, Fischer RP: Antacid therapy and nutritional supplementation in the prevention of Curling's ulcer. Surg Gynecol Obstet 148: 367–70, 1979.
55. Jones RH, Rudge CJ, Bewick M, Parsons V, Weston MJ: Cimetidine: prophylaxis against upper gastrointestinal haemorrhage after renal transplantation. Br Med J 1: 398–400, 1978.
56. Halloran LG, Zfass AM, Gayle WE, Wheeler CB, Miller JD: Prevention of acute gastrointestinal complications after severe head injury: a controlled trial of cimetidine prophylaxis. Am J Surg 139: 44–8, 1980.
57. Priebe HJ, Skillman JJ, Bushnell LS, Long PC, Silen W: Antacid versus cimetidine in preventing acute gastrointestinal bleeding. A randomized trial in 75 critically ill patients. N Engl J Med 302: 426–30, 1980.
58. Stothert JC Jr, Simonowitz DA, Dellinger EP, Farley M, Edwards WA, Blair AD, Cutler R,

Carrico CJ: Randomized prospective evaluation of cimetidine and antacid control of gastric pH in the critically ill. Ann Surg 192: 169–74, 1980.

59. Robert A: Prostaglandins and the digestive system. In: The prostaglandins, Volume 3, Ramwell PW (ed), Plenum Publishing Corp, New York, 1977, p 225–66.

60. Robert A, Nezamis JE, Lancaster C, Hanchar AJ: Cytoprotection by prostaglandins in rats. Gastroenterology 77: 433–43, 1979.

61. Baum S, Nusbaum M: The control of gastrointestinal hemorrhage by selective mesenteric arterial infusion of vasopressin. Radiology 98: 497–505, 1971.

62. Athanasoulis CA, Baum S, Waltman AC, Ring EJ, Imbembo A, Vandersalm TJ: Control of acute gastric mucosal hemorrhage. Intraarterial infusion of posterior pituitary extract. N Engl J Med 290: 597–602, 1974.

63. Conn HO, Ramsby GR, Storer EH, Mutchnick MG, Prakash JH, Philips MM, Cohen GA, Fields GN, Petroski D: Intraarterial vasopressin in the treatment of upper gastrointestinal hemorrhage: a prospective, controlled clinical trial. Gastroenterology 68: 211–21, 1975.

64. Chojkier M, Groszmann RJ, Atterbury Ce, Bar-Meir S, Blei AT, Frankel J, Glickman MG, Kniaz JL, Shade R, Taggart GJ, Conn HO: A controlled comparison of continuous intraarterial and intravenous infusions of vasopressin in hemorrhage from esophageal varices. Gastroenterology 77: 540–6, 1979.

65. Fogel MR, Knauer CM, Ljudevit AL, Mahal AS, Stein DET, Kemeny J, Rinki MM, Walker JE, Siegmund D, Gregory PB: Continuous intravenous vasopressin in active upper gastrointestinal bleeding. A placebo-controlled trial. Ann Intern Med 96: 565–9, 1982.

66. Laurence BH, Vallon AG, Cotton PB, Armengol Miro JR, Salord Oses JC, LeBodic L, Sudry P, Fruhmoren P, Bodem F: Endoscopic laser photocoagulation for bleeding peptic ulcer. Lancet 1: 124–5, 1980.

67. Kiefhaber P, Nath G, Moritz K: Endoscopic control of massive gastrointestinal hemorrhage by irradiation with a high-power neodymium-YAG laser. Prog Surg 15: 140–55, 1977.

68. Rutgeerts P, Vontrappen G, Broeckaert J, Janssens J, Coremans G, Geboes K, Schurmans P: Controlled trial of YAG laser treatment of upper digestive hemorrhage. Gastroenterology 83: 410–6, 1982.

69. Vallon AG, Cotton PB, Laurence BH, Armengol Miro JR, Salord Oses JC: Randomized trial of endoscopic argon laser photocoagulation in bleeding peptic ulcers. Gut 22: 228–33, 1981.

70. Papp JP: Endoscopic electrocoagulation of actively bleeding arterial upper gastrointestinal lesions. Am J Gastroenterol 71: 516–21, 1979.

71. Papp JP: Endoscopic electrocoagulation in the management of upper gastrointestinal tract bleeding. Surg Clin North Am 62: 797–806, 1982.

72. Crafoord C, Frenckner P: New surgical treatment of varicose veins of the esophagus. Otolaryngol 27: 422–9, 1939.

73. Clark AW, Westaby D, Silk DBA, Dawson JL, MacDougall BRD, Mitchell KJ, Strunin L, Williams R: Prospective controlled trial of injection sclerotherapy in patients with cirrhosis and recent variceal hemorrhage. Lancet 2: 552–4, 1980.

74. MacDougall BRD, Theodossi A, Westaby D, Dawson JL, Williams R: Increased long-term survival in variceal hemorrhage using injection sclerotherapy. Lancet 1: 124–7, 1982.

75. Graham DY, Smith JC: The course of patients after variceal hemorrhage. Gastroenterology 80: 800–9, 1981.

76. Briley CA, Jackson DC, Johnsrude IS, Mills SR: Acute gastrointestinal hemorrhage of small bowel origin. Radiology 136: 317–9, 1980.

77. Adler SN, Lyon DT, Sullivan PD: Adenocarcinoma of the small bowel. Clinical features, similarity to regional enteritis, and analysis of 338 documented cases. Am J Gastroenterol 77: 326–30, 1982.

78. Bridge MF, Perzin KH: Primary adenocarcinoma of the jejunum and ileum. A clinicopathologic study. Cancer 36: 1876–87, 1975.

79. Darling RC, Welch CE: Tumors of the small intestine. N Engl J Med 260: 397–408, 1959.
80. VonKnorring J, Hockerstedt, Holmstrom T, Salaspuro M, Scheinin TM: Severe gastrointestinal bleeding due to carcinoid tumour of the ileum. Ann Chir Gynaecol 70: 18–21, 1981.
81. DeCastro CA, Dockerty MB, Mayo CW: Metastatic tumors of the small intestine. Surg Gynecol Obstet 105: 159–65, 1957.
82. Richman A, Lipsey J: Melanoma of the small intestine and stomach. J Mt Sinai Hosp 17: 907–16, 1951.
83. Beirne MG: Malignant melanoma of the small intestine. Radiology 65: 749–52, 1955.
84. Chait MM, Kurtz RC, Hajdu SI: Gastrointestinal tract metastasis in patients with germ-cell tumor of the testis. Am J Dig Dis 23: 925–8, 1978.
85. DeCosse JJ, Rhodes RS, Wentz WB, Reagan JW, Dworken HJ, Holden WD: The natural history and management of radiation-induced injury of the gastrointestinal tract. Ann Surg 170: 369–84, 1969.
86. Cathcart PM, Carthcart RS, Rambo WM: Management of massive lower GI bleeding. Am Surgeon 43: 217–9, 1977.
87. Rigg BM, Ewing MR: Current attitudes on diverticulitis with particular reference to colonic bleeding. Arch Surg 92: 321–2, 1966.
88. Meyers MA, Alonso DR, Gray GF, Baer JW: Pathogenesis of bleeding colonic diverticulosis. Gastroenterology 71: 477–83, 1976.
89. Herzog P, Holtermuller KH, Preiss J, Fischer J, Ewe K, Schreiber HJ, Berres M: Fecal blood loss in patients with colonic polyps: a comparison of measurements with Chromium^{51}-labeled erythrocytes and with the Haemoccult test. Gastroenterology 83: 957–62, 1982.
90. Weaver GA, Alpern HD, Davis JS, Ramsey WH, Reichelderfer M: Gastrointestinal angiodysplasia associated with aortic valve disease: Part of a spectrum of angiodysplasia of the gut. Gastroenterology 77: 1–11, 1979.
91. Baum S, Athanasoulis CA, Waltman AC, Galdabini J, Shapiro RH, Warshaw AL, Ottinger LW: Angiodysplasia of the right colon: a cause of gastrointestinal bleeding. Am J Roentgenol 129: 789–94, 1977.
92. Boley SJ, Sammartano R, Adams A, DiBiase A, Kleinhaus S, Sprayregen S: On the nature and etiology of vascular ectasias of the colon. Gastroenterology 72: 650–60, 1977.
93. Sakurai Y, Tsuchiya H, Ikegami F, Funatomi T, Takasu S, Uchikoshi T: Acute right-sided hemorrhagic colitis associated with oral Ampicillin administration. Dig Dis Sci 24: 910–5, 1979.
94. Steinberg D, Gold J, Brodin A. Necrotizing enterocolitis in leukemia. Arch Intern Med 131: 538–44, 1973.
95. DelFava RZ, Cronin TG: Typhlitis complicating leukemia in an adult. Barium enema findings. Am J Roentgenol 129: 347–8, 1977.
96. Kies MS, Luedke DW, Boyd JF, McCue MJ: Neutropenic enterocolitis: two case reports of long-term survival following surgery. Cancer 43: 730–4, 1979.
97. Knutson CO, Max MH: Value of colonoscopy in patients with rectal blood loss unexplained by rigid proctosigmoidoscopy and barium contrast enema examination. Am J Surg 139: 84–7, 1980.
98. Tedesco FJ, Waye JD, Raskin JB, Morris SJ, Greenwald RA: Colonoscopic evaluation of rectal bleeding. Ann Intern Med 89: 907–9, 1978.
99. Bunker SR, Brown JM, McAuley RJ, Lull RJ, Jackson JH, Hattner RS, Huberty JP: Detection of gastrointestinal bleeding sites. Use of in vitro technetium Tc99m-labeled RBC's. JAMA 247: 789–92, 1982.
100. Markisz JA, Front D, Royal HD, Sacks B, Parker A, Kolodny GM: An evaluation of 99mTc-labeled red blood cell scintigraphy for the detection and localization of gastrointestinal bleeding sites. Gastroenterology 83: 394–8, 1982.
101. Casarella WJ, Galloway SJ, Taxin RN, Follett DH, Pollock EJ, Seaman WB: 'Lower' gastrointestinal tract hemorrhage: new concepts based on arteriography. Am J Roentgenol 121: 357–68, 1972.

102. Adams JT: The barium enemas as treatment for massive diverticular bleeding. Dis Colon Rectum 17: 439–41, 1974.
103. Wright HK, Pelliccia O, Higgins EF, Screenivas V, Gupta A: Controlled, semi-elective, segmental resection for massive colonic hemorrhage. Am J Surg 139: 535–8, 1980.

11. Nonsurgical biliary drainage in cancer

DAVID S. ZIMMON and ARTHUR R. CLEMETT

1. Introduction

The rapid evolution of nonsurgical techniques for drainage of the biliary tree first by the percutaneous route and more recently by the use of endoscopic retrograde cholangiopancreatography (ERCP) has raised important issues and questions. We now have three competing techniques for the diagnosis and management of patients with actual or incipient bile duct obstruction due to cancer. What is the role of each technique? In what way do they compliment or compete with each other? Can an algorythm for their use be developed? Can we balance the risk versus the benefits of these various techniques?

A further complicating factor is the rapid evolution of technique and skill, first in the area of percutaneous transhepatic cholangiography and drainage (PTCD) and then in the area of endoscopic retrograde cholangiography and drainage (ERCPD). Furthermore, we must not overlook the fact that alternative methods of surgical access to the biliary tree can be useful and of great assistance when combined with percutaneous or endoscopic techniques.

1.1. The concept of nonsurgical biliary drainage

Initially, when these techniques were primitive and poorly developed they were used to reduced the hazard of diagnostic percutaneous transhepatic cholangiography (PTC) or ERCP. This was particularly, important in PTC since bile leakage, hemobilia, hypotension, frank gram negative shock and serious cholangitis are common consequences. These important and frequent complications can be controlled by the use of sheathed needle duct puncture followed by a drainage catheter. To this end, more than 20 years ago, fine needle percutaneous transhepatic cholangiography was combined with attempts at drainage [1]. Although complications from diagnostic ERCP are much less common, long nasobiliary

J.J. DeCosse and P. Sherlock (eds), Clinical Management of Gastrointestinal Cancer.
© *1984, Martinus Nijhoff Publishers, Boston. ISBN 0-89838-601-2. Printed in The Netherlands.*

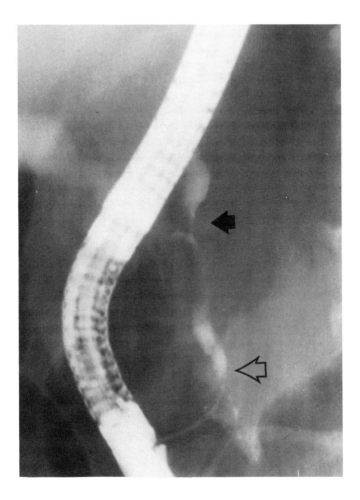

Figure 1A. This ERCP demonstrates stenosis of the proximal common bile duct and adjacent cystic duct (closed arrowhead) with a cannulating catheter (open arrowhead) in the distal common bile duct. The preceding pancreatogram showed pancreatic duct obstruction within 1 cm of the papilla typical of pancreatic cancer.

drains passed through the endoscope and brought out through the patient's nose after ERCP were used to believe cholestasis and cholangitis and to prevent impaction of stones after endoscopic sphincterotomy [2, 3]. Both techniques have evolved dramatically in the past 10 years and in sophisticated hands should now be routine alternatives to traditional surgical exploration. Particularly, in the deeply jaundiced patient or the patient who presents with cholangitis, drainage following an invasive diagnostic biliary tract procedure has become mandatory when technically possible [4] (Fig. 1).

The high operative and perioperative mortality associated with extensive curative or palliative surgery in patients with biliary obstruction from cancer long

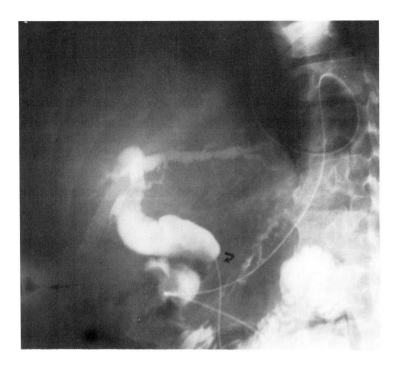

Figure 1B. After placement of the nasobiliary drain in the hepatic duct above the stenosis (curved arrow) the dilated left hepatic duct system is visualized with the patient prone. Gallstones are seen in the gallbladder at the left hand margin of the photograph (arrow). The nasobiliary drain is opacified by contrast draining from the biliary tree.

has been recognized [5]. An important surgical alternative was a two stage operation. Initially, percutaneous and endoscopic nonsurgical drainage were conceived as alternatives to the two stage operation. Nonsurgical drainage was achieved. Jaundice and infection were relieved. Then a curative or palliative operation was performed. Recently, numerous careful surgical studies have demonstrated the value of preoperative biliary drainage [6, 7, 8]. With this documentation, preoperative nonsurgical biliary drainage because an essential part of the surgeon's armamentarium [9]. Consequently, surgical exploration in the jaundiced patient without diagnosis or preparation is untenable (Fig. 2).

Temporary, nonsurgical drainage of bile duct obstruction may be useful during chemotherapy or radiation when this is the primary modality for treatment. In general, however, there is no great advantage to removing the drainage prosthesis. It is left in place until long term follow-up shows that an adequate stable lumen remains. These techniques are important before chemotherapy or radiation since they improve the patient's performance status and allow full therapy to be administered. The non-jaundiced patient is better able to tolerate chemotherapy and maintain resistance to infection.

Nonsurgical drainage of the biliary tree is an important alternative to surgery.

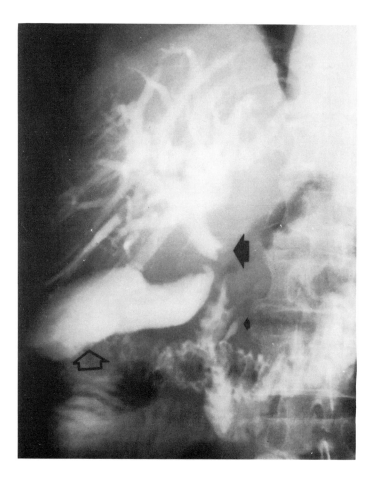

Figure 2. This ERCP shows marked dilatation of the intrahepatic biliary tree above a carcinoma of the pancreas compressing the distal hepatic duct (large closed arrowhead). At a prior abdominal exploration cholecystojejunostomy had been performed. The anastomosis between the gallbladder and jejunum is visible at the lower left (open large arrowhead). Contrast was forced through the common bile duct into both the intrahepatic biliary tree and gallbladder opacifying the jejunum. In the lower midportion of the photograph the obstructed pancreatic duct (small closed arrowhead) is visible establishing the diagnosis of pancreatic cancer. This failed surgical anatomosis could be salvaged by either a precutaneous or endoscopic stent.

It is as effective as palliative surgical drainage with less risk, discomfort and expense. Often, nonsurgical drainage can be applied when surgical palliation is impossible technically or difficult clinically because of the patient's age, high risk or associated diseases. It provides an alternative to surgery when surgery fails immediately or when progression of disease defeats surgical palliative drainage.

These alternatives raise important questions and drastically alter our approach to the jaundiced patient. A choice must be made between nonsurgical drainage preoperatively as temporary palliation or as permanent palliation. To answer

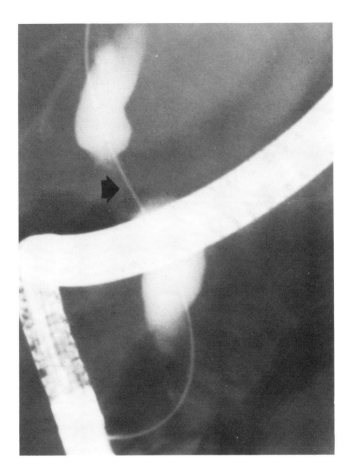

Figure 3A. This ERCP shows the stenting wire guide passing through a carcinoma of the distal hepatic duct (closed arrowhead). The pancreatic duct was normal. In the interval between pancreatography, a sphincterotomy, passage of the cannulating catheter and stenting wire the pancreatic duct drained of contrast.

these questions, a precise road map of the biliary and pancreatic pathologic anatomy is required. This demands direct cholangiography by either percutaneous or endoscopic routes which in general should be protected by drainage. Concomitantly a pathologic diagnosis should be established by biopsy.

In the ideal circumstance the jaundiced patient has a periampullary, mid bile duct or upper bile duct cancer. Drainage is established by passage of a plastic catheter through the obstruction. Histologic confirmation of the radiologic diagnosis is obtained either by direct endoscopic or percutaneous biopsy. Angiography and pancreatography confirm clinical resectability. The patient is then dismissed from the hospital and returns in 4 to 6 weeks for curative surgical resection when no longer jaundiced (Fig. 3).

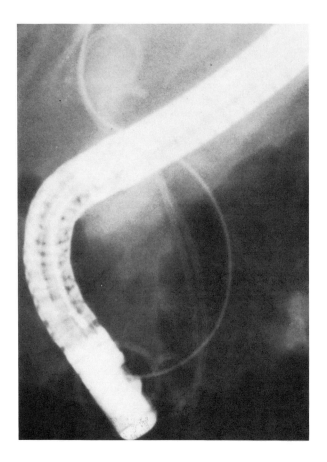

Figure 3B. Over the wire two 5 French double pigtail stents pass above the obstruction into the common hepatic duct. The distal pigtails are in the duodenum. The wire is passed for the third time in preparation for the last of three 5 French stents.

1.2. Aims of nonsurgical drainage

Nonsurgical drainage of the biliary tree achieves relief of symptoms. Pruritis and pain presumably due to dilatation of biliary structures are relieved when drainage is accomplished. Internal drainage, that is return of bile to the gastrointestinal tract, provides a stimulus for appetite, improves bile flow by re-establishing the enterohepatic circulation of bile acids and relieves the malabsorption associated with bile salt deficiency. Although patients tolerate external biliary drainage, optimal management is best accomplished by internal biliary drainage that relieves the malabsorption of cholestasis. Internal biliary drainage maintains liver function and relieves or prevents the development of cholangitis. Relief of cholestasis improves performance status, immunologic competence and with intake of adequate calories allows vigorous chemotherapy and radiation therapy.

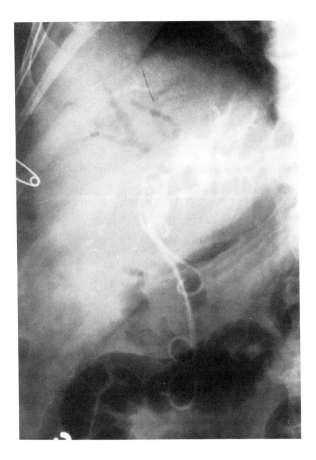

Figure 3C. Three stents are in place with proximal pigtails in the common hepatic duct and distal pigtails extending into the duodenum. In the prone position, the right hepatic duct system is drained of contrast and fills with air. The left hepatic duct system remains opacified by contrast and is markedly dilated.

Nonsurgical biliary drainage avoids the expense and disability of hospitalization or operative therapy which is only palliative and often associated with a high mortality. This is particularly important in the patient with carcinoma of the pancreas where life expectancy often is short when signalled by the onset of painless jaundice [10] (Fig. 4).

1.3. Diagnostic prerequisites

Complete radiologic anatomic and pathologic diagnosis including a microscopic diagnosis should be vigorously sought in patients before or at the time of non-surgical drainage. This can generally be achieved with less risk and expense than by the prior mode of laparotomy. Ultrasound and computerized scans are capable

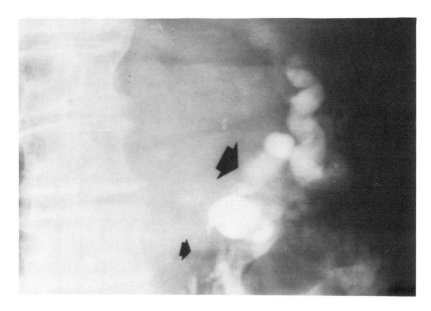

Figure 4A. Pancreatic duct stenosis in the head (small closed arrowhead) with marked dilatation of the proximal pancreatic duct (large closed arrowhead) establishes the diagnosis of pancreatic cancer. The bile duct could not be opacified (ERCP).

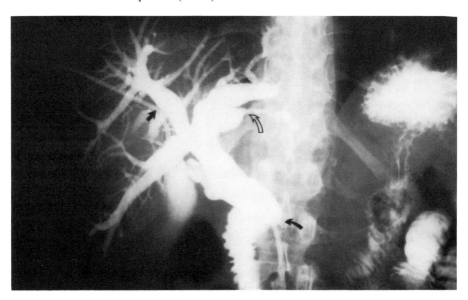

Figure 4B. After a percutaneous transhepatic cholangiogram, this percutaneous biliary stent was passed through the tumor into the duodenum. The transhepatic portion of the stent (closed straight arrow) enters the anterior division of the right hepatic duct. The stent (closed curved arrow) passes through a long distal bile duct stenosis into the duodenum opacified by contrast. Hepatic metastases are visible as compression in the medial division of the left hepatic duct (open curved arrow). The tumor mass compresses the horizontal duodenum.

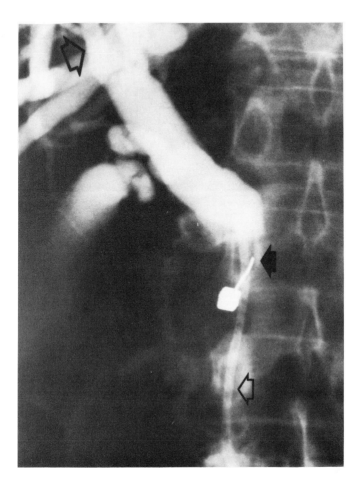

Figure 4C. A percutaneous biopsy with the stent as a target was positive for adenocarcinoma (closed arrowhead). A small segment of bile duct below the obstructing tumor is visible (open arrowhead).

of delineating mass lesions and the presence of bile duct obstruction. Often ultrasound cannot precisely indicate the level of duct obstruction. Furthermore, the presence of two sites of obstruction often confuses the ultrasonographer (Fig. 5). This circumstance is relatively common in carcinoma of the pancreas where the periampullary mass produces distal duct obstruction and metastasis produce obstruction of the common hepatic duct or intrahepatic ducts. Ultrasound or computerized scans may serve as aiming methods for percutaneous needle biopsy. Thus, the patient may present with jaundice or a mass be demonstrated by non-invasive techniques and a percutaneous needle biopsy show adenocarcinoma.

In this common circumstance nonsurgical drainage is appropriate. Relief of major obstruction in the right or left hepatic duct systems even the presence of

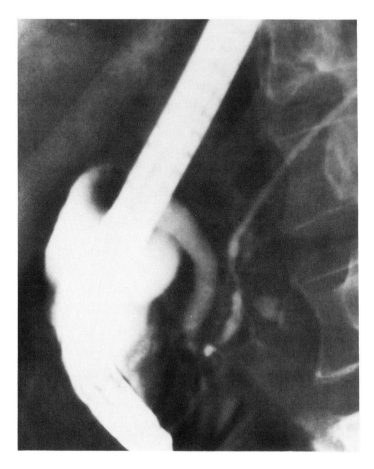

Figure 5A. This ERCP shows an irregular stenosis of the pancreatic duct within the head. Adjacent ducts in the uncinate are dilated indicating tumor invasion. Note the absence pancreatic duct dilatation. No mass was visible by ultrasonography or computerized tomography. The entire lesion is less than 1 cm in diameter. The distal common bile duct is normal.

diffuse metastasis within the liver or when combined with distal bile duct obstruction may yield a period of palliation with partial resolution of cholestasis and/or pruritis. Relatively modest improvement in excretory function by the liver will relieve pruritis (Fig. 6). In the circumstance where cholestasis is not intense and liver function preserved, hepatobiliary scanning may identify the level of duct obstruction. Caution must be exercised since (complete duct obstruction) with failure of isotope excretion into the biliary tree can occur with either extrahepatic obstruction or cholestasis due to hepatocellular disease. Furthermore, it is often difficult to identify the level of obstruction in a markedly dilated biliary tree.

In these circumstances it is wise to proceed to direct cholangigraphy for identification of the site(s) of obstruction and for determination of the mechanical

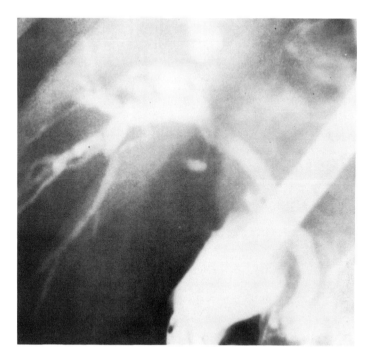

Figure 5B. Obstruction of the proximal hepatic duct with dilatation of the intrahepatic biliary tree could easily be mistaken for primary hepatic duct cancer in this patient without the information gained from the pancreatogram.

feasibility and potential clinical value of nonsurgical drainage. The best approach is ERCP because of its low diagnostic complication rate to be followed with PTC or operation if that is indicated by the anatomic findings. This is particularly important in patients with disease above the common hepatic duct or a pancreatic mass where metastasis or proximal extension is common. Without direct cholangiography it may be difficult to decide whether a high hepatic duct lesion should be approached from the left or right. Often it is technically unsatisfactory and clinically hazardous to attempt to obtain a diagnostic cholangiogram by puncturing the right hepatic lobe when it is diffusely involved with cancer. Local obstruction of ducts within the liver prevents the contrast from reaching the main duct system and the risk of producing complications is increased (Fig. 7). The left hepatic duct approach is extremely useful, but may be technically difficult [11]. The left hepatic duct can be approached through the umbilical fissure with a relatively modest surgical procedure as an alternative to the percutaneous method when this is required.

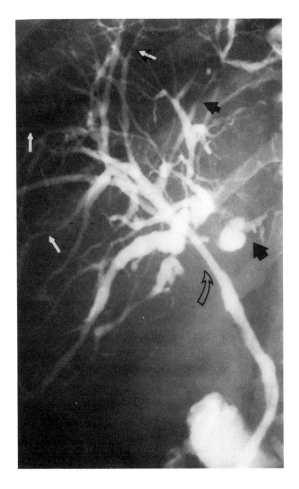

Figure 6. This percutaneous stent was placed for palliation in a patient with extensive hepatic metastasis from breast cancer. Liver scan had revealed multiple metastasis indicated by duct narrowing with proximal dilatation in many of the intrahepatic ducts visualized. A major factor in cholestasis was common hepatic duct obstructions (open curved arrow). The left hepatic duct was also obstructed (closed arrowhead). Dilatation of intrahepatic duct is not prominent in this patient. Mechanical feasibility and clinical appropriateness of this stent was determined by a prior ERCP showing common hepatic duct obstruction.

2. Technical considerations

2.1. Definition of terms

Soft plastic tubes with holes punched to fit the biliary tree are used. These plastic catheters are modified according to measurements made from the cholangiogram obtained before insertion of the catheter. The biliary stent functions because

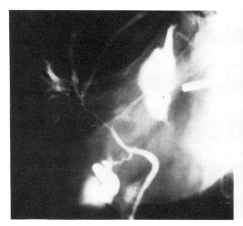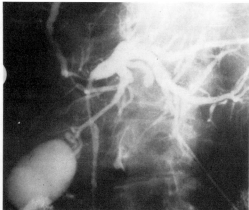

Figure 7. The left shows a percutaneous cholangiogram performed by the left hepatic duct approach in a patient with a sclerosing central hepatic duct tumor. The right hepatic duct system is encased and narrowed. On the right contrast injected through the left hepatic duct stent shows dilatation of the left hepatic system and limited communication between the common hepatic duct and right hepatic duct. The long common hepatic duct stenosis extended above the hepatic duct bifurcation necessitating the left hepatic duct approach. With this stent and radiation therapy, the patient survived five years from the time of diagnosis.

holes are positioned proximally in the liver above the site of obstruction and the tube then passes through the obstruction to carry bile distally in the bile duct or into the duodenum. A biliary drain carries bile outside the body. When placed percutaneously all bile flows externally if the drain is placed above the lesion. To achieve mechanical stability, percutaneous drains are usually placed through the obstructing lesion into the duodenum. In this case duodenal contents are aspirated and carried through the biliary tree. Undoubtedly, there is reflux and contamination of the biliary tree. In any case the procedure of passing the percutaneous drain or stent into the duodenum over a wire guide and then withdrawing the guide must contaminate the biliary contents with duodenal bacteria. Therefore, percutaneous procedures are not sterile.

When endoscopic drainage is used, the guide wire and drain are contaminated in passage through the endoscope and duodenum. Once they are placed in the biliary tree all biliary drainage is external. Continued contamination of intrahepatic bile no longer occurs. For this reasons, external biliary drainage by the endoscopic route minimizes the risk of continued biliary contamination. This is particularly important when drainage is achieved in the older patient where the upper gastrointestinal tract may harbor pathogenic bacteria.

The biliary 'stent' may be identical to the drain except that it is placed through the obstruction and allows bile to pass into the duodenum or duct system below the obstruction. Stents placed by either the percutaneous or endoscopic route are similar.

An 'endoprosthesis' refers to a stent which is free within the duct system and no longer connected externally. The endoprosthesis must be approached through the endoscopic or percutaneous route for manipulation since the external portion is absent.

Numerous devices of various sizes and shapes have been proposed and are used for both endoscopic and percutaneous biliary drainage. The diameter of the plastic tubes used ranges from 5 to 10 French external diameter. That is from approximately 1.6 mm to approximately 3.1 mm. These devices may be made of teflon, polyethylene or polyurethane. The ideal substance is not clear but most operators prefer polyethylene or polyurethane to teflon. The stiffness of teflon permits kinking and erosion of duct structures leading to bleeding and occasionally perforation. A similar debate exists over internal lumen diameter. The 5 French polyethylene tube has an internal diameter of 1.07 mm. This diameter is adequate for total bile flow from hepatic duct to duodenum at a normal bile secretory pressure. By increasing the external diameter to 6 French one obtains a lumen increase of only 0.12 mm. The 7 French tube has a lumen of 1.5 mm (40% larger). The commonly used 8.3 French catheter has a lumen of approximately 1.8 mm. The advantages of a lumen size greater than 5 French are not clear. We have approached this problem by using multiple small tubes. Two or three 5 French stents give a lumen diameter of 2 or 3 mm respectively and have the potential mechanical advantage of maintaining a space through the tumor by their continued motion and irregular combined shape. In special circumstances such as the dilatation of stenosis, it is useful to add individual 5 French tubes to stretch the stenosis to 15 or 20 French (Fig. 8).

2.2. Conversion of a percutaneous stent to an endoscopic stent

When it is not possible to pass an endoscopic stent for technical reasons and a percutaneous stent is placed, it is often useful to convert the percutaneous stent to an endoprosthesis which then is changed by the endoscopic route if necessary. This has the advantage of leaving the patient without an external device and substantially reduces the risk of pseudoaneurysm of a hepatic artery with hemobilia, displacement of the stent by accident, by a disoriented patient or by a patient attempting suicide. This is also valuable when life expectancy is short since the average stent requires replacement every 4 to 6 months. The use of multiple small stents (5 French) has the advantage of maintaining a lumen through the tumor when stents are being changed. One or two old stents may be removed and replaced with new stents leaving the third stent in place. Then the last stent is changed leaving the patient with three new stents. Procedures of this type can be performed on an ambulatory basis.

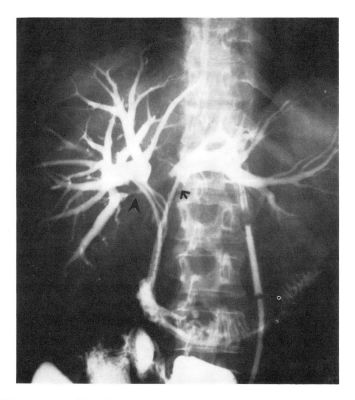

Figure 8. This carcinoma of the gallbladder progressed to invade the porta hepatis with separation of the left and right hepatic ducts. The left hepatic duct is drained by a single 8.2 French percutaneous stent (arrow). The right hepatic duct system drained poorly and required multiple stents because of intermittent hemobilia and detritis produced by the tumor (arrowhead). Two 7 French and one 8.3 French stents were placed to maintain bile flow. The two 7 French stents are free endoprostheses. The 8.3 French stent extends from the right chest allowing access. Intermittent bleeding and stent occlusion required irrigation and frequent stent changes.

2.3 Technique in PTC and PTCD

The intrinsic technical problems of PTC and PTCD are the result of the blind puncture required to enter the intrahepatic biliary tree. At each level complications may occur although meticulous technique reduces the incidence. At the skin, pain and wound infections may be troublesome. The intercostal space is occasionally difficult to penetrate, particularly, in the older patients where narrowing is present. Pain from the intercostal puncture may be severe. Occasionally, the neurovascular bundle is injured and bleeding results. With the right intercostal approach the pleural space is often transversed [11]. This raises the possibility of pneumothorax, hydro- or hemopneumothorax and empyema. Again in the older patients or in the patients with pulmonary disease and a deep costophrenic sulcus the risk of these complications is greater. They can be limited by approaching the anterior division of the right hepatic duct. Complications are increased by attempts to puncture the posterior division. Puncture of the diaphragm produces pain and the risk of subphrenic bile or infection. This may be manifest by splinting of the right diaphragm and atelectasis.

Laceration of the liver surface leads to bleeding and bile leakage with bile peritonitis or subhepatic abscess formation. Within the liver substance, hematoma may form and delayed bleeding or hemobilia may result. When bile is infected liver abscess may occur. The extensive blood supply of the liver under low pressure non results in a bile to blood fistula when the biliary tree is punctured. Even with the use of a fine needle the biliary tree is filled through a tract in the liver substance and bile leakage into the vascular compartment is common. Cholangitis with or without sepsis occurs in 20% of patients. This is the most likely cause of hypotension so often noted during percutaneous transhepatic cholangiography. If viable bacteria leak from the biliary tree, gram negative sepsis and shock may ensue. Even after prophylactic antibiotic therapy for 24 to 48 hours hypotension or shock may occur from the release of endotoxin by nonviable bacteria.

Hemobilia during percutaneous cholangiography is common. Clots produce an intraluminal filling defect in the biliary tree that may be mistaken for stone. Laceration of the hepatic arterty may lead to intrahepatic hematoma, intraperitoneal bleeding or pseudoaneurysm with late bleeding if an aneurysm ruptures into the biliary tree. In one-third of patients angiography after PTCD shows a gross vascular lesion such as a hepatic artery pseudoaneurysms (17%), arteriovenous fistula (8%) and hematoma (8%). Bleeding from these complications accounts for a 3% mortality [12]. These complications may occur after placement of the biliary stent and are difficult to manage.

In attempting to pass biliary stents or drains through obstructing lesions the wire guide may perforate the duct system or the duodenum. The forcing of a catheter through the papilla of Vater with compression of the pancreatic duct can produce pancreatitis.

Displacement of percutaneous stents and drains is common, in some series occurring in 20% of patients [13]. This again results in a communication between the biliary tree and the vascular system within the liver leading to sepsis and bile leakage into the subphrenic, subhepatic or pleural spaces. Bleeding is also common. If leakage occurs into the free peritoneal cavity, peritonitis or bilious ascites results. Since the biliary tree has been decompressed stent replacement may be difficult.

Finally even if a successful stent has been placed there may be delayed infection of the wound, migration or displacement of the stent and severe local pain. Over all severe life threatening complications occur in 20% of patients undergoing PTCD. Remedial surgery is necessary in 6% [14].

The advantage of a percutaneous stent is that it is easy for the operator to perform cholangiography and exchange stents by passing a soft tip wire guide

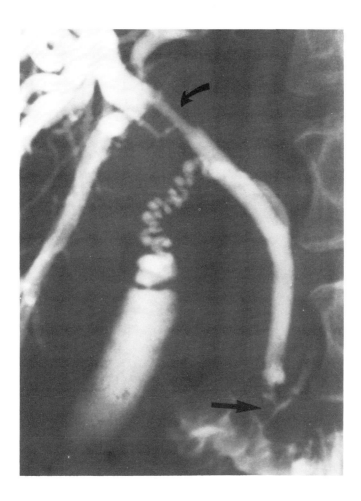

Figure 9A. This percutaneous transhepatic stent was placed in a 64 year-old female with a primary left hepatic duct cancer. Jaundice supervened when the right hepatic duct became obstructed (curved arrow). A small normal common channel joining the biliary tree and pancreatic duct (straight arrow) is avoided by maintaining the stent in the common bile duct above the sphincter. The left hepatic duct system is not visible. The prior ERCP showed only the right hepatic duct system indicating complete long standing obstruction of the left. After establishing drainage through the right hepatic duct, jaundice resolved. A percutaneous transhepatic cholangiogram confirmed the large obstructing tumor and technical impossibility of left lobe drainage.

through the stent into the duodenum, removing the stent leaving the wire in place and replacing a new stent (Fig. 9). It is also easy to institute biliary drainage by opening the stent if obstruction and cholangitis occur. Stents may be modified by conversion to an endoprosthesis that is then handled by the endoscopic route. The stent also provides easy access to other segments of the liver as tumor advances. Stents may be passed from the right hepatic duct into the left or into individual segment of lobes such as the posterior segment of the right or the

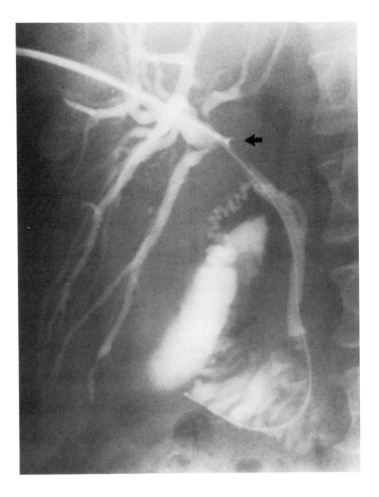

Figure 9B. After decompression forcep biopsy of the tumor (arrowhead) is obtained through the stent tract. Access is maintained by the soft wire guide passed into the duodenum. After the biopsy, the stent is replaced and the wire removed.

lateral segment of the left lobe (Fig. 10). The percutaneous stent also provides access for the placement of intraluminal radiation sources for direct treatment of tumors. Finally the stent cholangiogram is an ideal method for observing the evolution of the patient's tumor during chemotherapy or radiation therapy. Serial stent cholangiograms are easily obtained and allow excellent visualization of the intrahepatic biliary tree and the tumor.

2.4. Endoscopic stents and drains

The placement of a 5 French endoscopic stent or drain is a simple extension of

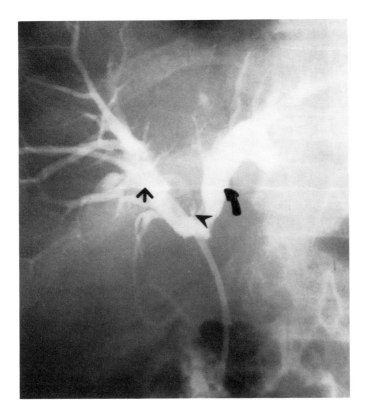

Figure 10A. This 78 year-old patient with carcinoma of the pancreas was initially treated with an endoscopic stent visible at the lower margin of the photograph. Extension of tumor into the porta hepatis required a right hepatic duct stent (straight closed arrow). The stent passes through the anterior division of the right hepatic duct and tumor into the duodenum. The right posterior hepatic duct (arrowhead) is obstructed and fills poorly. The left hepatic duct system (curved arrow) is dilated.

diagnostic ERCP with little added risk. After placing the cannulating catheter in the bile duct and injecting contrast to obtain a diagnostic cholangiogram, a wire guide with a soft spring tip is passed within the cannulating catheter through the stenosis into the proximal duct system. The cannulating catheter is then removed leaving the wire in place. The stent or drain is then passed over the wire into the proximal duct system and the endoscope and wire removed (Fig. 11). When a drain is used a small nasogastric tube is passed through the patient's nose and out the mouth. The drainage catheter is then placed within that tube and pulled out the patient's nose [15].

If the choice is made for a larger stent or for multiple 5 French stents it is wise to perform a small incision of the papilla of Vater to separate the pancreatic duct from the bile duct. Although there is some risk to incising the papilla, this small incision has less risk of hemorrhage or pancreatitis than the longer incision used for the removal of stones where the hazard of major hemorrhage is approximately

294

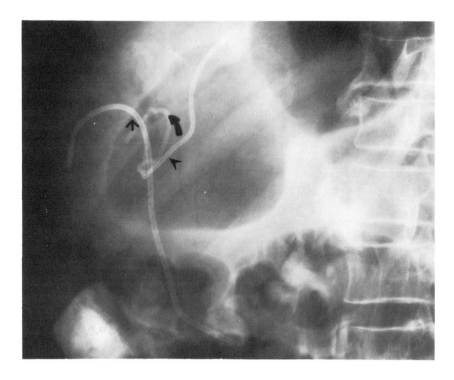

Figure 10B. Endoprostheses were placed in the left (curved arrow) and right posterior (arrowhead) ducts by using the stent path through the anterior division of the right hepatic duct (straight arrow) as seen in this lateral view.

2%. Incision of the papilla also facilitates changing the stent at a later time since the pancreatic duct opening remains at the margin of the papilla of Vater and the biliary orifice is now placed more proximally and is therefore, more easily cannulated selectively.

When only the terminal portion of the bile duct or the papilla of Vater itself is involved in periampullary cancer an endoscopic puncture of the intraduodenal bile duct above the obstruction is substituted for the sphincterotomy. A 2 mm puncture is made using cautery directly through the duodenal mucosal into the visualized distended intraduodenal bile duct. The stent is then placed above the papilla directly into the bile duct [16].

The risk of these procedures approaches that for the removal of stones by endoscopic sphincterotomy. In a large series of patients, there is 0.5% mortality and a 5% complication rate for endoscopic sphincterotomy and stone removal [17]. Major complications include bleeding from the sphincterotomy, pancreatitis from injury of the adjacent pancreatic duct or pancreatic tissue and cholangitis from stone impaction or manipulation within an infected biliary tree. This complication rate includes the risk of diagnostic ERCP. In expert hands the overall complication rate is approximately 1% [18] and a mortality of less than 0.2% [19].

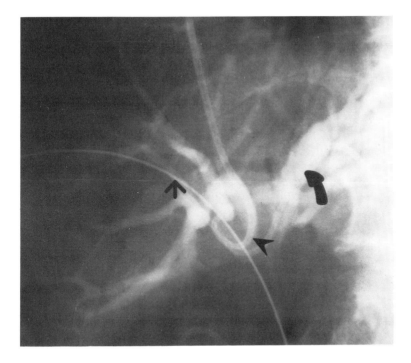

Figure 10C. With dilute contrast, the wire guide is seen in the anterior division of the right hepatic duct (straight arrow) with an endoprosthesis in both posterior division of the right (arrowhead) and left (curved arrow). All duct system are decompressed.

The risk of endoscopic diagnosis and drainage through ERCP is substantially less than that of the percutaneous techniques. Furthermore, failure by the endoscopic route had little risk. Failure generally results from inability to inject contrast into a completely obstructed duct system above a tumor mass. Hence, the complication rate for failure is low. Failure of cholangiography or pancreatography is proceeded by upper gastrointestinal endoscopy with its diagnostic value and appreciation of a periampullary mass with biopsy of duodenum or papilla of Vater malignancy if present.

2.5. Clinical pathological correlation

In periampullary lesions, the important differentiation is carcinoma of the pancreas from the other periampullary cancers where the potential for cure by resection is greater [20]. This requires the use of ERCP and visualization of the pancreatic duct. Carcinoma of the duodenum and the papilla of Vater are easily diagnosed by endoscopic biopsy where the percutaneous approach only confirms a diagnosis of bile duct obstruction. It is similarly difficult to differentiate terminal bile duct and mid bile duct primary neoplasms from carcinoma of the pancreas

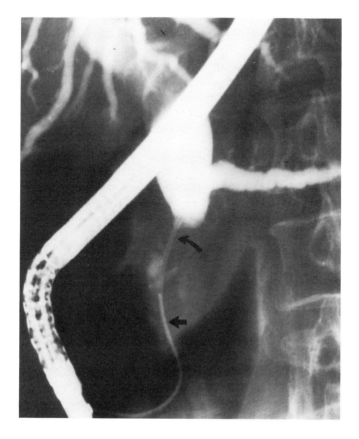

Figure 11A. This 5 French endoscopic stent (curved arrow) passes into the common hepatic duct above a carcinoma of the pancreas. The wire guide is partially removed (straight arrow). The dilated obstructed pancreatic duct is on the right. The hepatic duct and intrahepatic biliary tree are above. The irregular area with absent contrast between the arrows is the tumor mass.

with extension or metastasis by cholangiography alone. The same reasoning applies to nonsurgical drainage. The risk of prejudicing surgery by a complication of percutaneous nonsurgical drainage and the desire both on the part of the patient and the therapist for early resection and limited hospital stay dictate the use of a single 5 French endoscopic stent to achieve decompression and resolution of cholestasis followed by prompt surgery. In these patients we avoid the use of endoscopic sphincterotomy because of the risk of the bleeding from these vascular tumors.

Cancer involving the hepatic duct at the level of the bifurcation into the right and left system may be primary or metastatic. The radiologic differentiation of primary from metastatic lesions is not possible. A careful search for a primary cancer, particularly in the middle aged female patient where these lesions are common, may be fruitless, but is essential. Again a pancreatogram to exclude

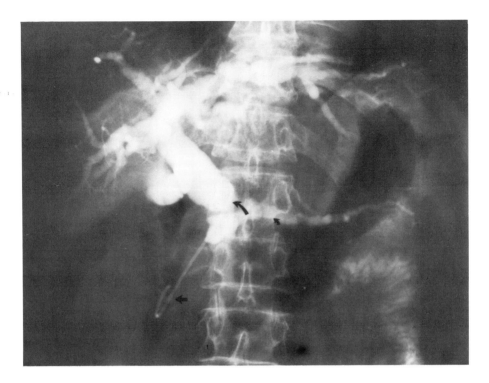

Figure 11B. Immediately after removal of the endoscope the proximal pigtail is in the bile duct (curved arrow) and the distal pigtail in the duodenum (straight arrow). The pancreatic duct remains opacified (right arrowhead).

carcinoma of the pancreas and a careful endoscopic examination to exclude upper gastrointestinal tract cancer is required. Breast and uterus should be examined by the appropriate techniques. These lesions can be stented endoscopically to relieve cholestasis at the time of diagnostic examination. This serves as a temporizing procedure to establish the absence of other intrahepatic lesions and reduce the risk of percutaneous draingae. Resectability for cure should be determined by angiography, but in our experience this is rarely possible. After percutaneous drainage and relief of cholestasis radiation therapy is generally indicated.

With rare exceptions adenocarcinoma of the pancreas can only be palliated [21]. In the majority of large bulky carcinomas of the head of the pancreas, endoscopic diagnosis and drainage is preferred with percutaneous drainage when the endoscopic approach fails technically. Even in the patients where angiography suggests the possibility of palliative resection, intra-abdominal and hepatic metastasis are common [5]. These findings are often signalled by failure of nonsurgical drainage to reduce the patient's bilirubin to a level considered acceptable for a safe surgical approach (6 mg/dl). In these patients, nonsurgical biliary drainage allows stratification as therapy proceeds. Burcharth has summarized the results of four publications comprising 166 patients and shown that only 63% achieved marked bilirubin reduction [14]. No change was found in 20%. The remaining 17% had only a moderate bilirubin reduction. Thus, more than one-third of patients responded poorly as a result of hepatic failure, advanced cancer or both. Nonsurgical biliary drainage identifies the patients with a poor prognosis and permits an appropriate therapeutic decision. Undoubtely, these failures of nonsurgical drainage comprise the patients who also failed to respond to surgical drainage with its greater trauma. In the group where angiography suggests resectability and cholestasis clears without evidence of intra-abdominal or hepatic metastasis, palliative resection may be undertaken with a relatively acceptable risk or chemotherapy elected.

2.6. Linkage between diagnosis and therapy

Although ERCP has a substantially lower risk than percutaneous diagnostic procedures concern about cholangitis in the patients with bile duct obstruction is well founded. Complications in diagnostic ERCP rarely occur if proper technique is followed in patients without an obstructed duct [22]. In patients with an obstructed duct system, a brief course of prophylactic antibiotic is appropriate. It is more effective to immediately achieve drainage. This can be accomplished either by a nasobiliary drain or by a endoscopic stent. The use of a single 5 French tube allows adequate biliary drainage. We place a stent or nasobiliary drain in patients with bile duct obstruction from cancer even when their ERCP has been performed on an ambulatory basis. This assures that cholangitis will not occur [22].

In the PTC the major complication risk of a diagnostic procedure alone is 5% to 10% [23, 24]. Of course no percutaneous transhepatic procedures are performed on an ambulatory patient. Prophylactic antibiotic therapy for at least 24 hours before a percutaneous transhepatic procedures is essential. With increasing skill in the use of percutaneous transhepatic biliary drainage, it has become fashionable to combined the diagnostic procedure with the drainage procedure. This has a number of advantages.

The volume of contrast and the effort required to achieve a diagnostic procedure in a patient with a markedly dilated duct system can be limited. One may accept a less than ideal initial diagnostic study and proceed directly with the introduction of a drainage catheter. After the catheter is placed comfortably within the duct system and the tract from the skin to the intrahepatic biliary tree is sealed with the plastic catheter, the diagnostic portion of the study is completed. It is usually wise to then advance the drainage catheter through the obstructing lesion as a permanent internal stent since this is a more stable mechanical position that tends to prevent dislodgement. Nevertheless, a substantial number of stents passing into the duodenum through obstructing lesions become dislodged (6%).

This leaves a difficult clinical situation often producing major complications. These misadventures account for the 25% complication rate and 3% mortality of percutaneous transhepatic biliary drainage (PTCE) [11, 14].

It should be apparent that some of the previously mentioned problems limit this approach. A prior choice between a right or left hepatic puncture must be made. The primary diagnostic information usually acquired by ERCP is lacking. Visualization of the pancreatic duct and the differential diagnosis of the periampullary disease is made difficult by the placement of a percutaneous stent through the papilla of Vater.

2.7. Technical factors

Certain extremely firm tumors, usually carcinoma of the pancreas, cannot be passed by the wire guide required to introduce the plastic stent. This is a more common failing by the endoscopic route since the mechanical difficulty of working 120 cm from the patient's mouth is substantial. Even in percutaneous approaches some lesions cannot be passed and must be managed by external drainage. These constitute approximately 5% of the total. Occasionally, lesions cannot be passed percutaneously but can be managed endoscopically and vice versa. In general, however, the percutaneous approach is more likely to succeed technically. The experience of the operator is an important factor in the success of these techniques.

The extent and length of the lesion as well its rate of growth are important factors in both the mechanical and clinical success of nonsurgical biliary drainage. Lesions with great bulk in the duodenum cannot be managed well endoscopically. Even if an initial success is achieved it is unlikely that it will be possible to exchange the stent at a later date. In these patients it may be wise to supplement the initial endoscopic approach with a percutaneous stent. Similarly lesions at the bifurcation of the hepatic duct may be palliated only for short periods by a single catheter. As the tumors grows to obstruct the right or left hepatic duct, a second stent is required.

The character of the lesion, the patient's intrinsic resistance to infection and the amount of proximal ductal dilatation influence the success of biliary stents. Some tumors produce a large quantity of debris which occludes the catheter, requires irrigation and often demands continued external drainage. Similarly, patients who have bleeding either from the manipulation required to pass the stent or from the tumor itself will repeatedly occlude the stent and require irrigation and frequent changes. When the duct system is markedly dilated, even gravity drainage may not return the duct to normal caliber. Dilatation gives a large reservoir for infection with poor bile flow. Once infected such a biliary system rarely clears spontaneously. Extremely debilitated patients may also be unable to clear the biliary tree of infection despite external drainage to gravity; they may have recurrent cholangitis as soon as internal drainage is attempted.

A number of these complicating factors could potentially be solved by a large surgical biliary drainage procedure. This should be considered, but unfortunately, the majority of these patients have very large tumors or are in clinical circumstances that preclude a surgical approach.

A number of other factors often have overriding significance in the outcome of nonsurgical biliary drainage and yet are difficult to identify in the individual patient. Extensive hepatic metastasis or vascular comprise of the portal vein, hepatic artery or tumor embolization within the liver may be responsible for unrelieved cholestasis despite what appears to be adequate drainage. In certain patients liver failure with cholestasis has reached a point where resolution is impossible. Renal dysfunction with hepatorenal syndrome and complicating primary or secondary infection as well as extreme malnutrition may not be reversible.

Complicating disease of other organs, particularly, lung and liver raise the risk of percutaneous procedures substantially. An unpleasant and poorly managed complication of percutaneous stent, particularly by right transpleural approach, is pain with impaired respiration and atelectasis of the right lower lobe. This is accentuated by subphrenic or subhepatic leakage of bile or infection [11]. Therefore, in patients with pulmonary disease a greater effort to achieve endoscopic drainage should be made. Liver disease with portal hypertension may also be an important complicating factor.

3. Conclusions

Nonsurgical biliary drainage is accomplished by a diverse series of techniques and manipulations that provide an important alternative to the traditional surgical approach. They allow a rapid determination of pathologic anatomy and, when combined with endoscopic or percutaneous aspiration biopsy, yield a tissue diagnosis. These techniques are not without hazard and a substantial portion of these patients fail to respond even when satisfactory drainage is achieved without complication. In general, they should be applied before surgical therapy. The concept of immediate surgical exploration of the jaundiced patient is no longer tenable. Endoscopic examination of the upper gastrointestinal tract, biliary and pancreatic ducts should be a prerequisite for any further intervention. In comparison to PTC, ERCP has the advantage of a minimum diagnostic risk combined with visualization of the upper gastrointestinal tract and pancreatic duct. In the presence of an obstructed duct system, endoscopic drainage should be instituted when technically possible. When endoscopic techniques fail a prompt shift, preferably during the same procedure, to the percutaneous route is indicated. Both these techniques should be combined with percutaneous cytological diagnosis using the direct cholangiogram or pancreatogram as a target. Aspiration using anatomic landmarks derived from prior cholangiography, pancreatography or angiography may be useful if the initial biopsy is unsuccessful [25].

The relatively high risks of diagnostic PTC may be limited by PTCD. However, information to date indicates that PTCD in and of itself has substantial risks and, therefore, should only be undertaken in appropriate clinical circumstances [14]. The decision for surgical management, particularly with the hope of curative resection in the small percentage of patients where this is feasible or for long term successful palliation should remain a sought after goal. The morbidity and mortality of surgical management in these patients can be substantial reduced by preoperative nonsurgical drainage. These techniques provide an important alternative to two stage operations and are useful in stratifying patients. The large segment of this population (one-third) who do not response to nonsurgical drainage and undoubtedly correspond to the high mortality group of patients who previously underwent surgical exploration must be identified if appropriate therapy is to be undertaken and the results of these therapies evaluated successfully.

References

1. Shaldon S, Barber KM, Young WB: Percutaneous transhepatic cholangiography: A modified technic. Gastroenterology 42: 371–379, 1962.
2. Nagai N, Toki F, Oi I, *et al.*: Continuous pancreatocholedochal catheterization. Gastrointest Endosc 23: 78–81, 1976.
3. Cotton PB, Burney PCJ, Mason RR: Transnasal bile duct catheterization after endoscopic sphincterotomy. Gut 20: 285–287, 1979.
4. Zimmon DS: New uses of endoscopic retrograde cholangiopancreatography (ERCP) in the management of biliary and pancreatic disease. In: Progress in Gastroenterology. Grune and Stratton, New York. CH23, pp. 447–503, 1983.
5. Buckwalter JA, Lawton RL, Tidrich RT: Bypass operations for neoplastic biliary tract obstruction. Am J Surg 109: 100–106, 1965.
6. Nakayama T, Ikeda A, Okuda K: Percutaneous transhepatic drainage of the biliary tract: Technique and results in 104 cases. Gastroenterology 74: 554–559, 1978.
7. Pitt HA, Cameron JL, Postier RG, *et al.*: Factors affecting mortality in biliary tract surgery. Am J Surg 141: 66–72, 1981.
8. Denning DS, Ellison EC, Carey LC: Preoperative percutaneous transhepatic biliary decompression lowers operative morbidity in patients with obstructive jaundice. Am J Surg 141: 61–65, 1981.
9. Hazards of biliary surgery. (Editorial). Br Med J 282: 2077–2078, 1981.
10. Beall MS, Dyer GA, Stephenson HE, Jr: Disappointments in the management of patients with malignancy of pancreas, duodenum, and common bile duct. Arch Surg 101: 461, 1970.
11. Jaques PF, Mandell VS, Delany DJ, Nath PH: Percutaneous transhepatic biliary drainage: Advantages of the left-lobe subxiphoid approach. Radiology 145: 534–536, 1982.
12. Hoevels J, Nilsson U: Intrahepatic vascular lesions following nonsurgical percutaneous transhepatic bile duct intubation. Gastrointest Radiol 5: 127–135, 1980.
13. Pollock TW, Ring FR, Oleaga JA, *et al.*: Percutaneous decompression of benign and malignancy biliary obstruction. Arch Surg 114: 148–151, 1979.
14. Burcharth F: Nonsurgical drainage of the biliary tract. Seminars in Liver Disease 2: 75–86, 1982.

15. Zimmon DS, Clemett AR: Endoscopic stents and drains in the management of pancreatic and bile duct obstruction. Surg Clinics of North Am 62: 837–844, 1982.
16. Osnes M: Endoscopic choledochoduodenostomy for common bile duct obstruction. Lancet 1: 1059, 1979.
17. Safrany L, Cotton PB: Endoscopic management of choledocholithiasis. Surg Clinics of North Am 62: 825–836, 1982.
18. Belohlavek D, Kock H, Rösch W, et al.: 5 Years experience in endoscopic retrograde cholangio-pancreatography (ERCP). Endoscopy 8: 115–118, 1976.
19. Kessler RE, Falkenstein DB, Clemett AR, et al.: Indications, clinical value and complications of endoscopic retrograde cholangiopancreatography. Surg Gynec Obstet 142: 865–870, 1976.
20. Bismuth H, Malt RA: Current concepts in cancer: Carcinoma of the biliary tract. NEJM 301: 704–705, 1979.
21. Hermann RE, Cooperman AM: Current concepts in cancer: Cancer of the pancreas. NEJM 301: 482–484, 1979.
22. Zimmon DS, Falkenstein DB, Riccobono C, et al.: Complications of endoscopic retrograde cholangiopancreatography: Analysis of 300 consecutive cases. Gastroenterology 69: 303–309, 1975.
23. Kreck MJ, Balint JA: 'Skinny Needle' cholangiography. Gastroenterology 78: 598–604, 1980.
24. Mueller PR, VanSonnenberg E, Simeone JF: Fine needle transhepatic cholangiography. Ann Intern Med 97: 567–572, 1982.
25. Kline TS, Hunter HS: Needle aspiration biopsy: A critical appraisal eight years and 3,267 specimens later. JAMA 239: 36–39, 1978.
26. Ihre T, Pyk E, Raaschou-Nielsen T, et al.: Percutaneous fine-needle aspiration biopsy during endoscopic retrograde choangio-pancreatography. Scand J Gastro 13: 657–662, 1978.

12. Nutritional repletion after major gut excision

MAURICE E. SHILS

1. Introduction

Because of the intimate relationship between alimentary tract function and nutrition, it is obvious that any disease process, including malignancies, which results in resection, abnormal continuity or by-pass of any part of that tract, may interfere with normal function. Such changes in turn have the potential for deleterious effects on nutritional status. Gastrointestinal malignancies are among the more common types of tumors with gastric, pancreatic and colon and rectal carcinomas occurring among the 10 most frequent primary sites in the United States [1]. In addition, the liver is a major target for metastases.

Malnutrition – primarily protein-calorie undernutrition – is particularly common in patients with alimentary tract cancer [2–4] and weight loss has significant prognostic implications for patients with colon cancer [4]. Understanding the nutritional and metabolic consequences of such surgery will alert the physician to initiate preventive measures to prevent insofar as possible undesirable changes and to maintain as optimum a quality of life as possible in the patients. Where malnutrition and metabolic changes have already occurred when the patient presents to the physician, a knowledge of the underlying issues permits a more rational application of necessary nutritional and dietary intervention modalities.

This chapter reviews the basis for the development of nutritional problems and their treatment related to excision of various parts of the alimentary tract. The primary concern is related to the effects of surgical intervention for the treatment of cancer. Many of these surgical procedures are also used in the treatment of non-malignant diseases and so the lessons are more universal. In addition, brief attention is paid here to some of the nutritional consequences of surgical procedures which have been or are being employed in the treatment of morbid obesity by modification of the gastric reservoir.

J.J. DeCosse and P. Sherlock (eds), Clinical Management of Gastrointestinal Cancer.
© 1984, Martinus Nijhoff Publishers, Boston. ISBN 0-89838-601-2. Printed in The Netherlands.

2. Head and neck cancer

Since patients, especially males, with malignancies in this area often have a history of chronic alcohol intake, they may be in a nutritionally depleted state prior to therapy.

Treatment of tumors in this area frequently combines surgery, radiation and chemotherapy. Surgery may include partial or total glossectomy and mandibulectomy and resection of portions of the hard or soft palate and muscles of the lower face and neck depending on the site and extent of the disease. Radiation complicates the mechanical problems of chewing and deglutition because of consequent loss of taste ('mouth blindness') [5], xerostomia as the result of salivary gland damage and injury to teeth. As the result of impaired swallowing, aspiration is a chronic danger and tube feeding may be required to assure adequate nutrition. In serious cases where salivary secretions cannot be managed, laryngectomy with physical separation of the respiratory and alimentary tracts is indicated.

2.1. Recommendations for nutrition and diet support

Where nutritional status is significantly impaired, (e.g. more than 10% recent weight loss, albumin less than 3.1 g%, history of recent ethanol intake) there should be some rehabilitative pre-operative nutrition effort if time permits. This can be in the form of oral or tube feeding of palatable complete liquid formulas or supplements in addition to whatever oral intake the patient is capable of. In more extreme cases, parenteral nutrition in hospital may be necessary.

When prolonged serious post-operative swallowing difficulties are considered likely as a result of treatment, formation of a feeding gastrostomy should be considered. This route of feeding decreases the danger of aspiration with oral food intake, avoids the need for insertion and removal of naso-pharyngeal feeding tubes and allows immediate nutritional rehabilitation efforts or maintenance of pre-existing adequate nutritional status. Attention to proper management of gastostomy tubes results in controlling leakage, skin maceration and pain. Initial insertion of a mushroom catheter is followed by replacement after healing with a soft Foley catheter. The patient and family member are instructed to place 4 × 4 gauze pads half-transected around the catheter, tape the pads to the skin with paper tape, pull the catheter hub moderately tightly against the abdominal wall and tape onto the gauze pad so that the catheter does not move to and fro from the stomach.

Post-treatment attention to providing attractive foods with pleasant aroma, lubricated by gravies and salad dressings of high caloric and nutrition content may be helpful in encouraging better food intake. Nutritious liquid formulas taken by mouth if they can be swallowed or by intermittent tube or gastrostomy feedings (if not tolerated by mouth) are often helpful as supplementing oral feeding.

Small caliber, flexible mercury-weighted tubes are available for nasogastric feeding which are easily inserted and removed on a daily basis or after each feeding by the patient or family member are very well tolerated by most patients and allow intermittent feedings. Such tubes often eliminate the need for indwelling naso-pharyngeal tubes and are an alternative to permanent esophagostomy or gastrostomy for feeding purposes. Listings and discussions of various tubes, infusion pumps, other equipment and formulas for oral and/or tube feeding are available [6].

Some patients are at serious risk of aspiration of regurgitated food because of absent gag reflex with a tendency to easy regurgitation or vomiting, especially in the presence of significant pulmonary disease. For such patients daily passage of a tube with its tip in the lower esophagus or stomach carries a certain hazard. The danger of aspiration may be reduced markedly by infusing the formula by slow drip over a number of hours using a pump to assure regular flow rate. The hazard may be further reduced by using tubes with somewhat heavier mercury weights which are allowed to be passed into the upper small bowel prior to initiating feeding. These tubes are very well tolerated and should be left in place unless there is an important reason for their temporary removal.

Minimizing cost and assuring nutritional adequacy are important considerations for those long term patients dependent in large part or totally on tube feedings. Blended formulas of food available at home in proper types and amounts (e.g. formula MSKCC) [6, 7] tend to be nutritionally adequate and less expensive than most commercial formulas. Unfortunately ordinary kitchen blenders do not disperse meats and vegetables finely enough to pass through small-bore feeding tubes. This problem can be overcome by the use of pureed food or passing blenderized food through fine mesh strainers.

3. Esophageal resection

Whether it be because of benign stricture or carcinoma, a significant number of affected patients will have lost weight as a result of decreased intake secondary to progressive dysphagia. Where obstruction is not complete, instruction and attention to ingestion of adequate amounts of nutritionally adequate liquid foods or formulas are often beneficial in preventing malnutrition. When pre-operative malnutrition (as defined above) exists and serious anorexia is also present, passage of a fine-bore feeding tube should be considered if occlusion is only partial and total parenteral nutrition where the obstruction is functionally total. However, in the experience of this author oral or tube feeding in the period of radiation and chemotherapy are usually inadequate to meet to need, either because of interference with feeding, nausea, pain or combinations thereof. In such instances adequate parenteral feeding is indicated to maintain nutritional status.

Radiation to the lower neck and mediastinum may induce esophagitis but this usually disappears following cessation of therapy. However, some patients may develop fibrosis with resultant esophageal stricture.

Chemotherapy (presently a combination of drugs increasingly being tested in high dose and with one or more cycles) induces nausea, anorexia, sore mouth and diarrhea further inhibiting food intake in those without severe dysphagia and decreasing the possibility of tube feeding, especially in the presence of serious thrombocytopenia.

Surgical treatment for carcinoma of the esophagus usually involves total or distal esophagectomy associated with bilateral vagotomy, proximal gastrectomy and gastric pullup into the chest. Such surgery is usually associated with a tendency to regurgitation, rapid satiety, decreased rate of gastric emptying of solid food despite pyloroplasty, diarrhea (intermittent or continuous) and steatorrhea (mild to moderate) [9]. The causes of the diarrhea and steatorrhea are unknown. They often occur together but may exist as separate entities. The combination of decreased fat absorption, impaired appetite with rapid satiety, and fear of eating because of diarrhea predisposes to weight loss.

Total vagotomy has been associated with as increase in basal serum gastrin levels in man but post prandial gastrin output is only slightly elevated. GIP levels are increased in basal serum concentration and in response to glucose. The plasma pancreatic polypeptide response in insulin hypoglycemia is markedly reduced as is the response to a meal [10].

Vagotomy and pyloroplasty (V and P) modify the absorption of a glucose load. Compared to normal controls, those with V and P when given 90 g glucose load orally had a more rapid appearance of glucose in the blood followed by a fall in glucose with hypoglycemic levels being attained and the peak plasma insulin values were more than four times higher [11]. In addition, only about $60 \pm 7\%$ of ingested glucose appeared in the systemic circulation in those with V and P as compared to $92 \pm 2\%$ in the controls. These changes are explainable on the basis of a markedly shorter absorption period with malabsorption occurring presumably as the result of an overwhelming of the glucose absorptive mechanisms; the hyperosmolarity of the oral glucose solution (40%) may have been a contributing factor. Similar mechanisms may operate in patients with subtotal gastrectomy with V and P who are given a large glucose load.

3.1. Recommendation for nutritional and dietary support

Post-operative dietary and nutritional intervention involves provision of frequent small meals moderately high in carbohydrate and protein since these are well tolerated. If steatorrhea is marked, restriction of large amounts of long chain fats is advisable, with substitution in part by medium chain triglycerides (MCT).

True, 'dumping' is not likely to occur in such patients since there is a normal gastric-duodenal continuity; furthermore there is usually slow gastric emptying of solid food despite pyloroplasty. However, such patients often have rapid passage of liquids; hence dumpting symptoms may occur if large amounts of solutions of concentrated carbohydrates are taken rapidly by mouth. Post-operative fistulas are much less common now as compared to the period when colon or jejunal interposition was used more frequently; however, stricture is not uncommon and may require periodic dilatation or futher surgery.

MCT is a bland oil similar in appearance to other vegetable oils. It is derived from coconut oil which is specially processed so that almost all of the triglycerides present are as C6–C12 fatty acids [12]. These fatty acids do not follow the abosorptive pathway of the long chain fats but, instead, enter the portal vein and are rapidly metabolized into the liver. Because some patients develop intestinal distress when suddenly given large amounts of MCT, it is advisable to start with approximately 20–30 ml distributed over the day and increase volume as tolerated. The oil can be used in liquid formulas, in cooking and as a salad dressing. Since the fatty acids are rapidly metabolized, a mild acidosis may occur which is managed in the administration of sodium bicarbonate. Its use in cirrhotics with or without portocaval shunting may exacerbate encephalopathic changes because the concentration of fatty acids of MCT have been found to increase in spinal fluid to levels 4 to 5 times that observed in noncirrhotic controls [13]; such fatty acids have been found to cause abnormal central nervous system effects in experimental animals.

Carcinoma of the esophagogastric junction creates physiologic and nutritional problems which are similar to those of the patient with an esophagogastrostomy. Because a larger portion of the proximal stomach is resected, early satiety may be more marked and gastric secretions and intrinsic factor production may be reduced with resultant additional malabsorptive problems, i.e. overgrowth of the small bowel with fecal organisms and impaired vitamin B_{12} absorption. The same dietary approach is recommended for those with a lesser degree of gastric resection but the possibilities must be considered of the development of a blind loop syndrome and of B_{12} malabsorption.

4. Surgical modification of the stomach

4.1. Gastric cancer

Although the rate of occurrence of gastric cancer has shown a steady downward trend in the United States for more than 20 years [1] it is still a major cause of death equal in new cases to that of pancreatic cancer and exceeded along the gastrointestinal tract only by colon and rectal malignancies.

4.2. Gastrectomy

Surgical treatment for gastric cancer involves either high subtotal gastrectomy with a gastro-jejunal anastamosis or total gastrectomy with esophago-jejuno-stomy. Removal of most or all of the stomach serves to reduce or delete its reservoir, metering, secretory and digestive functions as well as altering the normal continuity of the tract. This modification from the normal has both physiologic and nutritional consequences which may vary from mild to severe depending upon the extent of resection, the individual patient response and the effectiveness of preventive intervention by the physician. The nutritional problems of patients with high subtotal or total gastrectomy have a different physiologic basis than those resulting from esophagogastrostomy.

In those patients with a high subtotal or total gastrectomy a variety of signs and symptoms may occur in association with ingestion of food – especially those high in soluble carbohydrates – which have been termed the 'dumping syndrome'. When it occurs this syndrome usually appears at the end of a meal or 10 to 15 minutes after its completion and then subsides at a rate depending on its severity and on the behavior of the patient. Objective findings include tachycardia, tachypnea, elevation of blood pressure, increased small intestinal intraluminal pressure and motility, decreased plasma volume, decreased plasma potassium and phosphate, hyperglycemia, decreased cardiac output and T-wave and ST segment changes in the electrocardiogram. In addition, there are manifestations of autonomic or adrenal medullary response such as apprehension, sweating and vascular instability. In some patients the symptoms may be so severe that the patient must lie down for fear of fainting. The intake of food may be chronically reduced in an effort to avoid or ameliorate the symptoms.

The dumping syndrome has been studied extensively since Machella established the fact that a large fluid volume shift into the bowel occurred after intraluminal introduction of a hyperosmolar meal [14]. The shift in fluid is associated with a release of humoral agents which account in part for some of the symptomatology. The incidence of clinically significant dumping after gastrectomy varies among various authors from 5 to 15 percent with perhaps 2 percent of the patient being incapacitated by these symptoms [15].

There is a rapid entry of carbohydrate into the upper small bowel with resulting hyperglycemia [16, 17]. Postprandial insulin levels are elevated above normal in all Billroth II patients and are even higher in those with the dumping syndrome [18]. Similarly the glucagon-like immunoreactivity is increased postoperatively [19]. In these patients serum basal gastric inhibitory peptide (GIP) is normal but the postprandial GIP is markedly increased [7]. Gastrojejunostomy is associated with decreased basal serum gastrin concentrations and absent release post prandially. Neurotensin [20], serotonin [21] and bradykinin [22] increase in gastrectomized patients with the dumping syndrome as compared to those that do not dump. It has been suggested that bradykinin is responsible for the early vasomotor symptoms with serotonin associated with delayed responses.

Because of the rapid passage of food down the upper alimentary tract and the markedly reduced or absent gastric reservoir of additional food, hypoglycemic symptoms may begin approximately one hour later in association with the increased insulin and other hormonal responses. These symptoms may be confused with those of the dumping syndrome but should be differentiated.

Following a subtotal or total gastrectomy, varying degrees of malabsorption of a number of nutrients may occur. Vitamin B_{12} (cobalamin) in animal-derived foods is tightly bound to proteins and is released in the normal stomach by the action of HCl and pepsin. Intrinsic factor is produced in the stomach and is essential for B_{12} absorption. Until recently it was commonly believed that co-balamin released from dietary protein in the stomach was then bound there by intrinsic factor. Newer evidence indicates that a B_{12}-binding protein in gastric juice designated as R protein has a much higher affinity for cobalamin than does intrinsic factor, particularly at acid pH, and that dietary B_{12} enters the jejunum bound to R protein. The cobalamin does not become bound to intrinsic factor until the R protein moiety is partially degraded by pancreatic proteases in the small intestine [23].

Partial gastrectomy with its resultant acid and pepsin secretion results in an impaired liberation of diet-bound cobalamin. In such patients the critical factor in B_{12} absorption is not lack of intrinsic factor since it is secreted in excess. Clinical B_{12} deficiency may occur in such patients but the time span may be 15 years [23]. Vitamin B_{12} absorption as measured by the Schilling test has been found to be impaired in 42.3% of 97 patients with a subtotal gastrectomy and gastrojejuno-stomy [24]. Total gastrectomy is associated with a complete absence of intrinsic factor. In these patients clinical evidence of B_{12} deficiency will occur in 3 to 5 years because these individuals malabsorb all forms of dietary B_{12} as well as that in the biliary secretion which is tightly bound to R protein.

Absorption of fat and protein has been studied in gastrectomized patients. Average levels of fat absorption after total gastrectomy are approximately 80% with much variation among individuals [15]. While there is considerable vari-ability among patients, increased fat malabsorption is associated with the degree of weight loss following total gastrectomy [25]. Although fat losses may be significant, it has been suggested that weight loss and the development of mal-nutrition are more directly related to factors affecting total intake [15]. Fat malabsorption may be related to relative pancreatic insufficiency. Lundh had suggested that the decreased enzyme activity in the jejunum in such patients was secondary to inadequate pancreatic response [26]. This was believed due in part to rapid entry of the food and a discrepancy between the time of enzyme secretion and mixing of the food (a condition termed 'pancreaticocibal asynchrony'). However, some investigators have found that administration of pancreatic ex-tract has been without effect [27]. Others have found that liquid meals in gastrec-tomized patients are associated with a normal response of the pancreas but that there is effective diminished enzyme activity as a result of dilution and of sequestration of trypsin and bile in the afferent loop [28].

The loss of gastric juice and the rise of pH in the upper small bowel predispose to growth of colonic organisms in the afferent loop and in any jejunal pouches that are prepared in an effort to slow transit of food into the upper jejunum. Bacterial overgrowth is enhanced by failure of some of these loops to drain normally with a resultant blind loop syndrome with decreased utilization of vitamin B_{12}, formation of hydroxy fatty acids which may lead to diarrhea and fat and carbohydrate malabsorption.

The rapid entry into the intestine of significant amounts of milk or milk products is often associated with symptoms of lactose intolerance – presumably due to the high concentrations of lactose achieved in gastrectomized patients who have a latent lactase deficiency [29]. Similarly latent celiac disease may become active following gastrectomy because of the presence of higher than usual concentrations of gluten along the small intestine [30].

Gastrectomized patients absorb iron in reduced amounts with resultant iron deficiency anemia which becomes manifest after a number of years. This is secondary to impaired reduction of ferric ion to the ferrous form and to decreased ability to release organically bound iron from food. Chronic blood loss which has been noted in such patients is a contributory factor [31]. Decreased absorption of fat soluble vitamins, particularly vitamins A and D, leads to gradual depletion. An association between gastric resection and skeletal disease has been recognized for many years, particularly in England and Australia but also in the United States [32]. In a series of 342 patients with partial gastractomy, 30% had defects in calcium metabolism with 25% having osteomalacia diagnosed on bone biopsy. Only 5% of age and sex-matched patients with peptic ulcer disease without surgery had defects in calcium metabolism. There was a significant correlation with the degree of steatorrhea [28]. This presumably explains the vitamin D malabsorption which has been noted [33] and which leads to decreased efficiency of calcium absorption. Decreased intake of calcium as a consequence of reduction in milk and milk products with milk intolerance exacerbates the problem. With the decreased food intake and varying degrees of malabsorption, decreased levels of water-soluble nutrients are to be expected, in particular those of folate and zinc.

In an effort to minimize the severity of dumping syndromes, surgical procedures have been developed which include interposing antiperistaltic jejunal segments between the remaining stomach and duodenum [34] or constructing a pouch from a segment of jejunum as a substitute stomach [35]. Although clinical reports claim improvement following such surgery, experiments in dogs with total gastrectomy and anti-peristaltic jejunal segments resulted in failure to improve nutrition although transit time was markedly slowed [36].

For multiple reasons related in varying degrees to the occurrence of the dumping syndrome, pain, opiates, depression, or residual tumor and to unknown factors, anorexia is fairly common in patients with a 'radical' or total gastrectomy. Weight loss may be a serious and chronic problem. The increasing use of chemotherapy in such patients is an exacerbating factor. An additional anorexigenic factor in patients with a very major or total gastrectomy is the pain induced by bile reflux and associated esophagitis which is exacerbated by eating. A trial of cholestyramine (in an effort to bind bile salts) and of sucralfate (to coat the epithelium in an effort to reduce irritation) are warranted although usually only partially effective at best. If the condition is intractable, surgical intervention with a Roux-en-Y procedure is to be considered.

Resection in the treatment of peptic ulcer
The removal of much of the acid-secreting portion of the stomach with a gastro-jejunostomy of yesteryear has been succeeded by a combination of excision limited to the gastric-producing antrum in combination with total or selective vagotomy. As a consequence dumping is absent or minimal with the latter types of surgery and malabsorption problems would be expected to be markedly reduced. It has been found, however, that subdiaphragmatic vagotomy as well as certain selective procedures may be associated with diarrhea (usually intermittent) and some steatorrhea – usually mild [9]. For those patients who had major gastric resection in the past or for those where such resection had to be performed recently for benign disease, nutritional problems may occur similar to those reviewed above.

4.3. Recommendations for nutrition and dietary support of gastrectomized patients

The dumping syndrome can be greatly minimized or prevented by provision of and adherence to a dietary regimen termed the anti-dumping diet. This consists of a diet high in protein, low in soluble carbohydrates, restricted in fluid with the meal and served approximately 6 times per day. This regimen results in a decreased osmolar load in the upper jejunum because of decreased carbohydrate and meal size and a reduction in insulin output; together with decreased intervals between meals such a diet minimizes significant hypoglycemia. Additional measures for those who continue to be symptomatic include reclining for a period immediately after eating. The use of a pectin derivative has been reported to prolong gastric emptying and to decrease dumping, blood volume changes, hyperglycemia and serum insulin [37, 38].

Since such diets [e.g. 39] tend to be high in long-chain triglycerides, steatorrhea may be significant if the gastric resection is a major one. This can be reduced by progressive intake in the amount of medium-chain triglycerides (MCT) replacing long chain fats as tolerated. When steatorrhea is present, a trial of pancreatic extract is indicated to rule out luminal pancreatic enzyme insufficiency as the result of dilution or pancreatic secretory defect. Because gastric acid production is decreased or absent in these patients, the use of bicarbonate with uncoated pancreatic extract or of coated pancreatic enzyme preparations are not likely to be more effective than uncoated pancreatic extract preparations alone taken in adequate amounts. (vide infra)

Deficiencies of vitamins and minerals can be prevented or treated by their oral administration in adequate amounts. Supplementary iron with ascorbic acid, vitamin B_{12} injection (100 mcg once monthly is sufficient) and use of *complete* supplementary vitamins (high potency vitamin formulations are usually not necessary) should be considered. It should be noted that some supplementary and high potency vitamins may be lacking in folate. Vitamin D supplements may be useful when fat malabsorption is significant; the need can be determined by measurement of the levels of 25 hydroxyvitamin D. If in doubt about the need for oral vitamin and mineral supplements in a given patient, determination of levels of certain key vitamins is indicated (e.g. vitamin A and folate). Where there is a question of inadequacy of vitamin B_{12} absorption, a Schilling test performed without intrinsic factor is sufficient, providing that there is no blind loop syndrome and the distal ileum is intact. It should be noted that the Schilling test may be normal (since crystalline cobalamin is the test material) and there may be sufficient intrinsic factor produced by the residual stomach; nevertheless the patient may be unable to obtain sufficient B_{12} found in food because of lack of HCl and pepsin. In such an instance, oral supplementary B_{12} is useful.

Symptoms of milk intolerance may be prevented and adequate calcium, riboflavin and associated nutrient intake improved by a) having milk ingested in small amounts (e.g. small glasses) frequently over the day or b) pretreating milk with the lactase preparation lactaid which hydrolyzes lactose. If these procedures prove unsatisfactory, prescribe calcium salts in sufficient amounts to yield 1 gram of this ion. The calcium content varies greatly in different salts; e.g. the gluconate USP has about 9% calcium, the lactate USP 13% and the carbonate USP has 40%.

When the most careful dietary advice and the adherence to an anti-dumping diet does not enable the patient to either avoid serious dumping symptoms or to ingest a sufficient amount of food to maintain or gain weight, it is recommended that intermittent slow-drip tube feedings of a complete formula be instituted. Because of the very slow entry of food into the jejunum by this technique, dumping is not likely to occur. Such feedings may need to be given only during the anorectic period of chemotherapy; following cessation of treatment appetite may improve. On the other hand, there are patients who remain seriously anorectic following cessation of chemotherapy even though the tumor growth is well controlled; in such instances nightly tube feedings should be continued. It is my policy to start feedings at a volume of 50 ml per hour and increase the daily rate by 10 to 20 ml per hour as tolerated with a goal of 150–175 ml per hour over 10 hours with a caloric density of 1 to 1.5 kcal/ml depending on the nutritional status of the patients.

5. Gastric surgery in the treatment of obesity

Because of the high prevalence of nutritional and metabolic complications following jejuno-ileal bypass, the surgical approach has turned to reduction of the volume of the gastric reservoir as a means of limiting food intake. Gastric bypass was first performed in 1966 with total division of the stomach with the proximal small remnant of stomach anastamosed to jejunum. This was followed by partitioning of the stomach by stapling leaving a 50 ml pouch of proximal stomach with a gastrojejunostomy. Variations of gastric partitioning – at least 12 in number [40] – have followed. In an early procedure a 50 ml pouch was formed by stapling across the proximal stomach leaving a small opening for liquified food to enter distally. In efforts to prevent dilatation of the pouch surgeons have proceeded to employ silicon or marlex bands horizontally or vertically. One or another of these procedures has been widely performed in many hospitals – in most instances without close follow-up and evaluation. Even in major medical centers where there has been short and long term evaluation, I am not aware of any published report on detailed nutritional assessment including periodic evaluation of body composition and various nutrient levels. One would have thought that the experiences with jenuno-colonic and jejuno-ileal by-pass would have led to such studies. Presumably, the possibility of nutritional deficiencies occurring was not considered seriously because the small bowel was intact.

The ingestion of small volumes of liquids by mouth or by tube is a key factor in allowing weight loss and minimizing dilatation of the pouch. Inadequate dietary advice and supervision may lead to deficiencies. One study employed reasonably close follow-up behavioral modification and dietary instructions for patients with gastric exclusion with emphasis on 'mostly protein foods' in volumes of 1 to 2 tablespoons twice daily and multiple vitamin and mineral tablets. Nevertheless, 5 of 50 patients had 'hair thinning' and four had dumping [41]. Zinc was added because of the hair changes but without evidence that such a deficiency was occurring. A contrary opinion is that the cause of hair loss is 'probably not zinc but probably lack of sulfur-containing amino acids' since improved protein intake was associated with restoration of hair [42].

In another series, 43 by-pass patients had intraoperative and postoperative liver biopsy 1 year later. While 58% had improvement, 12% showed worsening of histologic grading with increased fatty infiltration in some and increased fibrosis in others [43]. No mention is made of other nutritional assessment. Nausea and vomiting was the primary postoperative problem with an incidence of 10% but were found to disappear after several weeks.

More general experience is not yet available concerning incidence of vomiting and its accompanying nutritional problems, too rapid weight loss and its untoward metabolic consequences and failure to meet all nutritional needs. The need for careful attention to the needs of such patients is exemplified by the development of Wernicke's encephalopathy following persistent nausea and vomiting in two young women after gastric 'plication' – presumably meaning gastric partition. Neither of the patients had been given vitamin supplements at home or on periodic hospitalizations until encephalopathy was obvious [44]. It would be expected (and it has occurred) that iron deficiency and/or vitamin B_{12} depletion would occur in patients with gastric by-pass [45–47]. Data on kinetics of these deficiencies are not available. Additional iron with ascorbic acid orally and periodic B_{12} injections should solve these problems, with periodic nutritional assessment to assure that such nutrients are being absorbed and utilized.

The medical problems of the morbidly obese are significant and chronic, and non-operative success over a period of a year or more is less than 5%. Despite the occurrence of variable and significant failures in weight loss in some patients by these surgical techniques, they appear to offer a significantly better prognosis than conservative management or jejuno-ileal by-pass. However, it is incumbent on all surgeons performing such procedures to provide the necessary follow-up and expertise to assure that a good overall nutritional status is maintained. This includes avoidance of too rapid weight loss, provision of all essential nutrients in adequate amounts (including high quality protein, vitamins, minerals and trace elements) in association with periodic nutritional assessment to assure that such nutrients are being absorbed and utilized and a reasonable metabolic status is being maintained.

6. Pancreatic and associated organ resection

6.1. Pancreatic carcinoma

Weight loss is a very common feature of carcinoma of the pancreas no matter where the lesion is located [48]. Warren et al. recorded preoperative weight losses, averaging 12 to 16 pounds, depending on the site, in 253 patients with periampullary cancer [49]. Weight loss in patients with ductal carcinoma of the pancreas commonly occurred in 39% [50]. Twenty-six per cent of patients with pancreatic cancer lost more than 10% of their weight within two months [4]. Eating may aggravate the pain which is of frequent occurrence. Jaundice occurs in approximately 75% of patients with carcinoma in the head of the pancreas and periampullary areas.

Carcinoma of the pancreas may cause digestive enzyme deficiency, especially when there is extensive involvement of this organ particularly in the head region or when a major portion of the duct is obstructed. A marked decrease results in maldigestion and consequent malabsorption of fats particularly, but also, to a lesser degree, of protein and of long-chain carbohydrates [50]. Nine per cent of patients with ductal carcinoma had steatorrhea [50]. The resulting malabsorption combined with the anorexia which is so common in such patients contributes to the progressive weight loss.

Bile insufficiency: Conjugated bile salts play an important role in the absorption of fat; hence, any condition that reduces their concentration below the critical level for adequate micellar formation will lead to steatorrhea. This may occur with obstruction by tumor at the ampulla of Vater, in the common duct behind the pancreatic head or at the porta hepatis. Bile insufficiency reduces intestinal absorption of vitamin K and leads to reduction in plasma levels of the vitamin K dependent coagulation factors as well as of other fat-soluble vitamins.

6.2. Pancreatoduodenectomy

This operative procedure was described by Whipple *et al.* in 1935 for the surgical treatment of carcinoma of the ampulla of Vater [51]. Other carcinomas of the periampullary region that are amenable to treatment by this operation include those of the distal common bile duct and duodenum. Some surgeons utilize it for carcinoma of the head of the pancreas. In the usual operative procedure the distal portion of the stomach is removed; the pancreas is transected (usually at its neck but varying amounts may be removed or even the entire organ), and the duodenum and a few inches of jejunum distal to ligament of Treitz are excised.

Three options are available to the surgeon in dealing with the pancreatic stump: (a) inversion of the transected end of the pancreas into the jejunal lumen as an end-to-end anastomosis; (b) suturing the cut end of the duct of Wirsung to the jejunal or gastric mucosa; or (c) ligation of the pancreatic duct with oversewing of the transected pancreas. There appear to be major differences of opinion among surgeons on the value of performing pancreatic duct anastomosis. Goldsmith *et al.* found no difference in post-operative morbidity and mortality or in histological appearance of the remnant at postmortem examination in patients who had the pancreatic duct reimplanted at pancreatoduodenectomy and those who had the duct ligated and the cut end of the pancreas closed. The decision on the management of the pancreatic stump has nutritional implications, inasmuch as ligation of the pancreatic duct with oversewing of the transected end of the pancreas will lead to complete pancreatic exocrine insufficiency.

Malabsorption secondary to exocrine enzyme insufficiency following pancreatoduodenectomy is appreciable, i.e. 25–50% [49, 53–57]. Fat malabsorption occurred in 50% of patuents surviving this procedure is whom the pancreatic stump was anastomosed either to the stomach [56] or jejunum [56]. Even in those undergoing resection for cancer of the ampulla, pancreatic exocrine insufficiency occurred in 27.7% [55]. The probability of pancreatic enzyme deficiency should be considered and checked in any patient with pancreatoduodenectomy even with ductal reanastomosis.

Diabetes: Another aspect of this surgical procedure concerns the endocrine function of the residual pancreas. Decreased glucose tolerance has been noted in pancreatoduodenectomized patients in whom fasting blood sugar levels were within normal limits [54, 56]. In pancreatoduodenectomized patients in whom at least the caudal half of the pancreas was preserved, fasting levels of glucose, nonesterified fatty acids, and immunoreactive insulin were within normal limits; however, following glucose ingestion the blood sugar levels of those with partial pancreatectomy were appreciably higher than those of gastrectomized and normal individuals while the insulin levels were lower [58]. Hence, insufficient insulin response from the remnant of the pancreas appears to be a major cause of glucose intolerance in these patients. This problem is complicated by the fact that approximately 10 to 12% of patients presenting with carcinoma of the pancreas are overtly diabetic [50, 59] and 10 to 35% (depending on the site of the tumor) have asymptomatic glycosuria or hyperglycemia [49].

6.3. Total pancreatectomy and regional pancreatectomy

Total pancreatectomy has been recommended because it eliminates the danger of pancreatic fistula without significantly increasing the surgical risk and because it eliminates the possibility of failure to remove carcinoma existing more distally either because of spread or multifocal tumor [50, 60]. This procedure poses a difficult metabolic situation with its resultant exocrine and endocrine insufficiency. Even with the optimum use of pancreatic extract, there tends to be loss of some fat soluble vitamins and nitrogen in stool. The usual diabetic-type diet with its increased protein and fat tends to exacerbate malabsorption. Replacing dietary fat with glucose to decrease steatorrhea increases the requirement for insulin. In a series of 48 totally pancreatectomized patients followed and evaluated for their control of diabetes, Pliam *et al.* found that 50% were easily managed, 8% were managed with difficulty when there was concomitant illness, 19% had occasional hypoglycemic reactions managed with oral carbohydrate, 4% did poorly with persistent glycosuria, and 20% were found to be very difficult to control with ketoacidosis or hyperglycemic episodes requiring hospitalization [61].

More radical surgery termed regional pancreatectomy has been develop in an effort to improve the poor survival by removing en bloc the pancreas, adjacent tissues and primary lymph drainage [62, 63]. In the type 1 procedure there is a total removal of the pancreas, pancreatic segment of portal vein, transverse mesocolon with middle colic vessels, surrounding soft tissues, regional lymph nodes, distal stomach, duodenum, spleen, gallbladder, and common bile duct with skeletonizing of the porta hepatis, celiac exis and superior mesenteric artery, vena cava and aorta. Tumor involving the celiac axis, superior mesenteric atery or hepatic artery is managed with arterial resection and reconstruction in addition to the Type 1 operation.

Because of marked anorexia and severe diarrhea and malabsorption occurring usually in combination after surgery, total parenteral nutrition has been employed in maintaining a number of these patients postoperatively and has proved to be a very valuable – even lifesaving – technique. I have relied upon high-glucose infusions as the major source of calories, with insulin added to the total parenteral nutrition solutions usually up to levels of 4 or 5 units of regular insulin for every 100 carbohydrate calories. Fractional coverage with a sliding scale for regular insulin is given as needed every six hours depending upon the level of glucose in blood or urine. The insulin in the TPN is then adjusted upward or downward as indicated. Intravenous fat may be used to replace a large portion of the glucose, but in my experience this is usually not necessary provided there is proper supervision of the parenteral feeding program and a progressive cautious increase in glucose and insulin.

A xylose tolerance test has been performed preoperatively and postoperatively in a number of patients, in some cases with serial follow-up. Almost all of these patients have had depressed xylose absorption postoperatively; absorption returned to normal after a period of 4 to 9 months [62]. Weight loss associated with depressed appetite and malabsorption has been significant; surviving patients are approximately 30% below their preoperative weight. Watery diarrhea has been frequent and has been associated with magnesium depletion and acidosis in some patients. The reason for this diarrhea and malabsorption of xylose is not apparent but may be related variably to a number of factors including gastractomy and duodenectomy, denervation, severance of lymphatics, small bowel resection in some instances, and bacterial overgrowth of small bowel. Five of six bowel fistulas closed spontaneously with total parenteral nutrition.

6.4. Recommendations for nutritional and dietary support

With cessation of parenteral support, anorexia, diabetes mellitus, pancreatic insufficiency and other types of malabsorption continue to present serious nutritional problems to the pancreatectomized patient. Frequent small meals are better tolerated than the usual 3 meals.

There must be administration of adequate amounts of pancreatic extract with all meals and snacks. Recent evaluations indicate positive adjunctive effects of ingestion of antacids, sodium bicarbonate or Cimetidine with oral pancreatic enzymes [64]. Despite earlier claims, there appears to be no advantage in treating with enteric-coated pancreatic extract as compared to uncoated preparations provided similar amounts of digestive enzymes are provided [65]. Patients with pancreatic resection and distal gastrectomy would be expected to have decreased gastric acid in any case.

Good control of the diabetes maximizes carbohydrate utilization and minimizes fluid and sodium losses secondary to osmotic diuresis caused by glycosuria. Medium-chain tryglycerides are more efficiently absorbed with inadequate or absent pancreatic enzyme replacement than are the usual long-chain dietary fats.

MCT is also absorbed much more efficiently than long-chain fats when there is an insufficiency of conjugated bile salts or when there are impaired intestinal absorptive mechanisms. Glucose oligosaccharides may also be helpful in increasing the caloric intake and absorption of pancreatically insufficient patients since there relatively short-chain glucose polymers are hydrolyzed to glucose by the brush-border enzyme sucrase-a-dextrinase. This commercially-available white powdery material is not sweet and may be used in a variety of ways to supplement intake.

When nutritional problems are severe following parenteral nutrition, intermittent tube feeding using formulas with protein hydrolysate, oligosaccharides, MCT, minerals and vitamins is useful [6, 7]. Such a formula does not require pancreatic extract. Slow drip infusion improves absorption and minimizes insulin requirement. Precautions in the use of MCT have been mentioned earlier.

Impaired absorption of vitamin B_{12} has been observed in a significant proportion of patients with chronic pancreatic insufficiency [66] or in those with total pancreatectomy [67] with improvement upon administration of pancreatic extract. The defect appears to be related to the role of pancreatic proteases in degrading the gastric R protein to which cobalamin is bound so that the vitamin is transferred to intrinsic factor to which it remains bound until it reaches the distal ileum [23].

7. Liver resection

With a description of a controlled technique for resection of the right lobe of the liver in 1952, major hepatic resection became frequent [68]. Advances in precise location of the tumor and hepatic artery branches, anesthesia and operative techniques, blood replacement, antibiotics and understanding of metabolic derangements caused by massive liver resection have appreciably decreased morbidity and mortality.

Major resection for cancers has been performed for the most part in 4 situations: primary malignant liver tumors in adults and children, cancer metastatic to liver from other sites; to permit en bloc excision of cancer of adjacent organs in stomach and colon; and to palliate the malignant carcinoid syndrome. Up to 90% of the liver may be resected with survival of the patient. In addition, resections are done in nonmalignant tumors such as benign hepatomas, cholangiomas, hamartomas, angiomas, teratomas and cysts.

7.1. Preoperative nutritional care

Many patients with primary of secondary liver involvement are undernourished; there may also be a history of alcoholism and the combination may result in extensive fatty infiltration. This state imposes increased surgical risk in terms of normal metabolic response to surgical stress and increases mortality. McDermott and Ackroyd have stressed the importance of delaying surgery if possible until some degree of nutritional repletion can be accomplished in malnourished patients [69]. The mode of nutritional rehabilitation may involve oral, tube, or parenteral feedings, with the route and nutrient composition depending upon the clinical situation.

7.2. Postoperative care

Normal liver tissue is endowed with a tremendous capacity for regeneration. Nevertheless, after major hepatic resection the early biochemical and metabolic changes than can occur can be serious and life-threatening. Appropriate steps are necessary to manage these changes to permit recovery and rapid regeneration. Glucose infusion is necessary to prevent a significant drop in blood sugar following resections of 70% or more (70) and the severe hypoglycemia which has been noted in patients following total hepatectomy and liver transplantation. Often following oral carbohydrate ingestion, blood sugar may be elevated for several weeks.

Since the liver is the site of albumin synthesis, hypoalbuminemia will occur to a significant degree unless replaced by parenteral administration. The need for supplementary albumin persists for approximately 1 week.

Postoperatively, fibrinogen, prothrombin and other coagulation factors (V, VII, IX, X) that are synthesized by the liver will fall following major resection [70, 71]. Despite the postoperative administration of vitamin K, prothrombin levels remained depressed in the postoperative phase; such depression is not reflected in any clinical disorder. These factors gradually return to normal as hepatic regeneration progresses.

Decreased total serum calcium reflects the decline in serum albumin. Transient low serum sodium and potassium have been reported in some patients after liver resection [72], while others have reported low level of serum inorganic phosphate following major hepatic resection and hepatic transplantation [73].

Evidence of liver decompensation has been observed in cases of extended right hepatic lobectomy [71]. In such instances reduction of oral protein intake (or institution of a modified amino acid regimen such as hepaticaid or its equivalent) in addition to initiation of other medical procedures for hepatic precoma are indicated. These disturbances disappear in a short period.

8. Intestinal resection

Major resection of the small bowel because of primary gastrointestinal malignancies is relatively uncommon. Resection only of the jejunum is also a relatively rare event in cancer patients. When it does occur, the ileum will adapt – if nutrition is well-maintained – and absorption usually becomes adequate.

8.1. Ileal dysfunction

The ileum is either bypassed, removed or damaged in varying degrees in cancer patients because of involvement with metastatic disease, fistula development or radiation enteritis. Resection, bypass or damage to the ileum leads to certain physiological and nutritional problems. Since the distal ileum is the site of the absorption of physiological amounts of vitamin B_{12}, provision of this vitamin intramuscularly once every month or two is necessary to prevent development of B_{12} deficiency. If the ileal resection is not extensive (usually less than 100 cm), sufficient bile salts enter the large bowel to induce a brown watery diarrhea (so-called cholereic diarrhea) which can be quite distressing to the patient [74]. Fecal aqeous dihydroxy bile acid concentrations and fecal pH have been noted to be significantly higher in patients with small ileal resection (100 cm) than in healthy controls or in those with large ileal resection (100 cm) or jejunoileal bypass. The pH is important since the solubility of these bile acids increases rapidly above pH 7.0 [75].

Cholestyramine ingestion may be dramatically effective in controlling this diarrhea through its mechanism of binding bile salts. It is my policy to prescribe a relatively large dose, e.g. four times daily, in order to demonstrate to the patient that effective control of the diarrhea can occur quickly. Following control of diarrhea the doses may be reduced to one-half or less. It is of interest that a significant proportion of patients with such cholereic diarrhea find that they can reduce the cholestyramine to very low doses or to intermittent doses once they are certain that they can control the problem. This suggests that there is an important psychological component to this diarrhea once it has begun.

The loss of bile salts with larger resections may be so great that very little of the amount entering the normal enterohepatic circulation is reabsorbed. The synthetic capacity of the liver to synthesize sufficient new bile salts is exceeded and the concentration of bile salt in the intestinal lumen may fall below the critical micellar concentration necessary for fat absorption. In such a situation the patient may be helped by the feeding of a diet restricted in long chain triglycerides and by the use of medium chain triglycerides which do not require bile salts for their absorption [74]. The use of water soluble forms of vitamin K, increased amounts of other fat soluble vitamins and of calcium, magnesium and zinc are indicated to prevent deficiency of these nutrients. It is important to remember that there must be provision of sufficient polyunsaturated fats (which are not provided by MCT) to assure adequate intake of essential fatty acids; in quantitative terms this would require absorption of approximately 6 to 10 grams of linoleic acid per day for an adult.

Another consequence of ileal resection is hyperoxaluria with increased incidence of renal oxalate stone formation. Ordinarily, oxalate in the intestinal lumen is precipitated to a very insoluble form by reacting with calcium ions. With bile salt deficiency there is a significant amount of unabsorbed free fatty acids in the lower small bowel as a result of impaired absorption. Free calcium ions bind to these unabsorbed fatty acids. Consequently, there is a shortage of calcium ions to bind oxalate. Soluble oxalate is then absorbed in the colon and appears in the urine in increased concentrations with the resultant probability of precipitation as the oxalate salt in the renal tubule [76]. Magnesium ions also tend to be lost in increased amounts in the stool as the result of their binding to free fatty acids. The dietary prescription designed to minimize oxalate stone formation includes: 1) a decrease in the intake of long chain triglycerides and an increase in MCT; 2) an increase in calcium intake to assure sufficiency to precipitate oxalate and improve calcium absorption; 3) an increase in magnesium because malabsorbers tend to have low urinary magnesium, and since this ion tends to solubilize calcium in the urine; 4) increase citrate by oral intake because malabsorbers tend to have low citrate in the urine and because citrate complexes with and solubilizes calcium. Increased magnesium intake also tends to decrease toward normal the abnormally elevated tubular reabsorption of citrate [77].

8.2. Major bowel resection or damage

Serious malabsorption in cancer patients with reasonable life expectancy usually results from the effects of radiation enteritis and its complications. Obstructions or fistulas may develop requiring resection. If such excisions are extensive or repeated the short bowel syndrome may result in part as a consequence of resection and in part because of radiation damage in remaining intestinal segments. Massive bowel resection may have to be performed in patients with low grade sarcomas (e.g. Gardner's Syndrome) which have progressed to the point where there is unresectable obstruction to the intestinal blood supply. Because of radiation enteritis or tumors, obstruction may be so persistent that food intake is seriously compromised.

The resulting malabsorption or inadequate food intake may be so serious that nutritional status can be maintained only by long-term slow drip feedings of special formulas or by total parenteral nutrition. This author has found the D-xylose tolerance test useful prognostically in deciding which feeding route is likely to be necessary on discharge. A five hour urinary excretion of xylose of less than 0.8 gm is generally incompatible with maintenance of adequate nutrition by means other than parenteral. It is desirable to apply this test when the patient has been on oral and enteral supplementary feedings for some weeks. Patients with excretion in the range of 1.2–1.6 grams may be able to be sustained by slow-drip tube feeding overnight of special formulas; those at the lower range may need periodic intravenous infusion of fluids and electrolytes, especially in the early period. Entry of food into the small bowel is essential if hyperplasia of the villi is to occur [78, 79]. In addition, a good nutritional statement must be attained. These techniques can be performed at home as well as in the hospital with appropriate training of patient and family. Criteria for home total parenteral feeding of such patients [80] and their management have been given elsewhere [80, 81]. An example of long-term home enteral feeding of a patient with severe radiation enteritis and intestinal resection has been published together with more detail on this technique [82]. There are a number of companies which will supply the TPN solution, enteral feedings and equipment on prescription of the physician.

9. Colectomy

Resection of the right colon with the ileal cecal valve and a portion of the distal ileum may be associated with watery diarrhea in large part because of entry of bile salts into the colon resulting from loss of distal ileum as discussed above. Loss of the ileo-cecal valve may also play a role [79]. Increased diarrhea with some malabsorption may also occur when, in addition to the colectomy, there was been prior radiation damage to the small bowel.

Following total colectomy and ileostomy performed on a patient with an otherwise intact small bowel, there may be significant losses of water and sodium within the first 7–10 days. However, most patients adapt and decrease the fluid and electrolyte losses. Generally, these stabilized individuals will lose 300–600 ml of water daily with 40–100 mEq of sodium and 2.5 to 10 mEq of potassium, emphasizing the physiologic role of the colon in absorbing water and sodium and in exchanging potassium for sodium. A small portion of patients fail to adapt; these include those with some underlying disease of the ileum. Such patients require special care in assuring adequate water and electrolyte intake to meet their needs. In those who adapt well, an episode of gastroenteritis, partial intestinal obstruction or prolonged excessive sweating pose additional losses and may cause dehydration. Studies of man and dogs during sodium depletion have demonstrated reduction of sodium concentration of ileostomy material as depletion progressed accompanied by increased potassium concentration [83].

References

1. Devesa SS, Silverman DT: Cancer incidence and mortality trends in the United States 1935–1974. J Natl Cancer Inst 60: 545–571, 1978.
2. Shils ME: Nutritional problems associated with gastrointestinal and genitourinary cancer. Cancer Res 37: 2366–2372, 1977.
3. Nixon DW, Heymsfield SB, Cohen AE, et al.: Protein-calorie undernutrition in hospitalized

cancer patients. Am J Med 68: 683–690, 1980.

4. DeWys WD, Begg C, Lavin PT, *et al.*: prognostic effect of weight loss prior to chemotherapy in cancer patients. Am J Med 69: 491–497, 1980.

5. MacCarthy-Leventhal EM: Post-radiation month blindness. Lancet 2: 1138–1959.

6. Shils ME, Bloch AS, Chernoff R: Liquid formulas for oral and tube feeding. pp 10 2nd ed. Memorial Sloan-Kettering Cancer Center, New York, New York 10021, 1979.

7. Shils ME, Bloch AS: Liquid formulas and defined formula diets; Section in Appendix in: Modern Nutrition in Health and Disease, Goodhart RS, Shils ME, (eds). Philadelphia, Lea and Febiger, 1980 2nd ed. pp. 1312–1330.

8. Barcia RM: Selection of enteral equipment. Nutr. Support Svces 3: 15–23, 1983.

9. Shils ME: The esophagus, the vagi and fat absorption. Surg Gynecol Obstet 132: 709–715, 1971.

10. Becker HD: Hormonal changes after gastric surgery. Clinics in gastroenterology. 9: 755–771, 1980.

11. Radziuk J, Bondy DC: Abnormal glucose tolerance and glucose malabsorption after vagotomy and pyloroplasty. A tracer method for measuring glucose absorption rates. Gastroenterology 83: 1017–25, 1982.

12. Greenberger NJ, Skillman TG: Medium Chain Triglycerides. New Engl J Med 280: 1045–1058, 1969.

13. Linscheer WG, Blum AL, Platt RR: Transfer of medium chain fatty acids from blood to spinal fluid in patients with cirrhosis. Gastroenterology 58: 509–515, 1970.

14. Machella TE: The mechanism of post gastrectomy 'dumping' syndrome. Ann Surg 130: 145–159, 1949.

15. Lawrence W Jr: Nutritional consequences of surgical resection of the gastrointestinal tract for cancer. Cancer Res 37: 2379–2386, 1977.

16. Breuer RS, Moses H III, Hagen TC *et al.*: Gastric operations and glucose homeostasis. Gastroenterology 62: 1109–1119, 1972.

17. Ralphs DNL, Thomson JPS, Haynes S *et al.*: The relationship between the rate of gastric emptying and the dumping syndrome. Br J Surg 65: 637–641, 1978.

18. Leichter SB, Arnold AC, Lewis SB: Glucose tolerance, insulin secretion and glucose utilization in subjects after gastric surgery. Am J Clin Nutr 30: 2053–1060, 1977.

19. Rehfeld JF, Heding LG, Holst JJ: Increased gut glucagon as a pathogenetic factor in reactive hypoglycemia? Lancet 1: 116–118, 1978.

20. Bloom SR, Blackburn AM, Ebeid FH *et al.*: Neurotensin and the dumping syndrome. Scand J Gastroenterology 13: suppl 49, 23, 1978.

21. Silver D, McGregor FH, Porter JM *et al.:* The mechanism of the dumping syndrome. Surg Clin NA 46: 425–431, 1966.

22. MacDonald JM, Webster MM, Tennyson CH *et al.*: Serotonin and bradykinin in the dumping syndrome. Am J Surg 117: 203–213, 1969.

23. Allen RH: Cobalamin (vitamin B_{12}) absorption and malabsorption. Viewpoints and Digestive Dis. 14: 17–20 (Nov.) 1982. 333 Cedar St. New Haven, Conn. 06510.

24. Rejman F: Postgastrectomy syndrome. A clinical study based upon 100 patients. Ann Chir Gynecol Fenn 59 (suppl 1970): 1–63, 1970.

25. Bradley EL III, Isaacs J, Hersh T, *et al.*: Nutritional consequences of total gastrectomy. Ann Surg 182: 415–429, 1975.

26. Lundh G: The mechanism of postgastrectomy malabsorption. Gastroenterology 42: 637–640, 1962.

27. Schwartz MK, Bodansky O, Randall HT: Metabolism in surgical patients III. Effect of drugs and dietary procedures on fat and nitrogen metabolism in totally gastrectomized patients. Surgery 40: 671–677, 1956.

28. MacGregor I, Parent J, Meyer JH: Gastric emtying of liquid meals and pancreatic and biliary secretion after subtotal gastrectomy or truncal vagotomy and pyloroplasty. Gastroenterology 72: 195–205, 1977.

29. Spencer J, Welbourn RB: Milk intolerance following gastric operations with special reference to lactase deficiency. Brit J Surg 55: 261–264, 1968.
30. Hedberg CH, Melnyk CS, Johnson CF: Gluten enterotherapy appearing after gastric surgery. Gastroenterology 50: 796–804, 1966.
31. Holt JM, Gear MWL, Warner GT: The role of chronic blood loss in the pathogenesis of postgastrectomy iron-deficiency anaemia. Gut 11: 847–850, 1970.
32. Eddy RL: Metabolic bone disease after gastrectomy. Am J Med 50: 442–449, 1971.
33. Compston JE, Creamer B: The consequences of small intestine resection. Quart J Med 46: 485–497, 1977.
34. Sawyer JL, Herrington JL Jr: Antiperistaltic jejunal segment for control of the dumping syndrome and postvagotomy diarrhea. Surgery 69: 263–267, 1971.
35. Hunt CJ: Construction of food pouch from segment of jejunum as substitute for stomach in total gastrectomy. Arch Surg 64: 601–608, 1952.
36. Winchester DP, Randolph DA, Hohf RP: The role of rapid intestinal transit in postgastrectomy malnutrition. Surg Gynecol Obstet 132: 861–865, 1971.
37. Jenkins DJA, Gasull MA, Leeds AR et al.: Effect of dietary fiber on complications of gastric surgery; prevention of post-prandial hypogycemia by pectin. Gastroenterology 72: 215–217, 1977.
38. Leeds AP, Ebid F, Ralph DNL et al.: Pectin in the dumping syndrome: reduction of symptoms and plasma volume changes. Lancet 1: 1075–1078, 1981.
39. Am. Diet Assoc. Handbook of Clinical Dietetics. Yale Univ. Press, New Haven, Conn. 1981, pp D3–D8.
40. Carey LC: In discussion following ref. 41, p. 642.
41. Lechner GW, Callender A: Subtotal gastric exclusion and gastric partitioning; a randomized prospective comparison of one hundred patients. Surgery 90: 637–642, 1981.
42. Printen KJ: In discussion following ref. 41, p. 643.
43. Rucker RD Jr, Horstmann J, Schneider RD, et al.: Comparison between jejunoileal and gastric bypass operations for morbid obesity. Surgery 92: 241–247, 1982.
44. Haid RW, Gutmann L, Crosby TW: Wernicke-Korsakoff encephalopathy after gastric plication. J Am Med Ass 247: 2566–2567, 1982.
45. Griffen WO: In discussion following ref. 41, p. 643.
46. Mason EE: Gastroplasty. Major Prob Clin Surg 26: 386–408, 1981.
47. Linner JH: Comparative effectiveness of gastric by-pass and gastroplasty. Arch Surg 117: 695–700, 1982.
48. Cattell RB, Warren KW: Surgery of the pancreas, 1953 Saunders, Phila. pp. 267–268; 327–328.
49. Warren KW, Veidenheimer MC, Pratt HS: Pancreatoduodenectomy for periampullary cancer. Surg Clin North Am 47: 639–645, 1967.
50. Brooks JR, Culebras JM: Cancer of the pancreas: Palliative operation, Whipple procedure or total pancreatectomy? Am J Surg 131: 516–520, 1976.
51. Whipple AO, Parsons WB, Mullins CR: Treatment of carcinoma of the ampulla of Vater. Ann Surg 102: 763–779, 1935.
52. Goldsmith HS, Ghosh BC, Huvos AG: Ligation versus implantation of the pancreatic duct after pancreatoduodenectomy. Surg Genecol Obstet 132: 87–92, 1971.
53. Wollaeger EE, Comfort MW, Clagett OT, et al.: Efficiency of gastrointestinal tract after resection of head of pancreas. J Am Med Assoc 137: 838–848, 1948.
54. Christiansen J, Olsen JH, Worming H: The pancreatic function following subtotal pancreatectomy for cancer. Scand J Gastroenterology (Suppl) 9: 189–193, 1971.
55. Monge JJ, Judd ES, Gage RP: Radical pancreatoduodenectomy. A 22 year experience with the complications, mortality rate and survival rate. Ann Surg 160: 711–719, 1964.
56. Fish JC, Smith LB, Williams RD: Digestive function after radical pancreatoduodenectomy. Am J Surg 177: 40–45, 1969.
57. Aston SJ, Longmire WP Jr.: Management of the pancreas after pancreatoduodenectomy. Ann

Surg 179: 322–327, 1974.

58. Miyata M, Takao T, Uozumi *et al.*: Insulin secretion after pancreatoduodenectomy. Ann. Surg 179: 494–498, 1974.

59. Gray LW Jr, Crook KN, Cohn J Jr.: Carcinoma of the pancreas, *in* 7th Nat. Cancer Conf. pp. 503–519. Lippincott, Phila. 1973.

60. ReMine WH, Priestly JR, Judd ES, *et al.*: Total pancreatectomy. Ann Surg 172: 595–604, 1970.

61. Pliam MB, ReMine WH: Further evaluation of total pancreatectomy. Arch Surg 110: 506–511, 1975.

62. Fortner JG, Kim DK, Cubilla A, *et al.*: Regional pancreatectomy: en bloc pancreatic, portal vein and lymph node resection. Ann Surg 186: 42–50, 1977.

63. Fortner JG: Surgical principles for pancreatic cancer: Regional, total and subtotal pancreatectomy. Cancer 47: 1712–1718, 1981.

64. Durie PR, Bell L, Linton W, *et al.*: Effect of cimetidine and sodium bicarbonate on pancreatic replacement therapy in cystic fibrosis. Gut 21: 778–786, 1980.

65. Dutta SK, Rubin J, Harvey J: Comparative evaluation of the therapeutic efficacy of a pH-sensitive enteric coated pancreatic enzyme preparation with conventional pancreatic enzyme therapy in the treatment of exocrine pancreatic insufficiency. Gastroenterology 84: 476–482, 1983.

66. Toskes PP, Hansell J, Cerda J, Deren JJ: Vitamin B_{12} malabsorption in chronic pancreatic insufficiency. New Eng J Med 284: 627–632, 1971.

67. Morishita R, Fujii M, Yamamoto T *et al.*: Effect of pancreatin on vitamin B_{12} malabsorption in patients with total pancreatectomy. Digestion 11: 240–248, 1974.

68. Lortat-Jacobs JC, Robert HG: Hepatectomie droite reglee. Presse Med 60: 549–000, 1952.

69. McDermott WV Jr., Ackroyd FW: Nutrient demands imposed by surgery of the liver. Am J Clin Nutr 32: 652–656, 1970.

70. McDermott WV Jr. Greenberger NJ, Isselbacher KJ, *et al.*: Major hepatic resection: diagnostic techniques and metabolic problems. Surgery 54: 56–64, 1963.

71. Pack GT, Molander DW: Metabolism before and after hepatic lobectomy for cancer. Arch Surg 80: 685–692, 1960.

72. Aronson KF, Ericcson B, Pihl B: Metabolic changes following major hepatic resection. Ann Surg 169: 102–110, 1969.

73. Fortner JG, Beattie EJ Jr., Shiu M, *et al.*: Surgery in liver tumors in Ravitch MM, Julian OC, Scott HW Jr., *et al.* (ed) Current problems in Surgery. Year Book Med. Publishers Chicago, June 1972, pp 56.

74. Hofmann AF, Poley JR: Role of bile acid malabsorption in pathogenesis of diarrhea and steatorrhea in patients with ileal resection I. Response to cholestryamine or replacement of dietary long chain triglycerides by medium chain triglyceride. Gastroenterology 62: 918–934, 1972.

75. McJunkin B, Fromm H, Sarva RP, *et al.*: Factors in the mechanism of diarrhea in bile acid and malabsorption: fecal pH – a key determinant. Gastroenterology 80: 1454–64, 1981.

76. Dobbins JW, Binder JH: Importance of the colon in enteric hyperoxaluria. N Eng J Med 296: 298–301, 1977.

77. Rudman D, Dedonis JC, Fountain MT, *et al.*: Hypocitraturia in patients with gastrointestinal malabsorption. N Eng J Med 303: 657–662, 1980.

78. Williamson RCN: Medical progress: intestinal adaptation. N Eng J Med 298: 1393–1402, 1444–1450, 1978.

79. Weser E, Fletcher JT, Urban E: Short bowel syndrome. Gastroenterology 77: 572–579, 1979.

80. Shils ME: A program for total parenteral nutrition at home. Am J Clin Nutr 28: 1429–1435, 1975.

81. Shils ME: Cancer and home parenteral nutrition. Proc Symp Home Parenteral Nutr Am Soc Enteral Parenteral Nutr 1025 Vermont Ave. NW, Suite 810, Wash. DC 20005, 1981 pp 18–21.

82. Shils ME: Enteral nutrition by tube. Cancer Res 37: 2432–2439, 1977.

83. Gallagher ND, Harrison DD, Skyring AP: Fluid and electrolyte disturbances in patients with long established ielostomies. Gut 3: 219–223, 1962.

13. Intraoperative radiation therapy for gastro-intestinal malignancy

MITSUYUKI ABE

1. Introduction

Although the development of anesthesia and antibiotics now permits extended operations of an increasingly radical nature, the possibility always exists that microscopic malignancy will be left behind even after what is believed to be a curative operation. Moreover complete elimination of cancer nests around major blood vessels is hard to attain by a surgical procedure. On the other hand, a cancercidal dose of external irradiation cannot be delivered to tumors adjacent to critical radiosensitive organs. In order to overcome these limitations of surgery and radiotherapy, intraoperative radiotherapy has been developed [1, 2, 3, 4].

Intraoperative radiotherapy is a technique in which resectable lesions are removed surgically and the remaining cancer nests are sterilized by irradiation during a surgical procedure. The potential benefit of this procedure results from direct visualization of the lesions, allowing a more accurate determination of the site which needs to be irradiated and physical removal of potentially dose limiting normal tissues from the field. Therefore a cancercidal dose can be delivered to unresectable lesions with less normal tissue morbidity. The principal disadvantage of intraoperative radiotherapy is that an adequate dose must be given in one session. Deciding the proper dose level is difficult.

2. Intraoperative irradiation techniques

2.1. Selection of electron energy

Intraoperative irradiation can be performed adequately with an electron beam, since the beam can be chosen to produce a desired depth of tissue penetration with sharp fall-off, thereby minimizing the exposure of normal tissue under the tumors. Figure 1 shows depth dose curves for ^{60}Co γ-ray and 4 MV X-ray beams, and for 6, 10 and 15 MeV electron beams. With electrons the fall-off in dose is

J.J. DeCosse and P. Sherlock (eds), Clinical Management of Gastrointestinal Cancer.
© 1984, Martinus Nijhoff Publishers, Boston. ISBN 0-89838-601-2. Printed in The Netherlands.

328

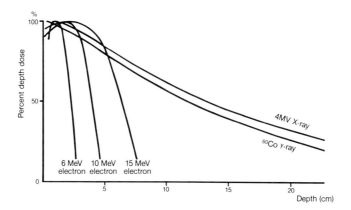

Figure 1. Depth dose curves for ^{60}Co γ-ray and 4 MV X-ray beams, and for 6, 10 and 15 MeV electron beams. With electrons the fall-off in dose is sharp beyond the 80% point.

sharp beyond the 80% point. Figure 2 demonstrates the isodose distribution with 18 MeV electrons in a patient with gastric cancer. The stomach is covered by an 80% dose range, while the spinal cord is not exposed to electron beams.

As much tumor tissue as possible should be extirpated, since larger tumors require higher doses of radiation than smaller ones to produce the same degree of regression. The electron energy is selected so that the entire tumor is included in an 80% depth dose distribution. The size and shape of the treatment cone which allows for at least a 1–2 cm margin of normal tissue are determined by palpation and measurement of the visualized lesion.

2.2. Radiation dose

Of particular importance in intraoperative radiotherapy is the determination of an optimal cancercidal dose given in a single treatment. Based on many experimental and clinical investigations on cellular lethality, it is clear that the dose required to eradicate a tumor depends upon the number of tumor cells, the fraction of anoxic cells and their pathologic type [5, 6]. In fractionated irradiation, the anoxic portion of the tumor decreases after each irradiation thus making successive irradiation effective. This is because of improved vascularization following tumor regression and the increased availability of oxygen because of its reduced consumption by the damaged cells. In single dose irradiation, one cannot utilize this reoxygenation effect. Accordingly, a single dose cannot be extrapolated from a simple time-dose graph, such as Strandqvist curves [7].

On the other hand, radiobiology does not, at present, give us the necessary information for determining a reasonable single dose for intraoperative irradiation. The optimal single dose must therefore be estimated from an analysis of

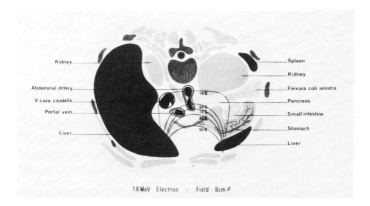

Figure 2. Isodose distribution with 18 MeV electrons in a patient with inoperable gastric cancer. The stomach is covered by an 80% dose range, while the spinal cord is not exposed to electron beams.

clinical results and postmortem examinations. For adenocarcinoma, single doses of 30 Gy–40 Gy, increasing with tumor size, are considered potentially curative [4]. A somewhat smaller dose may be sufficient to eradicate microscopic or clinically undetectable lesions because they have fewer cells and a lesser, if any, anoxic component.

2.3. Anesthesia during intraoperative irradiation

Intraoperative radiotherapy is performed easily if all surgical procedures can be carried out in a radiation therapy room. When an operating theater is separated from a radiation suite, the abdomen is temporarily closed with nylon stay sutures, and then the patient is covered with sterile sheets and transported under general anesthesia to the radiation therapy room. The abdomen is re-opened and a treatment cone is inserted which encompasses the area of gross tumor with adequate margins. All small intestine is packed out of the radiation field. During radiotherapy, the patient is observed by anesthesiologists outside the radiation room on closed circuit television. Remote monitoring of the patient is carried out. The ECG is monitored continuously on an oscilloscope and the adequancy of ventilation is monitored by respiratory movement of the thorax.

3. Intraoperative radiotherapy for gastric cancer

Recent advances in diagnostic radiology of the stomach in Japan have led to more gastrectomies at an early stage and higher survival rates. However, the percentage of patients with early gastric cancer in which tumor invasion is limited to the mucosa or submucosa is still very small. In the large majority of patients, the tumor has already reached the muscularis propria and extends to or through the serosa, and has produced perigastric lymph node metastases. For the treatment of these advanced gastric cancers, surgeons have exerted much effort in performing larger, more extensive resections [8, 9]. However, the prognosis following surgery of gastric cancer has not been improved for many years. The 5-year survival rate of patients subjected to curative operation is only about 40% [10].

The main reason why the success of gastric cancer surgery remains poor is that the incidence of metastases to the lymph nodes along the left gastric and common hepatic arteries and around the celiac axis is high [11, 12], and complete elimination of the tumor around these blood vessels is hard to attain by a surgical procedure. The possibility also exists that microscopic lesions remain in the tumor bed.

On the other hand radiotherapy has not played a major role in the treatment of gastric cancer, because adenocarcinoma is radioresistant and high dose external irradiation to the gastric region can cause intestinal damage. This damage is often a serious limiting factor in the delivery of a complete course of radiotherapy. In intraoperative radiotherapy, a cancercidal dose can be delivered safely to the unresectable remnants, because normal organs such as the small intestine or the liver can be shifted from the field so that the lesion is exposed directly to radiation.

3.1. Methods

To cure gastric cancer, the primary tumor must be removed surgically. This is because a large dose is required to eradicate a large tumor and radiation tolerance decreases quickly with increasing volume. In intraoperative radiotherapy of inoperable gastric cancer, a large volume dose is required and hence it is impossible to sterilize all the tumor cells in one exposure within the tolerance limit of the normal structures supporting or surrounding the tumor.

At first, gastrectomy is performed. A treatment cone should be inserted over unresectable disease or sites suspicious for containing residual tumor cells before gastroenterostomy, because at this stage, the site to be irradiated can be adequately exposed and the organs to be protected pulled aside. When intraoperative irradiation is applied in a curative operation, the radiation field is positioned toward the lymph node groups around the celiac axis, which most frequently contain metastatic cancer, and are hard to eliminate by a surgical procedure. If the posterior wall of the stomach is grossly adherent to the pancreas, this part must be adequately encompassed by the radiation field (Fig. 3).

The pentagonally shaped treatment cones which fit the costal arch and encompass the area stated above were especially made for this procedure (Fig. 4). These cones must be of various sizes and shapes so that various anatomic situations can

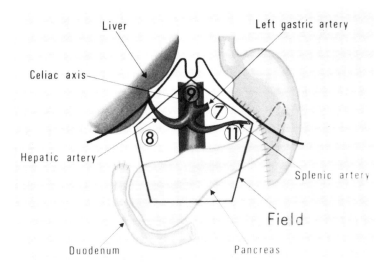

Figure 3. Field for a case of gastric cancer with invasion of the pancreas. The field covers the lymph node groups which most frequently contain metastatic cancer and are poorly eliminated by surgery.

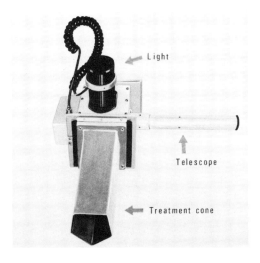

Figure 4. Pentagonally shaped treatment cone with an electric lamp and telescope to observe the field.

be adequately covered. Obviously, they should be designed so that they will not shatter if subjected to stress. The field is clearly illuminated by an electric lamp fixed to the telescope attached to the treatment cone. The cone is inserted into the abdomen inclining about 15°, so that the celiac axis is sufficiently covered (Fig. 5).

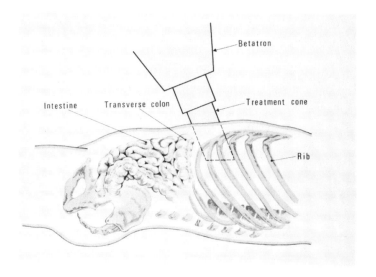

Figure 5. Intraoperative radiotherapy for gastric cancer. A treatment cone is inserted into the abdominal cavity, inclining about 15 degrees so that the celiac axis is sufficiently covered.

Figure 6 demonstrates intraoperative irradiation with an electron beam for a patient with gastric cancer.

All patients were classified according to the rules for gastric cancer studies in Japan [13]. These rules have been widely accepted in most medical centers in Japan and the international gastric cancer registration with WHO is also conducted using descriptions based on these rules. The rules related to the descriptions in this chapter are summarized below.

3.1.1. Location of gastric cancer and primary cancer site
The stomach is separated into the upper, middle and lower portions by drawing lines between the corresponding trisecting points on the greater and lesser curvatures (Fig. 7). If the lesion extends across these lines, the primarily involved portion(s) is listed first, followed by the less involved portion(s).

3.1.2. Classification of serosal invasion based on gross findings
S_0 No serosal invasion;
S_1 Suspected serosal invasion;
S_2 Definite serosal invasion;
S_3 Invasion to contiguous structures.

3.1.3. Classification of lymph nodes based on gross findings
The regional lymph nodes of the stomach are designated as shown in Table 1 and Figure 8. The lymph nodes of Groups 1, 2 and 3 (Table 1) are referred to as N_1, N_2

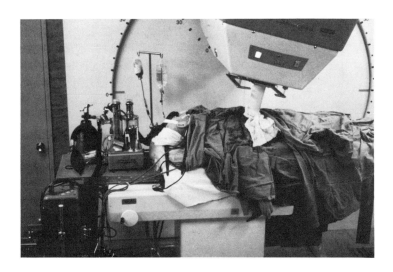

Figure 6. Intraoperative electron beam irradiation to a patient with gastric cancer under general anesthesia.

and N_3, respectively. Distant lymph nodes located beyond Group 3 (N_3) are referred to as N_4.

N $(-)$ No suspected lymph node metastasis;

N $(+)$ Metastasis to lymph nodes of Group 1;

N_1 $(-)$ No metastasis to lymph nodes of Group 1;

N_2 $(+)$ Metastasis to lymph nodes of Group 2;

N_2 $(-)$ No metastasis to lymph nodes of Group 2;

N_3 $(+)$ Metastasis to lymph nodes of Group 3;

N_3 $(-)$ No metastasis to lymph nodes of Group 3;

N_4 $(+)$ Metastasis to lymph nodes located beyond Group 3;

N_4 $(-)$ No metastasis to lymph nodes located beyond Group 3.

Use of the designation Group 1, 2, 3 (N_1, N_2, N_3) indicates the anatomical position of the lymph nodes. These designation do not imply that the respective lymph nodes are primary, secondary or tertiary lymph nodes. For example, lymph nodes 8, 10 and 11 of Group 2 and Group 3 are primary regional lymph nodes.

3.1.4. Classification of disseminating peritoneal metastasis based on gross findings

P_0 No disseminating metastases to the gastric serosa, greater and lesser omentum, mesentery, visceral and parietal peritoneum, and retroperitoneum.

P_1 Disseminating metastasis to the adjacent peritoneum (above the transverse colon and including the greater omentum) without metastasis to the distant

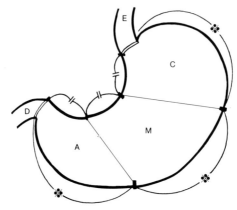

Figure 7. Location of gastric cancer [13].

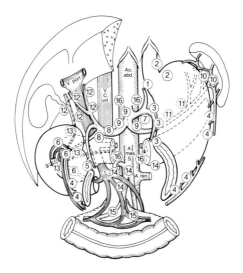

Figure 8. Lymph node designations used in the Japanese Research Society for Gastric Cancer [13].

peritoneum, i.e. the peritoneum below the transverse colon and the abdominal surface of the diaphragm.

P_2 A few to several scattered metastases to the distant peritoneum. This classification is applicable to cases in which there is only ovarian metastasis.

P_3 Numerous metastases to the distant peritoneum.

3.1.5. Classification of liver metastasis based on gross findings

H_0 No liver metastasis;

H_1 Metastasis is limited to one of the lobes;

H_2 Few scattered metastases to both lobes;

H_3 Numerous scattered metastases to both lobes.

Table 1. Grouping and lymph node designations used in the Japanese Research Society for Gastric Cancer [13]

Group \ Location	AMC, MAC MCA, CMA	A, AM	MA, M, MC	C, CM
Group 1 (N$_1$)	1	3	3	1
	2	4	4	2
	3	5	5	3
	4	6	6	4s
	5		1	
	6			
Group 2 (N$_2$)	7	7	2	4d
	8	8	7	7
	9	9	8	8
	10	1	9	9
	11		10	10
			11	11
				5
				6
Group 3 (N$_3$)	12	2	12	12
	13	10	13	13
	14	11	14	14
	110	12		110
	111	13		111
		14		

1	right cardial lymph node
2	left cardial lymph node
3	lymph node along the lesser curvature
4	lymph node along the greater curvature
	4s (left group) lymph node along the left gastroepiploic artery and short gastric arteries
	4d (right group) lymph node along the right gastroepiploic artery
5	suprapyloric lymph node
6	infrapyloric lymph node
7	lymph node along the left gastric artery
8	lymph node along the common hepatic artery
9	lymph node around the celiac artery
10	lymph node at the splenic hilus
11	lymph node along the splenic artery
12	lymph node in the hepatoduodenal ligament
13	lymph node at the posterior aspect of the pancreas
14	lymph node at the root of the mesentery
110	lower thoracic paraesophageal lymph node
111	diaphragmatic lymph node

3.1.6. Stage grouping of gastric cancer

The cancer stage is expressed according to Table 2. The stage to be recorded is that under which there is the highest degree of metastasis or invasion. For example, P_0, H_0, N_3, S_1 is to be recorded as Stage IV.

3.2. Results

At the start of our investigations, patients with no hope of cure because of liver or peritoneal metastases were treated in an effort to determine the effectiveness and safety of this form of radiotherapy. The total number of patients treated was 14 and resections could not be or were not performed, since all patients had advanced stage disease. The diameter of the primary tumors of these patients was more than 6 cm. The radiation field was limited to the primary tumor and regional lymph node metastases in order to alleviate symptoms.

A single dose ranging from 18 Gy to 40 Gy was delivered. The following information was obtained: (a) Marked palliation, such as relief from a large tumor mass obstructing the stomach was obtained about two weeks after irradiation in patients who received more than 20 Gy. All patients died and the mean survival time was 6.2 months. (b) Postmortem examination revealed that a single dose of more than 40 Gy is necessary to erradicate gross gastric cancer, since remaining cancer cells were still sporadically found by histological examination in the radiation field in patients who received 40 Gy. However it was demonstrated that lymph node metastases which were about 3 cm in diameter were eliminated by a single dose of 35 Gy. Figure 9a shows a histological section of a metastatic lymph node about 3 cm in diameter before irradiation. Figure 9b demonstrates a histological section of the same tumor taken 6 months after intraoperative irradiation with 35 Gy. No malignant cells were found. (c) No harmful side effects such as diarrhea, bloody stools, abdominal pain or infection resulted from intraoperative irradiation procedure were observed.

Based upon the information stated above, intraoperative radiotherapy was performed on patients in whom distant metastases were not found and the primary tumor was surgically removed. A single dose ranging from 25 Gy to

Table 2. Cancer stage based on gross findings [13]

Stage	Peritoneal metastasis	Liver metastasis	Lymph node metastasis	Serosal invasion
I	P_0	H_0	N $(-)$	S_0
II	P_0	H_0	N_1 $(+)$	S_1
III	P_0	H_0	N_2 $(+)$	S_2
IV	P_1, P_2, P_3	H_1, H_2, H_3	N_3 $(+)$, N_4 $(+)$	S_3

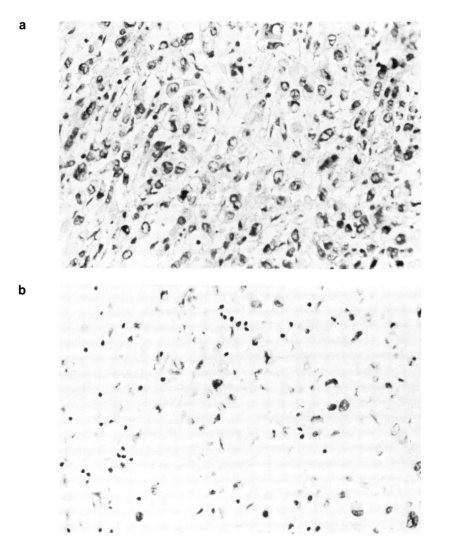

Figure 9a. Histologic section of metastatic lymph node of gastric cancer before irradiation.
Figure 9b. Histologic section of the same tumor which was irradiated with a single dose of 35 Gy. No malignant cells are found.

40 Gy, increasing with tumor volume, was delivered.

The total number of patients treated was 184; 96 patients (52.2%) are alive. In order to evaluate the effectiveness of intraoperative irradiation, a sequential study was performed on the survival rates between patients treated by intraoperative radiotherapy and those treated by surgery alone. Patients who were admitted to the Kyoto University Hospital on Tuesday received an operation alone and those who were admitted on Friday received intraoperative radiotherapy.

Figure 10a–d demonstrates the actuarial survival rates based on an analysis of

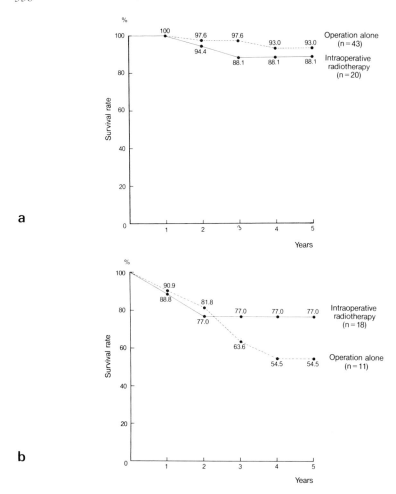

Figure 10. Actuarial survival curves of gastric cancer patients treated by intraoperative radiotherapy and those treated by surgery alone.
Figure 10a. Survival rates of Stage I gastric cancer.
Figure 10b. Survival rates of Stage II gastric cancer.

110 patients treated by operation alone and 84 patients treated by intraoperative radiotherapy. The five-year survival rates of the patients treated by operation alone was 93.0% for Stage I, 54.5% for Stage II, 36.8% for Stage III and 0% for Stage IV. On the other hand, the five-year survival rates of patients treated by intraoperative radiotherapy was 88.1% for Stage I, 77.0% for Stage II, 44.6% for Stage III and 19.5% for Stage IV [14]. With few exceptions chemotherapy was not used in either group of patients. It is clear from these results, that intraoperative radiotherapy has a definite effect on locally advanced gastric cancer.

The reason that the prognosis of Stage IV gastric cancer treated by intraoperative irradiation is promising is that this radiotherapy was selectively applied to

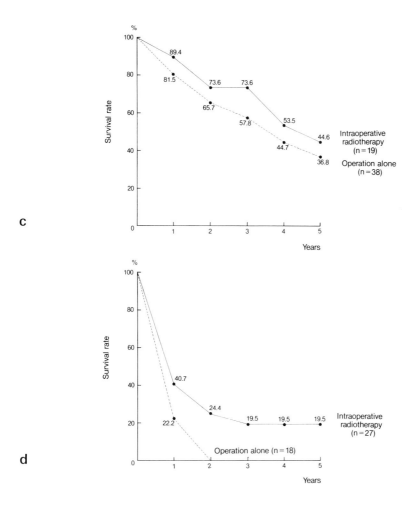

Figure 10c. Survival rates of Stage III gastric cancer.
Figure 10d. Survival rates of Stage IV gastric cancer.

patients who had no distant metastases and in whom the primary tumor was removed by gastrectomy. It is important to note that although all patients with Stage IV gastric cancer in this group received gastrectomy, 15 out of the 19 patients received a non curative operation because of an incomplete removal of lymph node metastases and/or of lesions invading directly to the pancreas. The results in the 19 patients are shown in Table 3. The details of three patients who underwent non curative surgery as a result of incomplete excision of neoplasms but have survived more than 5 years after intraoperative radiotherapy are described below:

Case 17: A 60-year-old female. The primary tumor was located in the antrum and penetrated through the serosa with direct invasion of the head of the pancreas. Metastases were found in the lymph nodes $N_{7, 8, 11}$, and $_{13}$. The primary tumor was removed by subtotal gastrectomy and a single dose of 30 Gy with 8 MeV electron was given through a pentagonal cone which encompassed the invaded part of the pancreas and the unresectable lymph node metastases. The patient is well and free from recurrence 7 years after treatment.

Case 18: A 64-year-old male. The primary tumor was located in the portions of M and A. The metastatic lesions were found around the celiac axis and they invaded directly into a part of the liver. The patient was classified as P_0, H_1, N_2, S_3, Stage IV. The primary tumor and the invaded part of the liver was removed, but the removal of the metastatic lymph nodes around the celiac axis was incomplete. A single dose of 30 Gy with 8 MeV electrons was delivered through a cone which encompassed the residual tumor. The patient has survived more then 6 years after treatment with no evidence of disease.

Case 19: A 64-year-old male. The primary tumor was located in the portions of A and M and invaded into the pancreas. Metastases to the lymph nodes of $N_{7, 8, 9, 11}$ and $_{13}$ were evident (Fig. 11a). The patient was classified as P_0, H_0, N_3, S_3, Stage IV. The primary tumor was removed by subtotal gastrectomy and a single dose of 35 Gy with 12 MeV electrons was given to the unresectable lymph node metastases (Fig. 11b). The patient is well and free from recurrence 7 years after intraoperative radiotherapy.

Table 3. Results of intraoperative radiotherapy for patients with Stage IV gastric cancer

Case	Age	Sex	PHNS classification	Operation	Dose (Gy)	Survival time
1	67	M	$P_0H_0N_1S_3$	Relative curative op.	30	2 year 2 mo dead
2	35	F	$P_0H_0N_2S_3$	,,	30	3 year 8 mo dead
3	50	F	$P_0H_0N_2S_3$	,,	28	4 year 8 mo dead
4	32	F	$P_0H_0N_3S_3$	,,	30	3 mo dead
5	60	M	$P_0H_0N_2S_3$	Absolute non curative op.	20	2 mo dead
6	24	M	$P_1H_0N_2S_2$	,,	20	8 mo dead
7	60	M	$P_1H_2N_2S_3$	,,	20	2 mo dead
8	56	M	$P_1H_0N_3S_3$	,,	20	5 mo dead
9	38	M	$P_0H_0N_2S_3$	,,	27	1 year dead
10	42	F	$P_0H_0N_2S_3$	,,	27	1 year 2 mo dead
11	66	M	$P_0H_0N_2S_3$	,,	30	1 year 5 mo dead
12	72	M	$P_0H_0N_2S_3$	,,	30	2 year 4 mo dead
13	66	M	$P_0H_0N_3S_3$	,,	30	1 year 5 mo dead
14	59	M	$P_1H_0N_3S_1$	,,	30	3 mo dead
15	70	F	$P_2H_0N_1S_3$	,,	30	6 mo dead
16	52	F	$P_1H_0N_2S_2$	,,	30	1 year 10 mo dead
17	60	F	$P_0H_0N_3S_3$	,,	30	7 year 1 mo alive
18	64	M	$P_0H_1N_2S_3$	,,	30	6 year 6 mo alive
19	64	M	$P_0H_0N_3S_3$	,,	35	7 year 10 mo alive

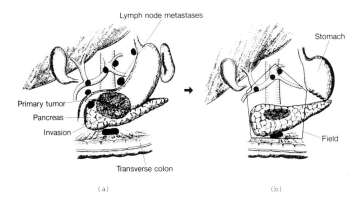

Figure 11. A case of a patient with gastric cancer who underwent intraoperative radiotherapy as a result of incomplete removal of neoplasms. The primary tumor located in the antrum penetrated through the serosa with invasion of the pancreas. Lymph node metastases were found mainly around the celiac axis. The invaded part of the pancreas and unresectable lymph node metastases were covered by a pentagonal treatment cone.

3.3. Indications of intraoperative radiotherapy for gastric cancer

1. The primary tumor is located in the portions of M and/or A.
2. The primary tumor is removed surgically.
3. No metastases to the peritoneum.
4. No liver metastases except for direct invasion of the liver from the lesion.
5. All lymph node metastases must be encompassed by one radiation field.

3.4. Complications

The organ to which irradiation cannot be avoided in intraoperative radiotherapy of gastric cancer is the pancreas where less than 40% of the whole pancreas is included in the radiation field. Acute and late damage to the pancreas was therefore examined by the changes of serum amylase and blood sugar after irradiation of 11 patients. Figures 12 and 13 demonstrate the changes of serum amylase and blood sugar respectively. The pre-irradiation levels of serum amylase and blood sugar were determined and the changes in the mean values of the 11 patients after irradiation were demonstrated as percentage of pre-irradiation levels. A transient increase in serum amylase and blood sugar ocurred after intraoperative irradiation, but they returned to the pre-irradiation level within a week. Neither significant late complications nor deviation from the usual post-operative course were observed. A definite difference from conventional radiotherapy is that almost no patients develop leukopenia following intraoperative irradiation. This seems to be due to the reduced treatment volume to irradiate.

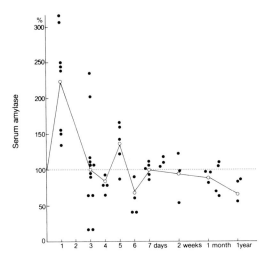

Figure 12. Changes in serum amylase after intraoperative radiotherapy.

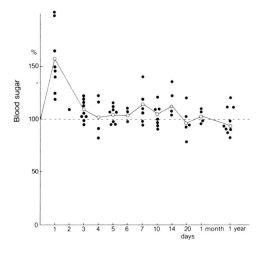

Figure 13. Changes in blood sugar after intraoperative radiotherapy.

4. Intraoperative radiotherapy for colorectal cancer

The abundant subserous network of lymphatics of the colon is drained mostly by the paracolic lymph nodes and continues to the intermediate group of lymph nodes or directly to the mesenteric or para-aortic nodes. In these lymphatic systems, en bloc excision of lymph nodes up to the intermediate group is possible together with the primary tumor of the colon, but complete eradication of cancer nests around the mesenteric arteries or the aorta is hard to attain by surgery. In addition, the incidence of local recurrence is high when the lesion penetrates through the wall of the colon with invasion into the nearby structures such as the bladder or muscles in the retroperitoneum.

Little attention has been given to the adjuvant role of radiotherapy in the management of unresectable lymph node metastases or invasion into the retroperitoneal structures. This is because external irradiation with large cumulative doses to the abdomen causes severe intestinal damage. In intraoperative radiotherapy, a cancercidal dose can be delivered safely to unresectable remnants since the intestine is removed from the field. Various clinical and pathologic studies have indicated that spread via lymphatics does not occur in many cases of colon cancer. Therefore, cure may be expected by intraoperative irradiation when the primary tumor is removed surgically but elimination of regional lymph node metastases or of invasion into the nearby structures is incomplete.

In rectal cancer, despite radical abdominoperineal resection, local recurrence in the absence of distant metastases continues to be a major reason for treatment failure. Although external beam radiotherapy in the range of 45 Gy – 50 Gy can be effective in controlling microscopic residual tumor, treatment of gross residual or inoperable cancer requires higher doses. At such levels the problem of irradiation-induced small bowel injury can become significant if loops are fixed within the treatment field. The use of intraoperative radiotherapy is a technique to increase significantly the tumor dose without any increase in radiation dose to the small intestine. Intraoperative radiotherapy can also be used as a boost dose in conjunction with external beam treatment.

4.1. Methods

Intraoperative irradiation is delivered after tumor resection but before anastomosis is accomplished. Irradiation before performing an anastomosis allows wide exposure of the resected bed and avoids irradiating normal portion of the intestinal tract. The treatment cones must be of various sizes and shapes so as to conform to various anatomic situation in the patient. A single dose of 30 Gy– 40 Gy depending upon the tumor size is delivered to the unresectable tumor.

4.2. Results

Figure 14 shows the results of intraoperative radiotherapy for colorectal cancer in the Kyoto University. Cases 1–6 are patients who developed recurrence after an operation. Except for case 6, the tumor could not be extirpated by surgery. All these patients were irradiated with single doses of 20 Gy–40 Gy but four of the six patients died without local control. Cases 7–13 were patients who had not received any previous treatment. In cases 8–13, the primary tumor was removed surgically and intraoperative irradiation with single doses of 25 Gy–30 Gy was

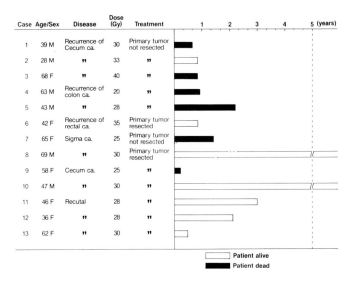

Case	Age/Sex	Disease	Dose (Gy)	Treatment					
1	39 M	Recurrence of Cecum ca.	30	Primary tumor not resected					
2	28 M	"	33	"					
3	68 F	"	40	"					
4	63 M	Recurrence of colon ca.	20	"					
5	43 M	"	28	"					
6	42 F	Recurrence of rectal ca.	35	Primary tumor resected					
7	65 F	Sigma ca.	25	Primary tumor not resected					
8	69 M	"	30	Primary tumor resected					
9	58 F	Cecum ca.	25	"					
10	47 M	"	30	"					
11	46 F	Recutal	28	"					
12	36 F	"	28	"					
13	62 F	"	30	"					

□ Patient alive
■ Patient dead

Figure 14. Results of intraoperative radiotherapy for colorectal cancer.

delivered to the unresectable remnants. In case 7 the primary tumor was too large to be removed and a single dose of 25 Gy was given. Five out of the 7 patients (cases 7–13) are alive and 2 have survived more than 5 years without evidence of recurrence. The details of these two patients are described below.

Case 8: The patient was a 69-year-old man with carcinoma of the sigmoid colon. The tumor was about 7 cm in diameter with lymph node metastases around the inferior mesenteric artery which infiltrated the retroperitoneal structures. The primary tumor was removed by left hemicolectomy. The infiltrated tissue and lymph node metastases were irradiated with 30 Gy. He is well without evidence of recurrence more than 7 years after treatment.

Case 10: The patient was a 47-year-old man with carcinoma of the cecum. Laparotomy revealed a tumor about 6 cm in diameter with retroperitoneal invasion and lymph node metastases along the ileocolic artery. The primary tumor was removed by right hemicolectomy but elimination of the metastatic disease was incomplete. Therefore, preceding anastomosis, a single dose of 30 Gy was delivered to the infiltrated retroperitoneal tissue including the lymph node metastases through an 8 × 8 cm field (Fig. 15). The patient is symptom free more than 9 years after treatment and has returned to work with no evidence of recurrence.

4.3. Indications

As in gastric cancer, cure cannot be expected if the primary tumor is not extirpated surgically. When there is metastatic disease around the superior

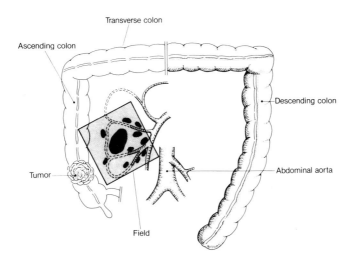

Transverse colon

Ascending colon

Descending colon

Abdominal aorta

Tumor

Field

Figure 15. A case of a patient with colon cancer treated by intraoperative radiotherapy as a result of non curative operation. The primary tumor located in the ascending colon was removed by right hemicolectomy. The infiltrated part of the retroperitoneal tissue and unresectable lymph node metastases were irradiated with a single dose of 30 Gy.

mesenteric artery, it is hard to deliver a large dose, since exposure of the radiosensitive duodenal loop near this artery cannot be avoided. By contrast, if surgical removal of the tumor around the inferior mesenteric artery is incomplete, intraoperative irradiation is indicated, because there are no radiosensitive structures in this area. When there is deep extraserosal invasion to the retroperitoneal structures, especially near the ureter, inferior vena cava, or colonic artery, radical surgery is difficult, hence the incidence of local recurrence is high. The 2 surviving patients are good examples of the difficulty of surgical resection and the subsequent cure of visible residual disease by intraoperative radiotherapy.

5. Intraoperative radiotherapy for pancreatic cancer

Pancreatic cancer rarely yields to curative measures, regardless of the treatment modality. Some fine results have been obtained in the treatment of this disease by external beam irradiation [15, 16], but the role of radiotherapy has been largely palliative. The deep location of the pancreas and its proximity to dose-limiting structures have limited the delivery of the high doses of external beam radiation necessary for curative intent. Intraoperative radiotherapy affords a more radical outcome than external irradiation.

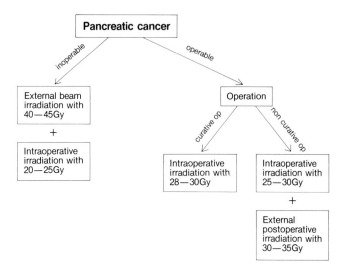

Figure 16. Treatment policy for pancreatic cancer.

5.1. Methods

Pancreatectomy has been reserved for a minority of patients, mostly because few pancreatic cancers are diagnosed in an operable stage. For patients who are diagnosed as inoperable, intraoperative radiotherapy is performed as a boost type of radiotherapy which is delivered as an adjunct to a conventional large field external beam radiotherapy. Namely, external photon radiation with cumulative doses of 40 Gy–45 Gy is delivered in an attempt to reduce a tumor size. Two to 4 weeks thereafter, laparotomy is performed and a single dose ranging from 20 Gy to 25 Gy depending upon the residual tumor size is given intraoperatively.

For patients who are diagnosed as operable and receive a gross resection of the tumor but have gross residual disease at the end of the surgical procedure, intraoperative irradiation with single doses of 25 Gy–30 Gy is given to the unresectable tumor followed about 4 weeks later by conventional postoperative irradiation to doses of 30 Gy–35 Gy. If patients receive curative operation, intraoperative irradiation with 28 Gy–30 Gy is given to the tumor bed or sites suspicious for containing residual tumor cells and no external postoperative irradiation is employed (Fig. 16). In all patients with pancreatic cancer it is recommended that a routine gastroenterostomy bypass procedure be performed in order to avoid a prepyloric or duodenal ulcer or obstruction secondary to the irradiation.

5.2. Results

The results of pancreatic cancer treated by intraoperative radiotherapy at different institutions are summarized in Table 4. At Kyoto University and Howard University Hospitals, all patients had unresectable pancreatic cancer and about 40% of the patients had liver metastases. Intraoperative irradiation was given to the primary tumor and its regional lymph nodes without adjuvant use of surgical resection or postoperative chemotherapy. Therefore long term survivals were not obtained. The most conspicuous effect of intraoperative radiotherapy on inoperable pancreatic cancer is relief of pain. About 80% of patients who complained of severe abdominal pain experienced relief of severe pain within a week after intraoperative irradiation with a single dose of more than 20 Gy. Matsuda *et al.* [18] have reviewed the experience with their 12 patients with locally advanced pancreatic cancer treated by intraoperative radiotherapy combined with postoperative external beam radiotherapy. The median and the longest survival times were 12.6 months and 50 months respectively. The clinical results of

Table 4. Results of intraoperative radiotherapy of advanced pancreatic cancer

Institution	Year	Treatment	No. of patients	Median survival (months)	Longest survival (months)	Reference
Kyoto University Hospital	1980	IOR* (20–30Gy)	6	4.0	8 died	[2]
Howard University Hospital	1981	IOR (15–30Gy)	19	5.5	15 died	[17]
Tokyo Komagome Hospital	1982	IOR (18–30Gy) + Postop external radiotherapy (9–41Gy)	12	12.6	50 died	[18]
Massachusetts General Hospital	1982	Preop external radiotherapy (10Gy) + IOR (20Gy) + Postop external radiotherapy (40Gy)	21	13.5		[19]

* IOR: Intraoperative radiotherapy.

348

intraoperative radiotherapy performed as a boost in conjunction with large field external beam radiotherapy seems to be promising for the treatment of advanced pancreatic cancer.

5.3. Complications

In the case of pancreas head cancer, exposure of the duodenum is difficult to avoid. Approximately 30% of patients with pancreas head cancer who received a single dose of more than 25 Gy experienced diarrhea and/or bloody stool and about 10% of the patients developed duodenal ulcer.

References

1. Abe M, Fukuda M, Yamano K, Matsuda S, Handa H: Intraoperative irradiation in abdominal and cerebral tumors. Acta Radiol 10: 408–416, 1971.
2. Abe M, Takahashi M, Yabumoto E, Adachi H, Yoshii M, Mori K: Clinical experiences with intraoperative radiotherapy of locally advanced cancers. Cancer 45: 40–48, 1980.
3. Abe M, Takahashi M, Yabumoto E, Onoyama Y, Torizuka K, Tobe T, Mori K: Techniques, indications and results of intraoperative radiotherapy of advanced cancers. Radiology 116: 693–702, 1975.
4. Abe M, Yabumoto E, Takahashi M, Tobe T, Mori K: Intraoperative radiotherapy of gastric cancer. Cancer 34: 2034–2041, 1974.
5. Suit HD: Radiation biology – A basis for radiotherapy. In: Textbook of radiotherapy. Fletcher GH (ed). Lea & Febiger, 1973, pp 65–114.
6. Nice CM, Kurz J: Relation of the tumor size to radioresistance. Radiology 60: 555–557, 1957.
7. Strandqvist M: Studien über die Kumulative Wirkung der Röntgenstrahlen bei Fraktionierung. Acta Radiol [suppl.] 55, 1944.
8. Appleby LH: The coeliac axis in the expansion of the operation for gastric carcinoma. Cancer 6: 704–707, 1953.
9. Gilbertsen VA: Results of treatment of stomach cancer – An appraisal of efforts for more extensive surgery and a report of 1983 cases. Cancer 23: 1305–1308, 1969.
10. Maruta K, Shida H: Some factors which influence prognosis after surgery for gastric cancer. Ann Surg 167: 313–318, 1968.
11. Berry REL, Rottschafer W: The lymphatic spread of cancer of the stomach observed in operative specimens removed by radical surgery including total pancreatectomy. Surg Gynecol Obstet 104: 269–279, 1957.
12. Sunderland DA, McNeer G, Ortega LG, Pearce LS: The lymphatic spread of gastric cancer. Cancer 6: 987–996, 1953.
13. Japanese Research Society for Gastric Cancer: The General Rules for Gastric Cancer in Surgery and Pathology. Tokyo. Kanehara. 1968.
14. Abe M, Takahashi M: Intraoperative radiotherapy: The Japanese experience. Int J Radiation Oncology Biol Phys 7: 863–868, 1981.
15. Dobelbower RR, Borgelt BB, Suntharalingam N, Strubler KA: Pancreatic carcinoma treated with high-dose, small-volume irradiation. Cancer 41: 1087–1092, 1978.
16. Haslam JB, Cavanaugh PJ, Stroup SL: Radiation therapy in the treatment of irresectable adenocarcinoma of the pancreas cancer.

17. Goldson AL, Ashaveri E, Espinoza MC, Roux V, Cornwell E, Rayford L, McLaren M, Nibhanupudy R, Mahan A, Taylor HF, Hemphil N, Pearson O: Single high dose intraoperative electrons for advanced stage pancreatic cancer: Phase I pilot study. Int J Radiation Oncology Biol Phys 7: 869–874, 1981.

18. Matsuda T: Radiotherapy for pancreatic carcinoma by combination of intraoperative radiotherapy and conformation radiotherapy. Paper presented at the 'High LET Particle Irradiation and Other Approaches to Increasing Effectiveness of Radiation Therapy for Cancer'. Seminar under the US-Japan Cooperative Research Program, October 2–5, Kyoto University Club House, Kyoto, Japan, 1982.

19. Tepper JE: Intraoperative radiation therapy in the United States. Paper presented at the 'High LET Particle Irradiation and Other Approaches to Increasing Effectiveness of Radiation Therapy for Cancer'. Seminar under the US-Japan Cooperative Research Program, October 2–5, Kyoto University Club House, Kyoto, Japan, 1982.

14. Antimarker antibodies for the external imaging of gastrointestinal cancer*

DAVID M. GOLDENBERG and FRANK H. DELAND

Introduction

Much effort has been made over the past fifteen or more years to identify a unique cancer antigen, since it has been thought that this could serve as an indicator, or 'marker', in the blood for the diagnosis and monitoring of cancer. Such antigens could be restricted to a particular tumor, distributed among tumors of a specific organ or type, or common to a larger group or to all cancer types. They might share characteristics with parts or products of normal adult or of fetal cells, or even of tissues undergoing pathological changes distinct from cancer. Such substances may be secretory products, constituents of the cell surface, of the cytoplasm, or even of the cell nucleus. Examples of all these possibilities exist in the prolific literature of cancer immunology and tumor markers [1, 2], and the recent introduction of hybridization techniques for the production of monoclonal antibodies has resulted in the resurgence of interest in thsis area. However, with few exceptions, such as human chorionic gonadotropin for choriocarcinoma, alpha-fetoprotein in the detection of hepatic or testicular cancer, prostatic acid phosphatase in prostatic carcinoma, and specific blood hormone levels for certain endocrine tumors [2], there are none that have the sensitivity or specificity needed for providing a definitive diagnosis of a particular cancer. In general, the major applications of tumor markers have been to determine the extent of disease, *i.e.*, to determine disease recurrence, to evaluate the patient's response to therapy, and as a prognostic indicator.

The gastrointestinal system represents a number of organs which have, collectively, received the greatest attention in efforts to identify a tumor-distinct and organ-specific antigen [3]. A list of the more prominent markers known for gastrointestinal tissues and tumors, excluding more recent observations made with hybridoma antibodies, is given in Table 1. The most clinical attention has

---

* Dedicated to Professor Kurt Elster, Bayreuth and Erlangen, Germany, on the occasion of his 65th birthday.

J.J. DeCosse and P. Sherlock (eds), Clinical Management of Gastrointestinal Cancer.
© 1984, Martinus Nijhoff Publishers, Boston. ISBN 0-89838-601-2. Printed in The Netherlands.

been given to CEA and AFP, while our own group has developed another gastrointestinal cancer marker called colon-specific antigen-p (CSAp). This chapter will review the current status of some clinical application of tumor-associated markers in gastrointestinal cancer. It will become apparent that these substances have as blood markers a limited role in the management of gastrointestinal cancers. Nevertheless, we have found that although they are not unique or specific for cancer, they are sufficiently increased quantitatively in the tumor, as compared to adjacent tissues, to serve as useful targets for radiolabeled antibodies in the external, scintigraphic detection of cancer, a method we have termed 'radioimmunodetection of cancer' [4, 5].

In vitro AFP, CEA, and CSAp assays in gastrointestinal cancers

AFP. AFP is a serum protein occurring during gestation and again expressed by certain neoplasms, particularly primary liver cancer and teratocarcinomas of the

Table 1. Tumor-associated markers in gastrointestinal cancer

	Antigen	Year	Investigator	Organ-specific	Cancer-specific
1.	AFP, α-fetoprotein	1963	Abelev *et al.*	No	No
2.	CEA, carcinoembryonic antigen	1965	Gold and Freedman	No	No
3.	FSA, fetal sulfo-glyco-protein	1968	Häkkinen *et al.*	Perhaps	No
4.	IMG, intestinal mucosa specific glycoprotein	1971	Kawasaki *et al.*	Cell-specific	No
5.	CMA, colonic mucoprotein antigen	1974	Gold and Miller	Cell-specific	No
6.	CSAs, colon-specific antigens	1976	Goldenberg *et al.*	Cell-specific	No
7.	SGA, sulfated glyco-peptidic antigen	1978	Bara *et al.*	Cell-specific	No
8.	GOA, goblet cell antigen	1979	Rapp *et al.*	Cell-specific	No
9.	ZGM, zinc glycinate marker	1976	Pusztaszeri *et al.*	No	No
10.	CSAp, colon-specific antigen-p	1977	Pant *et al.*	Cell-specific	No
11.	BFP, basic fetoprotein	1977	Ishii	No	No
12.	GT-II, galactosyltrans-ferase-isoenzyme	1978	Podolsky *et al.*	No	No
13.	POA, pancreatic oncofetal antigen	1978	Gelder *et al.*	No	No
14.	TennaGen	1979	Potter *et al.*	No	No

From Goldenberg [3].

testis and ovary [6]. AFP appears to be a very useful marker for the diagnosis and management of primary hepatocellular carcinoma, but elevations of serum AFP are by themselves not diagnostic of liver cancer, since elevations may occur in other diseases of the liver or in association with other tumor types. Up to 80–90% of patients with primary hepatocellular carcinoma have elevated serum AFP levels [7]. The normal concentration of AFP in adults is 10 ng/mL. Elevations between 30 and 400 ng/mL are found in patients with nonmalignant liver disease. Levels of AFP above 3000 ng/mL are virtually diagnostic of primary hepatocellu-lar carcinoma. With values between 400 and 3000 ng/mL, primary hepatocellular is very likely present if other types of AFP-producing tumors, such as teratocar-cinoma, can be ruled out [8]. Differentiating elevated AFP titers associated with nonmalignant conditions from those in patients with liver cancer is aided by serial determination of AFP, since elevations of serum AFP associated with hepatitis or cirrhosis are usually transitory while those associated with cancer persist or rise with time [9, 10]. In acute viral hepatitis, the degree of AFP elevation seems to reflect the extent of liver regeneration.

Animal and clinical data suggest that serial determinations of AFP may be useful for determining the effects of therapy. Curative surgery results in the AFP level falling to a normal range. When it does not return to normal or if the serum level drops with a half-life longer than 7–8 days, residual tumor is probably present. Chemotherapy of primary liver cancer is unsatisfactory. Nevertheless, sequential AFP measurements can be used to evaluate the effectiveness of drugs [11, 12].

Patients with tumors other than liver cancer and teratocarcinoma may also have elevated serum AFP titers, particularly tumors of the gastrointestinal tract with or without metastasis to the liver [7]. Most of these cases involve tumors of the upper gut, such as esophagus and stomach, but the low frequency of AFP positivity in non-hepatic, non-teratomatous tumors discourages its use in such disease categories (also see Chapter 1).

CEA. Carcinoembryonic antigen (CEA) was described in 1965 by Gold and Freedman as a protein(s) found in adenocarcinomas of the digestive tract and in the gut, liver and pancreas of the embryo and fetus during the first six months of gestation [13]. Subsequently, a radioimmunoassay was developed which detected as little as 1 ng of CEA per mL of serum. Values above 2.5 ng/mL were found in 35 of 36 patients with adenocarcinoma of the colon [14]. Although later studies showed that the CEA measured in such immunoassays is neither digestive tract-nor cancer-specific, the CEA test has become the most widespread blood assay used in the management of a number of cancer types [15]. Colorectal cancer, however, still represents its major applications [16]. A recent NIH Consensus Development Conference on the Clinical Use of CEA determined [17]:

1. The blood CEA assay cannot be used as a cancer screening test, since it lacks the necessary sensitivity and specificity. Although the CEA assay cannot be used independently to establish a diagnosis of cancer, in a patient with symptoms a

grossly elevated value graded in 5 to 10 times the upper limit of the reference normal range for the particular laboratory is considered significant in that particular patient. In these cases, further diagnostic workup to establish the presence or absence of cancer is indicated.

2. Serial monitoring of plasma CEA levels is considered the best noninvasive method for detection of disseminated recurrence of colorectal cancer. CEA is found to be elevated when residual disease is present or progressing. Following complete surgical removal of colorectal cancer, an elevated CEA value usually returns to normal within six weeks. Residual tumor is suggested when an elevated preoperative CEA titer fails to fall after surgery. It is best to obtain plasma samples for CEA assay preoperatively, four to six weeks postoperatively, and thereafter at regular intervals in order to best assess the possibility of recurrence. It has also been emphasized that preoperative CEA measurements are used as an adjunct to clinical and pathological staging of colorectal cancer.

3. In patients with known metastatic tumors, however, the CEA assay can complement other clinical measurements of tumor response to therapy. It is generally found that a marked steadily rising titer is indicative of a poor therapeutic response, although some patients may not show a rising plasma CEA titer despite advanced colorectal cancer being present. Thus, there is a discordance between CEA value and tumor size and change. By immunoassays that are currently available, CEA values greater than 2.5 or 5 ng/mL have been found in heavy cigarette smokers, in patients with benign liver disease, patients with benign tumors, and patients with inflammatory diseases such as ulcerative colitis, Crohn's disease, pancreatitis, and pulmonary infections. Only when CEA values are greater than 20 ng/mL is the presence of malignancy suggested. In this regard, it is important that serial assays of CEA, and not single determinations, be made.

CSAp. Colon-specific antigen-p (CSAp) was first isolated from a human colonic carcinoma propagated serially in golden hamsters, and identified with an

Table 2. CSAp elevations in patients with various diseases

Condition	Pos/total ≥10 units	& Positive
Gastric ca.	3/15	20
Colorectal ca.	27/44	61
Pancreatic ca.	3/15	20
Breast ca.	1/19	5
Ovarian ca.	0/24	0
Lung ca.	2/29	7
Cervical ca.	1/19	5
Colon adenomas	1/12	8
Benign GI diseases	11/62	18
Healthly controls	1/33	3

Adapted from Pant *et al.* [20].

antibody produced in the same animal species in which the tumor was grown, thus permitting the identification of the foreign, or human components [18, 19]. Later, goat antibodies to CSAp were produced, and a radiometric immunoassay for CSAp was developed [20]. In an analysis of 272 subjects, the distribution of blood CSAp values in each disease category indicated that the highest number of elevated CSAp values occurred in patients with colorectal cancer. This constituted a sensitivity of sixty-one percent in patients with colorectal cancer, but these were patients with advanced stages. Non-neoplastic gastrointestinal disorders showed an 18% abnormal titer frequency. Other results in this series are recorded in Table 2. It can be seen that in a small number of patients with gastric and pancreatic cancer, 20% had elevated CSAp titers. Thus, CSAp in the blood appears to discriminate quite well for patients with gastrointestinal disorders, and was elevated both to a higher extent and in a higher percentage of colorectal cancer patients than for any other disease categories studied. In a comparison of CEA and CSAp in the same patients, it was found that CSAp could increase the diagnostic accuracy of CEA in colorectal cancer by 14%. At a cutoff for CEA of 5 ng/mL, both markers were positive or negative in 48 or 4%, respectively, of the cases (52% concordance). Our studies suggested that the combined use of both CEA and CSAp assays would serve to differentiate malignant from benign colorectal neoplasms. Among patients with non-neoplastic, gastrointestinal disorders, 18% were positive for CSAp while 34% were positive for CEA (2.5 ng/ mL cutoff for CEA). At a higher cutoff for CEA (5 ng/mL), 18% were positive for CSAp and 21% for CEA. It must be noted, however, that most of the CSAp elevations in this disease group were only slightly above the cutoff level set for this marker in this study, so that raising the threshold slightly might decrease false positivity without sacrificing the assay's sensitivity. Our studies indicate that although the immunodiagnostic sensitivity of CSAp in colorectal cancer patients is less than that of CEA, it does appear to have a greater tumor- and colon-specificity than CEA. Patients with benign, non-neoplastic gastrointestinal diseases and with pancreatic cancer had elevated CSAp values in 18 and 20% of the cases, respectively. Similarly, CSAp was elevated in 20% of the gastric cancer cases studied, and these positive patients had the intestinal form of this tumor type. However, in all other cancers, including normal individuals, elevated CSAp values occurred in only 0–8% of the cases. On the other hand, CEA had a higher frequency of elevation in all of the disease categories studied, and the frequency obviously depended on the cutoff value used to determine the normal range for CEA. Thus, although CSAp falls short of CEA's sensitivity for detecting colorectal cancer (61 vs. 82–91%), its higher specificity for colorectal cancer suggests that it would be of value in combination with CEA. For example, in patients with benign colorectal neoplasms, the 25% positivity rate for CEA could be reduced to 0 if it were required that *both* markers be elevated simultaneously to warrant a diagnosis of cancer. This requirement, however, could likewise reduce the positive rate in colorectal cancer to 48%, using a 5 ng/mL cutoff for CEA, and to 55%

if a 2.5 ng/mL cutoff for CEA were used. The same principle holds true in patients with non-neoplastic gastrointestinal diseases. Other results have also indicated that CSAp can be used to monitor tumor response in patients under therapy for advanced colorectal cancer [20]. Further studies are required to assess its potential adjunctive role as an early diagnostic test for colorectal, gastric, and pancreatic cancers.

Radioimmunodetection of gastrointestinal cancers

Neither traditional immunological approaches nor the advent of hybridoma monoclonal antibody technology have as yet identified markers truly specific or distinct for cancer. Since the markers currently identified are quantitatively increased with certain neoplastic conditions, we undertook, beginning with experimental studies in 1972 with a CEA-producing human tumor model [21, 22], to determine whether such markers could serve as targets for radioactive antibodies, thus enabling the use of such antimarker antibodies for carrying diagnostic or therapeutic doses of radiation to neoplasms. The use of radioactive antibodies for tumor detection and localization by means of external scintigraphy has been termed the radioimmunodetection of cancer [4, 5]. We have recently reviewed the history and status of tumor imaging with radiolabeled antibodies [23]. Suffice it to say that although earlier clinical attempts at radioimmunodetection proved unconvincing, use of purified antibodies against CEA labeled with I-131, and the introduction of a computer-assisted subtraction method for substantially decreasing non-target background radioactivity, resulted in unequivocal imaging of tumors [23]. Our method of radioimmunodetection has been described in detail elsewhere [23–25]. Briefly summarized, purified CEA is used to immunize goats. The antiserum obtained several months later is purified by means of an automated affinity-chromatography system by which CEA crossreactive antigens are removed and the antibody is adsorbed onto a CEA-affinity column. This results in the CEA antibodies immunoreactivity increasing from approximately 25 to 70% [24]. The antibody IgG is isolated and then labeled with I-131 by the chloramine-T procedure. After appropriate evaluation for safety, the radioactive antibody is injected into the patient. Before doing so, however, the patient is skin-tested for hypersensitivity to the antibody and is thereafter placed on a daily oral dose of potassium iodide to reduce thyroid uptake of radioactive iodine. A dose of radioactivity of 2 mCi of I-131 is administered, comprising 2–3 μg of antibody IgG per Kg body weight. In order to compensate for circulating or interstitial nonspecific radioactivity, we employ a subtraction method involving the administration of technetium components a short while before imaging the patients [24, 26]. In this way, the 180 keV of Tc is subtracted from the 364 keV image of I-131, resulting in an I-131-tumor-image.

In addition to affinity-purified conventional goat antibody to CEA, we have employed several other antibody preparations for detecting gastrointestinal tumors (Table 3). Only the rabbit and goat antibodies against alpha-fetoprotein (AFP) were not affinity-purified. All of these preparations have been successful for imaging tumors containing the antigenic targets in question. Furthermore, no untoward reactions were observed in the patients included in these studies, even when repeat studies with the same antibodies were performed at different intervals.

Our experiences with CEA radioimmunodetection in colorectal cancer are summarized in Table 4 [27]. Ten of 12 patients with colorectal cancers showed positive radioimmunodetection results at the primary sites. Among the metastatic sites of tumor in these 51 patients, 47 of the 54 sites were defined by radioimmunodetection, of which only two could not be confirmed by other techniques. Among this series, false-positive results included two lung metastases (Patients nos. 21 and 39) that measured less than 2 cm diameter by chest roentgenogram, 1 liver metastasis (Patient no. 51), and one abdominal tumor (Patient no. 48). The patient whose liver metastasis was not defined by radioimmunodetection also has a negative liver scintigram. In the patient (No. 51) with liver metastasis not disclosed by radioimmunodetection, the primary tumor and a lumbar vertebral metastasis were localized with radioactive antibody to CEA.

On a site or lesion basis, these results demonstrate a sensitivity (true-positive rate) of 10 of 12 for primary tumors (83%) and 46 of 53 or 49 of 53 for metastases (87–92%), depending on whether or not the three equivocal findings are calculated as false-negative results [27]. The overall sensitivity for radioimmunodetection was 86 to 91% for this series of colorectal cancer patients. The false-negative rate on a patient basis was 5%, and between 9 and 14% on a lesion basis. Only two putatively false-positive radioimmunodetection results were found in this series, constituting a rate of less than 4%.

Followup of the patients in this series showed that 11 of the 51 had tumor sites revealed only by radioimmunodetection and later confirmed by other methods (Table 5). All eleven patients had elevated CEA titers in the blood at various intervals after resection of their primary tumors. Table 5 indicates the sites revealed by radioimmunodetection but at the same approximate time negative by

Table 3. Antibodies proven suitable for tumor localization by radioimmunodetection

Raised against	Source/Type	No. patients studied
CEA	Goat, affinity-purified polyclonal	322
CEA	Goat, affinity-purified, F(ab')$_2$	8
CEA	Mouse monoclonals	12
AFP	Goat polyclonal	46
AFP	Mouse monoclonal	4
CSAp	Goat polyclonal	26

other detection modalities. The lead time between disclosure of tumor by radio-immunodetection and confirmation by other methods appeared to range up to a maximum of forty weeks in this series [27]. From these and other studies with CEA radioimmunodectection, we have concluded that in colorectal cancer patients this method may 1) contribute to the preoperative clinical staging of the patients; 2) assist in the postoperative evaluation of tumor recurrence or spread; 3) complement other methods used to assess tumor response to therapy; 4) support the indication of a rising CEA titer, when other methods cannot detect tumor, for second-look surgery; and 5) confirm the findings of other detection methods that are less tumor-specific, such as liver/spleen scintigraphy, ultrasound, and computed tomography [27].

Our most recent gastrointestinal tumor marker, CSAp, has also been found to be a useful target for radioactive antibodies in colorectal cancer detection. As was the case with the in vitro CSAp assay, it seems that CSAp can complement the results obtained with CEA antibodies to be used for radioimmunodetection. CEA and CSAp radioimmunodetection in the same patient has shown a differential uptake of the two radioactive antibodies in two of the three sites of gastric cancer metastasis [28]. These results suggest that both CSAp and CEA antibodies should be used for disclosing colorectal and other digestive tract tumors by means of radioimmunodetection [28]. Studies are in progress to test this proposition.

Table 4. Tumor imaging with antibodies. CEA radioimmunodetection results by tumor site in 173 patients

Primary diagnosis	No. of patients	Sensitivity (true-positive rate)			
		Primary site	Secondary site	Total	Percent
Colorectal cancer	51	10/12	49/53	51/57	91
Ovarian cancer	19	10/10	11/14	21/24	88
Lung concer	30	18/25	5/8	23/33	70
Mammary cancer	6	2/5	7/9	9/14	64
Pancreatic cancer	6	3/6	1/2	4/8	50
Cervical cancer	15	6/8	13/13	19/21	90
Other uterine cancers	5	3/3	6/7	9/10	90
	4	2/3	3/3	5/6	83
Unknown origin	9	N.A.[a]	8/9	8/9	89
Miscellaneous cancers	26	9/21	8/9	17/30	57
Lymphoma	2	0/2	0/2	0/4	0

[a] N.A. = Not applicable.
CEA, carcinoembryonic antigen.
From Goldenberg and DeLand [23].

Table 5. Results in 11 patients where RAID detected tumor sites not revealed by other tests

No.	Patient No.	Primary tumor site	Plasma CEA (ng/ml)	Primary site	Secondary site(s)	Previous negative finding[b]	Confirmation	Time to confirmation (wk)
6	26	Rectum	92.0	0 → +[a]		IVP, BE	Proctosigmoidoscopy	0
11	60	Rectum	5600.0	+	+, liver	BE, IVP	Surgery	1
26	269	Colon	17.9	0	+, liver	L/S scan	L/S scan, CT scan	40
28	152	Colon	3150.0	0 → +	+, liver	BE, CT, US, L/S scan	Surgery	12
31	191	Colon	9.0	0	+, abdomen	IVP, US	Arteriogram, surgery	2
32	193	Colon	46.0	0	+, pelvis	CT, IVP	CT	28
33	195	Colon	12.2	0	+, abdomen	BE	Surgery	1–2
40	255	Colon	17.5	0	+, abdomen	BE, CT, Upper GI series	Surgery	5
44	292/270	Rectum	48.0	0	+, abdomen/pelvis	IVP, BE	Surgery	0
49	327	Colon	71.0	0	+, liver	L/S scan (partial), Surgery	Surgery	2
50	347	Colon	96.0	0	+, abdomen, +, abdomen	L/S scan, CT, BE	Surgery, Surgery	2

[a] 0 → +, recurrence at site of earlier tumor excision; +, tumor identified; 0, tumor excised. [b] Performed within 4 wk of RAID study, IVP = intravenous pyelography, BE = barium enema, CT = transmission computed tomography, US = ultrasonography, L/S = liver/spleen scan.
From Goldenberg et al. [23].

Conclusions

Despite the limited value of markers in the blood for cancer diagnosis, the evidence for radioimmunodetection shows that these same substances, with only quantitative increases in tumor tissues, selectively accrete radioactive antibodies for use as tumor imaging agents. It is also possible that such markers can serve as targets for antibody-mediated therapy. Although radioimmunodetection is still in early development as a cancer detection method, it has been used successfully to disclose occult sources of marker antigen production in patients with resected cancer. It is thus our view that this new detection modality will gain in importance among the diagnostic/detection modalities available in the management of cancer, and that its most immediate prospect appears to be in the *in situ* detection of gastrointestinal cancers. Whether radioimmunodetection methods can be refined to a sensitivity needed for the demonstration of early cancer will await advances in immunology (more tumor-specific antibodies), in radiochemistry (labeling with better imaging radionuclides), and in imaging (improved image processing and tomographic methods). Progress in all of these areas has been made since these were discussed at the first workshop on cancer radioimmunodetection held in 1979 [29].

With the poor response of colorectal cancer to curent anticancer agents, it would seem that the identification of metastases, even occult sites, such as can be achieved with in vitro assays of blood markers and with the *in vivo* application of radiolabeled antibodies for radioimmunodetection, would be of limited value for such patients. The solution is obviously not to ignore these detection efforts, but to improve our therapeutic armamentarium. Studies designed to assess the role of marker expression in the blood and tumor imaging by radioantibodies as pre- and post-therapy measures of predicting response and monitoring disease status, and to better stage extent of disease for stratifying patients for therapy, are needed.

Acknowledgements

We are grateful to S.J. Bennett, Ph.D., F.J. Primus, Ph.D., and E.Rouslahti, M.D., for collaborating in the area of antibody preparation, and to E.E. Kim, M.D., and M.O. Nelson, M.D., for clinical support and participation. Our studies have been supported by NIH grants CA-25584, CA-27742, and CA-31236, by a grant from the Veterans Administration, and by ACS grant IM-315.

References

1. Gold DV, Goldenberg DM: Antigens associated with human solid tumors. In: Cancer Markers. Diagnostic and Developmental Significance. S. Sell, ed. Humana Press, Clifton, New Jersey, pp. 329–369, 1980.

2. Herbermann RB, McIntire KR (eds.): Immunodiagnosis of Cancer, Parts 1 and 2. Marcel Dekker, Inc. New York and Basel, 1979.

3. Goldenberg DM: Immunobiology and biochemical markers of gastrointestinal cancer. In: Gastrointestinal Cancer. JR Stroehlein and MM Romsdahl (eds.), Raven Press, New York, pp 65–81, 1981.

4. Goldenberg DM: Immunodiagnosis and immunodetection of colorectal cancer. Cancer Bull 30: 213–218, 1978.

5. Goldenberg DM: An introduction to the radioimmunodetection of cancer. Cancer Res 40: 2957–2959, 1980.

6. Abelev GI: Alpha-fetoprotein as a marker of embryo-specific differentiations in normal and tumour tissues. Transpl Rev 20: 3–37, 1974.

7. McIntire KR, Waldmann TA, Moertel CG, Go VLW: Serum α-fetoprotein in patients with neoplasms of the gastrointestinal tract. Cancer Res 35: 991–996, 1975.

8. Silver HBK, Gold P, Feder S, Freedman SO, Shuster J: Radioimmunoassay for human alpha-fetoprotein. Proc Natl Acad Sci USA 70: 526–530. 1973.

9. Silver HKB, Deneault J, Gold P, Thompson WG, Shuster J, Freedman SO: The detection of α-fetoprotein in patients with viral hepatitis. Cancer Res 34: 244–247, 1974.

10. Bloomer JR, Waldmann TA, McIntire KR, Klatskin G: Relationship of serum α-fetoprotein to the severity and duration of illness in patients with viral hepatitis. Gastroenterology 68: 342–350, 1975.

11. Matsumoto Y, Suzuki T, Ono H, Nakasa A, Honjo I: Response of alpha-fetoprotein to chemotherapy in patients with hepatomas. Cancer 34: 1602–1606, 1974.

12. Purves LR, Bersohn I, Geddes EW, Falkson G, Cohen L: Serum alpha-fetoprotein: VI. Effects of chemotherapy and radiotherapy on alpha-fetoprotein levels in cases of primary liver cancer. S Afr Med J 44: 590–594, 1970.

13. Gold P, Freedman SO: Specific carcinoembryonic antigens of the human digestive system. J Exp Med 122: 467–481, 1965.

14. Thomson DMP, Krupey J, Freedman SO, Gold P: The radioimmunoassay of circulating carcinoembryonic antigen of the human digestive system. Proc Natl Acad Sci USA 64: 161–167, 1969.

15. Hansen HJ, Snyder JJ, Miller E, Vandevoorde JP, Miller ON, Hines LR, Burns JJ: Carcinoembryonic antigen (CEA) assay. A laboratory adjunct in the diagnosis and management of cancer. Human Pathol 4: 139–147, 1974.

16. Goldenberg DM: Carcinoembryonic antigen in the management of colorectal cancer. Acta Hepato-Gastroenerol 26: 1–3, 1979.

17. Goldenberg DM, Neville AM, Carter AC, Go VLW, Holyoke ED, Isselbacher KJ, Schein PS, Schwartz M: Carcinoembryonic antigen: Its role as a marker in the management of cancer. A National Institutes of Health Consensus Development Conference. Ann Intern Med 94: 402–409, 1981.

18. Goldenberg DM, Pant KD, Dahlman H: A new oncofetal antigen associated with gastrointestinal cancer. Proc Am Assoc Cancer Res 17: 155, 1976.

19. Pant KD, Dahlman HL, Goldenberg DM: A putatively new antigen (CSAp) associated with gastrointestinal and ovarian neoplasia. Immunol Commun 6: 411–421, 1977.

20. Pant KD, Shochat D, Nelson MO, Goldenberg DM: Colon-specific antigen-p (CSAp). 1: Initial clinical evaluation as a marker for colorectal cancer. Cancer 50: 919–926, 1982.

21. Primus FJ, Wang RH, Goldenberg DM, Hansen HJ: Localization of human GW-39 tumors in hamsters by radiolabeled heterospecific antibody to carcinoembryonic antigen. Cancer Res 33: 2977–2982, 1973.

22. Goldenberg DM, Preston DF, Primus FJ, Hansen HJ: Photoscan localization of GW-39 tumors in hamsters using radiolabeled anticarcinoembryonic antigen immunoglobulin G.

23. Goldenberg DM, DeLand FH: History and status of tumor imaging with radiolabeled antibodies. J Biol Response Modif 1: 121–136, 1982.

24. Goldenberg DM, DeLand F, Kim E, Bennett S, Primus FJ, van Nagell JR, Jr, Estes N, DeSimone P, Rayburn P: Use of radiolabeled antibodies to carcinoembryonic antigen for the detection and localization of diverse cancers by external photoscanning. New Engl J Med, 298: 1384–1388, 1978.

25. Goldenberg DM, Kim EE, DeLand FH, Bennett S, Primus FJ: Radioimmunodetection of cancer with radioactive antibodies to carcinoembryonic antigen. Cancer Res 40: 2984–2992, 1980.

26. DeLand FH, Kim EE, Simmons G, Goldenberg DM: Imaging approach in radioimmunodetection. Cancer Res 40: 3046–3049, 1980.

27. Goldenberg DM, Kim EE, Bennett SJ, Nelson MO, DeLand FH: Carcinoembryonic antigen radioimmunodetection in the evaluation of colorectal cancer in the detection of occult neoplasms. Gastroenterology 84: 524–532, 1983.

28. Nelson MO, DeLand FH, Shochat D, Bennett SJ, Goldenberg DM: External imaging of gastric cancer metastases with radiolabeled CEA and CSAp antibodies. N Engl J Med 308: 847, 1983.

29. Goldenberg DM (ed): Radioimmunodetection of Cancer Workshop. Cancer Res 40: 2957–3087, 1980.

15. Hyperthermia in the treatment of gastro-intestinal malignancy

F. KRISTIAN STORM* and DONALD L. MORTON

1. Introduction

This chapter is devoted to the potential role of hyperthermia in cancer therapy. This field is new and largely unexplored. Only recently has this technology produced a safe treatment for visceral disease. Thus, results of this type of treatment for specific gastrointestinal malignancies, while substantive, are sparce. We will review the history, the principles and the practice of hyperthermia and highlight those areas relating to GI cancer, in an effort to encourage further investigation of this promising therapy.

1.1. Historical background

The first recorded use of localized heat for treatment of cancer appeared in the writings of Ramajama (2000 B.C.); later Hippocrates (400 B.C.) and Galen (200 A.D.) told of the palliative effects obtained when *ferrum candens* (red-hot irons) were applied to superficial tumors. This practice continued throughout the Renaissance. In 1870, Busch observed several 'spontaneous' tumor regressions in patients whose infections were associated with high fever [1]. In 1893, Coley found that prolonged fevers of 39–41°C, induced with various bacterial toxins produced objective tumor regressions [2]. In 1898, F. Westermark found that hot-water-circulating cisterns caused palliative shedding of advanced carcinomas of the uterus but it was not until the turn of the century that the potential for localized hyperthermia was realized when reports from Germany in which d'Arsonval, Telsa and others described the healing effects of high-frequency currents.

After intense investigations, Nagelschmidt, in 1926, coined the term *diathermy* [3], 'to deep heat', and the widespread use of electromagnetic waves to heat tumors rapidly followed. In 1927, N. Westermark in Stockholm introduced the

---

* Clinical Fellow, American Cancer Society

J.J. DeCosse and P. Sherlock (eds), Clinical Management of Gastrointestinal Cancer.
© 1984, Martinus Nijhoff Publishers, Boston. ISBN 0-89838-601-2. Printed in The Netherlands.

concepts of dose/time response and histopathologic evaluation of thermal effects [4]. During the 1930's, Warren pioneered systemic hyperthermia with microwaves and infrared lamps. The patient was placed within a heating cabinet and Warren was able to show the tumoricidal effect of total-body hyperthermia [5]. In 1962, Crile reported partial local tumor control of spontaneous dog and human tumors after treatment with microwaves combined with low-dose radiation [6]. Then, in 1967, Cavaliere and his colleagues in Rome announced that tumor cells appeared to be selectively thermosensitive when compared to normal cells at temperatures between 42°C and 45°C (108°F to 113°F) [7]. These observations coupled with ever-increasing technological means to produce such temperatures provided the foundation for localized hyperthermia as therapy for cancer.

1.2. Mechanisms of thermal kill

Several investigators have found that damage to cancer cell respiration is a major factor in cell killing at $\geq 42°C$ [8, 9]. Although the exact mechanisms of heat destruction remain poorly understood, coincident alterations appear to take place in nucleic acid and protein synthesis which include a reduction of activity in many vital enzyme systems [10, 11]. These factors, associated with an increase in cell-wall membrane permeability [12, 13] and the liberation of lysozymes [14], probably account for autolytic cell destruction after hyperthermia.

The efficacy of thermocytotoxicity increases rapidly as temperatures are increased from 42°C to 45°C, the threshold of thermal pain in man. At such high temperatures, the differential thermosensitivity between malignant and normal cells is reduced and is replaced by a linear cell kill from progressive protein denaturation [15]. Thus, at $\geq 45°C$, host tissue tolerance becomes a prime concern in the design of clinical trials.

1.3. Histopathologic and gross morphologic effects of heat

In 1971 in Denmark, Overgaard treated mouse mammary carcinomas with localized radio-frequency hyperthermia at temperatures of 41.5–43.5°C and found distinct histologic changes in tumor cells, but not in stromal or vascular cells within the tumor or in adjacent normal tissues [16]. Rapid autolytic disintegration of heat-damaged tumor cells was observed, followed by a marked increase in connective stroma associated with progressive scar formation.

Progressive coagulation necrosis occurs at $\geq 45°C$ (15–17), although results appear to differ depending upon the location of the tumor [18]. In our experience superficial tumors generally sloughed off, whereas the volume of most visceral tumors did not change significantly after a transient increase in size during treatment. Serial biopsies showed early coagulation necrosis, edema, and vascular thrombosis, followed by a slow replacement of fibrous tissue over many weeks. It seems that these temperatures cause vascular thrombosis which slows or prevents the usual mechanisms of resorption. Therefore, biopsy or a careful assessment of tumor-doubling time (viz., stabilization of a previously progressive tumor) is necessary to determine the effects of high-temperature therapy for internal tumors.

1.4. Thermosensitivity of tumor cells

Throughout the late 1960's and early 1970's, evidence accrued to imply that at temperatures of 42–45°C tumor cells were slightly more sensitive to heat then their normal-cell counterparts. Cavaliere found that these temperatures caused irreversible damage to Novikoff hepatoma cells but not to normal or regenerating rat liver cells or to minimal deviation hepatoma 5123 [23]. Giovanella investigated thermal effects on normal (embryonic) and neoplastic (methylcholanthrene-induced sarcoma) mesenchymal cells. He found that 95% of all cultures of tumor-derived and tumor-producing cells died after 2 hours at 42.5°C, whereas only 43% of all cultured normal and non-tumor-producing cells died under similar conditions [19]. Of interest, when a cell subline derived from a non-tumor-producing line acquired high tumor-producing ability, it also acquired reduced thermotolerance. These and other investigations both *in vitro* and *in vivo* suggested that the acquisition of malignant potential was associated with increased thermosensitivity.

1.5. Selective tumor heating

It is well known from experiments on exposed tumors that the energy from interstitial implants, focused ultrasound, or microwaves when concentrated within a tumor provides enough local heat for potential tumor destruction. Less well known is the fact that non-focused microwaves and capacitive, inductive and magnetic-loop radio-frequency applicators can heat a *region* that contains the tumor by providing 'selective tumor heating', a remarkable implication for the treatment of deep-seated tumors.

In 1927, Westermark heated rat extremities bearing Flexner-Jobling carcinoma or Jensen sarcoma with high-frequency currents passed between lead electrodes. He found that tumor temperatures from 44–48°C could be attained without injury to normal surrounding tissues and postulated that differences in vascularity might account for the heat variations observed: 'It is a well-known fact that these rat tumors are poorly supplied with vessels. With regard to their temperature, therefore, they cannot derive any great influence through their circulation, their thermal regulation, therefore, being apparently bad' [4]. In 1962, Crile observed that since the blood supply of hepatic metastases in man was usually less than that of the liver itself, the heat generated in hepatic tumors tended to remain while the remaining liver was cooled by portal blood flow [6]. Since these early observations, the elegant studies by Mantyla [20] in Finland have confirmed that ambient tumor blood flow is generally less than that of normal host tissues.

When Le Veen heated tumors in three cancer patients with standard diathermy at 13.56 MHz he found that intratumor temperatures were 8–10° C hotter than those of adjacent normal tissues. He postulated that as a tumor grows it does not, or cannot, generate an integrated ramification of vessels as do normal tissues, which could cause a high resistance to blood flow and a reduced capability to exchange incident heat efficiently [21]. After extensive temperature measurements during hyperthermia therapy in spontaneous animal and human neoplasms, Storm [18] suggested that many tumors selectively retain more heat than normal tissues because their neovascularity is physiologically unresponsive to thermal stress and cannot regulate or augment blood flow.

Although these theories remain unproved, this phenomenon of 'selective tumor heating' after regional or volume energy deposition suggests that potentially effective independent tumor heating might be possible deep within the body, even without the ability to focus such energy.

2. Clinical instrumentation

2.1. Localized hyperthermia

2.1.1. Electrocoagulation

Electrocoagulation, or electrofulgeration, has been used for the palliative management of inoperable carcinoma of the rectum and has been part of the surgeon's armamentarium against exposed tumors for nearly 15 years. More recently, claims have been made for this method as a curative treatment of this disease [22]. The depth of heating depends upon the intensity of the current, size of the electrode (usually a wire-loop), resistance of the tissues, and the duration of exposure. The procedure is performed under spinal anesthesia in the operating room through a large proctoscope and takes 15 to 45 minutes. The tumor is partially resected over several weeks and frequently requires multiple procedures.

The effectiveness of therapy has depended upon the skill and experience of the operator. Most surgeons have reserved electrocoagulation for palliative management of low-lying obstructive tumors to avoid a colostomy in patients who have extensive metastatic disease beyond the pelvis, and for selected patients with small superficial non-ulcerating rectal cancers who are poor surgical risks for general anesthesia and abdominal-perineal resection [23].

2.1.2. Low-frequency current fields

Interstitial hyperthermia has been achieved by passing a LCF of 500 kHz between electrodes implanted directly into tumors [24, 25]. This method is essentially a form of resistive heating. The size and shape of the field can be manipulated by the number and position of the needles. Although invasive, this technique has been useful for the small accessible tumors where the full extent of the lesion was known (e.g., oropharynx, vagina, rectum) [26].

2.1.3. Ferromagnetic coupling

Liquid silicone impregnated with finely powdered iron particles has been used to occlude the vascular beds of tumors. The potential for selectively heating the metallic material that remains in the tumor in the vulcanized silicone offers promise.

Early experiments in dogs using an AC magnetic field at 20 kHz and hysteresis heating demonstrated significantly elevated temperatures (50–90° C) in injected organs and insignificant heating of non-injected organs [27]. Clinical trials will begin in the near future.

2.1.4. Ultrasound (US)

Ultrasound, a well-defined and spatially manipulative source of acoustic energy at 0.5–2 MHz and wavelengths of 3 mm to 0.75 mm, when focused, has potential for non-invasive selective heating of a target volume at depth [28]. As a result of insonation, the temperature rise in tissues can be controlled and reproduced [29]. However, unlike electromagnetic energy, ultrasound does not propagate effectively through air; the applicator must be coupled to the body surface with degassed saline and/or sound transmitting gel. Because of the high acoustic impedance mismatch between air and soft tissues, ultrasound is totally deflected at these interfaces and is ineffective near air-containing spaces (viz., oral-nasal cavity, respiratory and gastrointestinal tracts). Despite continued technical advances to overcome these problems by Lele at the Massachusetts Institute of Technology [30] and G. Hahn's group at Stanford, most clinical trials have been limited to superficial tumors at 43–45° C [31].

2.1.5. Microwaves (MW)

Microwaves at 433, 915, and 2450 MHz produced effective noninvasive localized hyperthermia to large areas of surface tissues and have been useful for treatment of superficial tumors. Most investigators employed specially constructed microwave waveguides that deposit energy into a defined area of tumor. This technique was popular for *in vitro* studies because of its easy application; however, penetration in man was limited to only a few centimeters because of extreme absorption by highwater-content overlying muscle. Guy found that these undesirable conditions could be partially eliminated by using lower frequencies (since the depth of penetration will increase as the fat and skin thickness become proportionally smaller compared to a wavelength) and a cooling applicator plate [32]. Recently, the University of Maryland organized multiple waveguides into a 'phase array' in an attempt to focus more energy within the deeper tumors. Although encouraging, only preliminary testing has been carried out [33].

2.1.6. Radio-frequency waves (RF)

Radio frequency at 13.56 and 27.1 MHz can be used for both local and regional in-depth noninvasive hyperthermia.

Capacitive electrodes: Capacitively-coupled parallel-opposed plates provide effective high-temperature heating in tumors. The field may be shaped by varying the size, contour and placement of the two electrodes. However, this method is usually reserved for surface or near-surface tumors because of the extreme energy absorption by any overlaying subcutaneous tissue [21, 34].

To a limited degree, injurious superficial heating can be lessened with cooled-contact electrodes, and intratumor temperatures as high as 57° C at a 10-cm depth have been achieved in selected patients who had minimal overlaying normal tissues [18]. Our investigations in dogs, sheep, and pigs revealed that 3–4 W/cm² was required to produce effective internal hyperthermia if surface tissue was cooled to 15° C; however, humans with equally thick tissues tolerated <1 W/cm² even with surface cooling to 3° C. It appears that surface cooling is only effective in man if skin and subcutaneous tissue are less than 1 cm in thickness [34].

In an effort to target RF energy to deeper tumors, multiple portals of entry and 'cross-fire' techniques have been studied in Wales. This method employs at least three pairs of sequentially activated contact capacitance electrodes placed on opposite sides of the body (Triport-222™, Life Extension Technology, Inc., Westport, Conn.). Using this device, Le Veen reported lung tumor temperatures of 45° C with minimal skin burns [35].

Induction coil: The so-called 'pancake' diathermy applicator is a compact coil/capacitor combination that induces circular eddy-currents in tissue by magnetic induction. This activity tends to be much less in the subcutaneous tissue [32]. Muscle heating to 44° C at 1 cm and 40° C at 4 cm have been achieved in the human thigh with a fat/muscle interface of 0.6 cm (Ultratherm 608™, Siemens Co., Erlangen, Germany). Modified coils (International Medical Electronics, Ltd., Kansas City, MO) have been useful for safely heating superficial tumors ≥42° C [36].

Magnetic-loop induction (Magnetrode™): Magnetic-loop applicators are self-resonant, non-contact circular structures composed of a single-turn coil with built-in impedance-matching circuitry operating at 13.56 MHz (Henry Medical Electronics, Inc., Los Angeles, CA). The element parameters are selected to produce very large circulating currents in the structure. These currents create a strong electromagnetic field into which the body or limb is immersed. Since the body is non-magnetic, interaction is restricted to the electric field, which consists of concentric circular flux lines. Although electrodynamic theory [37] and static phantoms [35] have shown a central 'dead spot', this null area has not been observed during tests in living animals (18,38) or in human cancer trials [18]. Muscle has been heated to 46°C at a 6 cm depth in the human thigh while skin and subcutaneous tissue temperatures remained at 36°C and 42.5°C, respectively, at the fat/muscle interface ≥1 cm [34].

This degree of penetration without surface tissue injury may be the result of a complex interaction in which current flow is parallel to layer boundaries in such a way that it is low in the highly resistant subcutaneous fat layer but high in the less resistant deeper tissues.

This approach permits safe and effective heating of human visceral tumors and provides most of the available knowledge about the effects of localized heat therapy on deep internal human tumors.

2.2. Systemic hyperthermia

2.2.1. Toxin therapy
With this method, exogenous proteins (often bacterial endotoxins) or chemical compounds are injected into the patient to cause systemic fever. Coley [2] first developed this now-historical method of fever therapy. It is no longer popular since individual patient response is quite variable and unpredictable, both in terms of the degree and duration of temperature elevation.

2.2.2. Paraffin-wax technique
This method, developed by Pettigrew in the early 1970's, uses the epidermal organ (viz., the skin) for heat exchange. The patient is immersed in molten wax (melting point 55°C; fusion point 43–45°C) and anesthesized with heated gases. This technique raises whole-body temperature 3–6°C per hour without burns and systemic temperatures of 41–42°C can be sustained for up to 20 hours, although the usual time of treatment is 3 to 6 hours [39, 40].

2.2.3. Water-blanket technique
Pioneered by Bull [41] and Larkin [42], this method enshrouds the patient in a hot-water-circulating suit after standard anesthesia. Feed-back loops and a microprocessor provide rather precise control of systemic hyperthermia; however, heating the body through the skin surface by this, or other means, causes profound cardiovascular stress.

2.2.4. Extracorporeal technique
Recently, Parks and Frazier [43] developed a technique for heating from the 'inside out', using an arterial/venous/femoral shunt connected to an external heat exchanger. The core temperature is elevated internally to systemic temperatures

of 41.5–42° within 30 to 90 minutes. The time to therapeutic temperatures is greatly reduced over the surface heating techniques, which lessens the potential for induction of thermotolerance that can occur with initial prolonged ineffective heating.

3. Tumor heating capacity

In 1975, Kim and Hahn of Memorial Sloan Kettering Cancer Institute were among the first to evaluate the heating patterns of cutaneous human cancers [44]. Hyperthermia was provided by a modified induction coil at 24 MHz. Twenty normal and 24 tumor tissue measurements were performed in 12 patients. At initiation of heating, both tumor and normal tissues averaged 35.9° C, but by 7 to 10 minutes, temperatures increased to about 40.5° C. The normal tissues stabilized there, whereas temperatures of most tumors rose to $\geq 42°$ C, where they too stabilized. Of 20 tumor measurements, temperatures $\geq 42°$ C (range 42–46° C) were possible in 17 (85%).

In 1977, we began clinical trials for patients with advanced cancer who did not respond to the standard methods of therapy, including surgery, radiation therapy, chemotherapy or combination therapy. Superficial tumors were treated with paired capacitance electrodes with or without surface cooling, and tumors with ≥ 1 cm of overlaying normal tissues or internal tumors were treated by magnetic-loop induction. Of 89 tumors evaluated in skin, subcutaneous tissue of muscle, intraabdominal viscera, intrathoracic viscera, or bone, temperatures $\geq 42°$ C were possible in 69 (78%) tumors, $\geq 45°$ C in 32 (36%) and $\geq 50°$ C in 22 (25%), while normal tissues remained within a physiologic temperature range of $\leq 45°$ C [34]. In 22 of these tumors, the central tumor temperature was compared to that of the normal tissue/tumor interface. In 2 (9%), no difference was observed, in 9 (41%) the difference was $\leq 1°$ C, in 5 (23%) the difference was $\leq 1.5°$, in 3 (14%) $\leq 2.5°$ C, and in 3 there was 3.5–9° C difference.

This capacity to heat tumors appears to be independent of tumor histology [45]. We recently measured temperatures in five varieties of human cancer, and achieved temperatures $\geq 42°$ C in 21/22 (95%) sarcomas, 18/24 (75%) melanomas, 24/36 (67%) adenocarcinomas, 3/4 epidermoid carcinomas, and 3/3 teratocarcinomas [34].

The capacity to heat tumors effectively also appears to be independent of location when employing magnetic-loop induction techniques. Baker [46] analyzed the tumor heating capacity in 99 patients with advanced tumors. He found therapeutic heating $\geq 42°$ C possible in 10/14 liver tumors, 7/11 intraabdominal tumors, 17/26 pelvic tumors, 6/9 chest wall tumors, 2/9 lung and mediastinal tumors, 2/9 head and neck tumors, and 6/11 extremity tumors.

Of the 89 tumors treated in our trial, 53 were ≥ 5 cm in *least* dimension and 36 were <5 cm. Effective heating to $\geq 42°$ C occurred more frequently in larger tumors (89%) than smaller tumors (61%) [34]. In 20 (22%) of the tumors studied, potentially tumoricidal temperatures could not be achieved without exceeding normal tissue tolerance. These tumors displayed thermal adaptation to constant or increased incident heat similar to that previously observed in normal animal muscle [18]. This intrinsic ability to adapt to thermal stress was also independent of tumor histology, but again appeared to be related to tumor size. Spontaneous cooling occurred in 14/36 (39%) tumors <5 cm, but in only 6/53 (11%) ≥5 cm in size [34].

These reports suggest that potentially effective hyperthermia can be achieved in most superficial and visceral human solid tumors regardless of histopathologic type or location, although it is most effective for large tumors. Some tumors cannot be safely heated ≥42°C and seem to retain their ability to regulate blood flow and dissipate heat. The cooler normal tissue/tumor interface observed in the majority of evaluable cases also suggests that the blood flow at the tumor periphery may have some bearing on the ability to effectively heat tumors.

4. Dose/response of thermal therapy

In 1975, Dickson, at the Royal Victoria Hospital at Newcastle-Upon-Tyne, plotted the thermal death times of all tumors studied to date. Included in these tables were *in vitro* investigations, induced tumors in animals, and some human cancers. He found that total tumor destruction by heat at 42°C would theoretically require 20 to 30 hours, at 45°C 3 to 4 hours, and at 50°C (122°F) only a few minutes. Based on these extrapolations and his own animal investigations, he subsequently concluded that for each degree centigrade rise in temperature above 42°C, the heating time for tumor destruction could be approximately halved [47].

In 1976, Le Veen reported his experience with standard RF capacitance hyperthermia and, although he concluded that this method was best for surgically exposed tumors to avoid surface tissue injury, he achieved temperatures >46°C in patients receiving 1–4 W/cm^2 for 30 minutes [21]. After one to nine treatments, he observed substantial tumor necrosis or regression of squamous carcinoma of head and neck (7), carcinoma of the lung (7), adenocarcinoma of colon and other tumors (4). Subsequently, Le Veen treated 32 patients with advanced lung cancer by the RF cross-fire technique [35]. Six of seven patients were alive and tumor free at 1 year, and two were tumor free at 3 years.

In 1977, Joines *et al.* at Duke University found 40% tumor regression within 4.5 weeks of five microwave treatments at 43.5°C for 30 minutes given every other day [48].

In 1979, Kim and Hahn reported their results from two to nine treatment times at 41–43.5°C for 30 to 40 minutes in 19 cutaneous human tumors [36]. Tumors under study were mycosis fungoides (6), melanoma (6), lymphoma cutis (2),

Kaposi sarcoma (2), and other less common tumors (3). They achieved complete responses in 4 (21%) tumors, partial responses in 6 (32%), and concluded that heat alone was partially effective, but transient. Luk subsequently treated 11 patients with recurrent breast, nasopharyngeal and anal carcinoma at 42.5° C for 60 minutes three times per week for 2 to 3 weeks and found two complete and two partial responses [49].

In 1980, Marmor and G. Hahn treated superficial tumors of <4 cm with ultrasound at temperatures of 43–45° C. Objective tumor responses were observed in 19/44 (43%), although most responses were partial and transitory [31].

In an attempt to evaluate the thermal death times of human cancers, we compared the net amount of tumor necrosis in 44 advanced malignancies after magnetrode-induced hyperthermia at various temperatures and fractionated exposure times [50]. We found that one treatment at ≥50° C for 17 to 45 minutes resulted in 20 to 100% tumor necrosis, whereas lower temperatures had no apparent effect. Two or three weekly treatments at 45–50° C for 30 to 72 minutes total treatment time produced 70 to 100% necrosis, whereas 40–45° C produced nearly equivalent necrosis but required more than twice the time. Five weekly and ten daily treatments for 135 to 600 minutes produced some tumor necrosis at 40–45° C; however, for similar amounts of treatment time, temperatures above 45° C were the most tumoricidal. Total tumor necrosis by the criteria employed (viz. total absence of cell nuclei) was rarely possible even at high temperatures. Although only minimal follow-up was possible in these patients with far advanced cancers, these findings suggested that human tumors might be less responsive to thermal therapy than predicted by models or induced tumors in animals.

The results of these studies to evaluate hyperthermia as a single agent suggested that higher temperatures, longer treatments and multiple treatments were the most effective. Optimal dose/time regimens and treatment fractionation schedules remain to be determined.

5. Hyperthermia toxicity

Local toxicity depends upon the dose of heat and the method of hyperthermia. Our initial investigations in dogs, sheep, and pigs revealed that the spontaneous cooling that maintained normal tissues at 43–44° C, well below thermal tolerance limits, could not be overcome without a substantial increase in heat dosage [18]. By increasing RF power from 1–10 W/cm^2, we made 13 separate thermal tolerance evaluations of dog skin and subcutaneous tissue. After 3 minutes of application, there were occasional transient first-degree burns (erythema) at 43–44° C and second-degree burns (edema, bullae) at 45–46° C. The extremities of nine dogs, one sheep and one pig were subjected to deep heat of 3 to 5 cm at temperatures of 41–44° C for 15 to 30 minutes to determine muscle, nerve and vessel thermal tolerance. Microscopic examination of these heattreated limbs did not reveal any histologic abnormalities, and in no instance was motor or vascular functional injury apparent over an observation period from 1 to 6 weeks. These findings were in accord with those of other researchers [51]. In the awake patient, Hardy found the upper limit of local tissue tolerance to be 45° C. Beyond this temperature pain and progressive protein denaturation occurred [15].

Subsequently, we subjected dogs to 42–45° C internal heat dosages over the thorax and abdomen for 15 minutes and observed the systemic effect for 2 to 3 weeks. During this interval, there was no clinical evidence of internal organ or spinal cord injury. Post-treatment, cardiac isoenzymes, hepatic transaminases and amylase were transiently elevated, but no abnormalities were apparent by electrocardiogram and there were no clinical symptoms or compromise to internal organs. However, sustained local hyperthermia at these temperatures universally resulted in fatal cardiac tachyarrhythmias and tissue injury. These findings confirmed other reports of injury during prolonged systemic hyperthermia [39–43] and regional limb perfusion [7, 52, 53].

Ultrasound, if allowed to dwell in normal tissues without continuous motion, will cause gas-bubble formation and injury and lose its potential therapeutic gain [29–31]. Ultrasound has also been associated with sustantial pain. The toxic effects of microwaves have been judged by normal tissue dose-time relations, with injury at temperatures ≥45° C as previously noted [32].

Employing standard capacitive RF heating at 1–4 W/cm^2, Le Veen reported that the energy was best transmitted to a surgically-exposed tumor in order to avoid undesirable heating of the skin and subcutaneous tissue [21]. He found that this method was successful only in patients who were so thin that there was almost no fat left on their bodies [35]. Subsequently, we confirmed these findings when surface cooling could not prevent preferential subcutaneous heat absorption ≥1 cm of subcutaneous tissue [34].

Our initial investigations with RF-cooled capacitance heating or magnetrode magnetic-loop induction deep-visceral hyperthermia at 13.56 MHz in dogs employed graded internal heat doses from 37–49° C. We took direct temperature measurements of heart, lung, esophagus, liver, stomach wall, stomach contents (solid and liquid), gallbladder, bile, spleen, pancreas, kidney, bladder and urine, small bowel wall and contents and colon and contents. Heating was remarkably uniform and there was no preferential heating or 'hot spots' of any of the normal organs evaluated [18, 34, 38]. We have yet to determine why high electrolyte solutions (e.g., bile, stomach contents) or avascular human contents (e.g., stool) are not selectively heated with these methods. In our experience of magnetrode hyperthermia in man, we have observed 10/2400 (0.004%) instances of local toxicity and no systemic toxicity. Awake patients undergoing deep visceral hyperthermia at 500–1000 watts absorbed power have displayed diaphoresis, skin flushing, a modest rise in core temperature (0.5–1° C), respiratory rate (2–12 rpm), systolic blood pressure (20–40 mm Hg), and a moderate to marked rise in pulse rate (20–60 beats/min).

Local toxicity occurred only in extraordinarily obese patients (2–3 cm sub-cutaneous tissue) or those with previously damaged normal tissues. In very obese patients, small local areas of subcutaneous fibrosis occurred at temperatures from 42–45° C, probably as a result of the extremely poor vascularity of such tissue. Second-degree burns occurred at ≤45° C in patients with split-thickness skin grafts, pedicle grafts, and radiation induced fibrosis and brawny edema. These results indicate that noncancerous tissues with inadequate blood supply are also thermosensitive.

Whole-body hyperthermia has been criticized because of the expertise required for its administration and its frequent complications. The cardiopulmonary system is subjected to extreme stess during the usual 8 to 10 hours of heating, and rapid and profound alterations can occur in body chemistries, fluids and electrolyte balance [39–43]. The liver is extremely susceptible to damage during systemic hyperthermia approaching 42° C, and precise monitoring within 0.1° C is mandatory to prevent hepatic necrosis.

Systemic hyperthermia is probably contraindicated for at least 3 months in patients who have been treated with radiation therapy over the spinal cord, because cases of transverse myelitis have occurred.

A rare complication of total-body heating has been hepato-renal shutdown due to rapid tumor dissolution and accumulated tumor breakdown products.

6. Immune correlations

Several investigators have implied that localized hyperthermia-induced tumor destruction may stimulate an immune-mediated abscopal response (an antitumor effect on distant untreated disease) as a result of an increase in circulating tumor antigen. Goldenberg [54] inhibited growth of GW-77 human colonic tumors in the hamster cheek pouch after radio-frequency heating, as well as of contralateral, presumably normothermic cheek pouch tumors. Marmor and G. Hahn found that EMT-6 sarcomas implanted in mice were highly sensitive to RF heating. However, cell kill as assessed by cloning efficiency of treated and immediately excised tumors was insufficient to account for the observed *in vivo* cure rate [55]. Among 42 of our patients who had far advanced cancer, none had regression of distant untreated disease even though an effect upon local treated disease was observed [34]. We suggest that an abscopal response, if such exists, may not occur or may be masked in patients with advanced systemic disease, and that further evaluations are needed in patients with a smaller tumor burden.

The potential for immune stimulation and in situ cell destruction from localized hyperthermia may not be realized with whole-body hyperthermia. In a recent review, Dickson [56], in fact, suggested that systemic heating may paralyze the immune system and lead to enhanced tumor growth. Moreover, others have found [57] that a slow heat induction period approaching 3 to 4 hours (frequently required with most wholebody heating techniques) may induce relative tumor thermotolerance and abrogate the effects of therapy. Clinical trials have yet to shed light on these important questions raised by *in vitro* investigations.

7. Hyperthermia as an adjuvant

7.1. Surgical adjuvant therapy

At temperatures >45°C, tumors display extensive vascular thrombosis [18]. Thrombosis may not be associated with the number or size of the vessels per se, but rather to the vessel's inability to augment blood flow in the presence of heat [31].

In selected patients (e.g., with locally advanced sarsoma) we administered high temperature hyperthermia preoperatively, and it was our impression that subsequent resection was facilitated in some instances by the avascular nature of the tumor [58].

7.2. Combination thermo-radiotherapy

In 1909, Schmidt postulated that heat sensitizes tissues to ionizing radiation. Since that time, hyperthermia has been combined with radiation therapy, both external beam and interstitial, in an effort to produce a synergistic or additive response [59]. Several investigations have concluded that hypoxic cells may be at least as sensitive to hyperthermia as oxygenated cells, forming one rationale for combination therapy [60, 61]. Others have suggested that the primary effect of hyperthermia is to inhibit cellular recovery from sublethal radiation injury [62].

In 1977, Kim treated the superficial tumors of ten patients with fractionated low dose radiation (800 to 2400 rads) and hyperthermia at 43.5°C [44]. Seven patients treated with combined therapy showed significant long-term benefits compared to those treated with radiation alone. In that year, Joines *et al.* [48] also treated superficial tumors for 30 minutes at 43.5°C for 30 minutes and 400 rads. Radiation and microwave heating were given alone or in combination every other day for a total of four treatments. In most instances the combined treatment caused complete tumor regression within 4.5 weeks, whereas the single agents applied to other tumors in the same patient caused only 40% regression during the same follow-up interval.

Hornbeck treated advanced cancer in 70 patients with combination 433 MHz microwave heating (Erbotherm™) (41°C at 7–8 cm) and standard dose-fraction radiation [63]. Of 21 patients who received a full course of therapy, 16 (80%) had a complete response and nine of the 16 remained disease free for 9 to 14 months. There was no complication from combined therapy, and no patient developed symptomatic or unusually sensitive skin reactions in or around the treatment area.

Recently, radiation therapists at the University of Kyoto treated 22 patients with 2450 MHz or 13.56 MHz hyperthermia alone or in combination with radiation [64]. Two weekly hyperthermia treatments at 41–43.5° C for 20 to 30 minutes were given immediately after radiation (2300–7000 rads). Remarkable regressions were achieved in patients receiving combination therapy, but no satisfactory results could not be obtained in patients treated with heat alone.

Haim Bicher at Henry Ford Hospital treated 57 superficial tumors in 43 patients with microwave hyperthermia and radiation in a unique fractionation protocol [65]. First, four fractions of 45° C for 60 to 90 minutes were applied at 72-hour intervals. After a one-week rest, a second series of four fractionated treatments was given that consisted of 400 rads followed within 20 minutes by 42.5° C for 60 to 90 minutes. These investigations found 64% complete regression and a 34% partial regression, with no response in only 2% of their patients. Only five local and two marginal recurrences have occurred at 6 months median.

The results of these preliminary radiation therapy trials indicate a potential beneficial effect for additive hyperthermia. Once dose/fraction schedules are more fully understood, it may be possible to achieve high rates of local disease control with reduced toxicity, or possibly enhance local cure over that possible with radiation alone.

7.3. Combination thermo-chemotherapy

In 1973, Johnson [66] reported that the tumoricidal effects of thio-tepa (5 g/ml) on V-79 Chinese hamster cells was enhanced two-fold by elevating temperatures from 37° C to 42° C. That year, Muckle and Dickson [67] reported that hyperthermia at 43° C combined with methotrexate at dosages of 0.4 mg/kg had more than double the effectiveness of drug alone on VX2 tumors in rabbits. In 1975, Hahn [68] found that an increase in temperature to 43° C would enhance the cell kill of adriamycin or bleomycin by three-fold in the EMT-6 sarcoma model compared to normothermic (37° C) temperatures. Equally interesting, he observed that adriamycin, usually unable to cross the membrane into the EMT-6 sarcoma cell, crossed the cell membrane under hyperthermic conditions. These observations supported the postulate that heat alters cell membrane permeability [12, 13]. Should this phenomenon occur in man, substantial preferential tumor kill might take place.

Using the clonogenic human stem cell assay, our group has compared cells treated with drug at normothermic (37° C) and hyperthermic (42° C) temperatures and results suggest that hyperthermia may significantly enhance tumor kill [69].

7.3.1. Regional thermochemotherapy
The best known clinical example of this synergism can be found in the regional hyperthermic chemotherapeutic limb perfusion for in-transit metastatic melanoma. Stehlin found that a 30% local disease control using L-PAM perfusion could be increased to 72% with additive hyperthermia at 40.5–42° C [52]. These results have been confirmed by others [53].

7.3.2. Local hyperthermia and systemic chemotherapy
During our Phase I trials of local hyperthermia, several patients were treated with combination thermochemotherapy, that included standard doses of 5-FU, methyl-CCNU, DTIC, high-dose methotrexate, cis-platinum or adriamycin after treatment failure from chemotherapy alone. Of 23 evaluable patients, 17 (74%) showed some response to additive heat; more importantly, there were no instances of increased toxicity. Most of these patients had visceral cancers, many of gastrointestinal origin.

7.3.3. Local hyperthermia and infusion chemotherapy for liver metastases
Since we found that intraarterial drug infusion therapy was superior to the intravenous route for some primary and secondary liver cancers [70], the idea that heat might enhance intracellular drug concentration led to combined-therapy clinical trials of intraarterial hepatic chemotherapy and hyperthermia at our institution.

7.3.4. Combination thermo-radio-chemotherapy
The largest trial of combined modalities is by Parks who frequently used whole-body hyperthermia in conjunction with chemotherapy and radiation [77]. A total of 102 patients received 371 treatments. Of 72 evaluable patients, objective regression occurred in 43, including 11 complete responses, even though nearly all of the patients (86%) had previously failed radiation and/or chemotherapy and had far advanced malignancy. Long-term responses occurred in 18% of patients from 7–28 months (10 months median).

7.4. Melanoma

In November 1978, we were pressed for a solution to a difficult problem – an alert but otherwise preterminal 29 year-old man with diffuse bilateral liver metastases of melanoma. We reviewed our experience with ten consecutive patients whose extensive disease had been treated with conventional intravenous (IV) imidazole-carboxamide (DTIC) 250 mgm/m^2/day × 5 days) and found no responders to therapy. All had expired of progressive liver metastases within 1 to 5 months (2.5 months median). A review of the history of six patients treated with intraarterial (IA) hepatic infusion therapy of similar doses of DTIC showed one partial response and two whose disease stabilized for 4 months. Based upon the more encouraging IA-DTIC treatment for melanoma [71] and the potential of hyperthermia enhancement, we treated this patient synchronously with the two modalities. Before treatment the patient was bedridden and required I.M. morphine for a markedly tender liver which was palpable down to the iliac crest. The DTIC (250 mg/m^2/day), infused by percutaneous hepatic artery catheter over 1 hour, was combined with simultaneous regional magnetic-loop induction hyperthermia to the liver daily for 5 days. By his third course of monthly treatments, the patient was pain free, off analgesics, and was skiing. At 5.5 months, his liver was of normal size with no evidence of metastases. Subsequently, this patient developed multiple distant metastases and he succumbed to brain metastases 1 year after the initiation of therapy.

This unexpectedly gratifying result led to a pilot study of combined infusion thermochemotherapy [72]. Ten consecutive patients with documented melanoma metastases to the liver but absence of brain metastases were treated with IA-DTIC and magnetic-loop induction hyperthermia at temperatures of 40.8–41.5° C. Eight patients achieved disease regression or stabilization of their disease from 3 to 14 months (6.5 months median). There was one complete response for 11 months, two partial responses for 7 to 14 months, and one minimal response for 3 months. Four patients had no progression of their disease associated with stabilization or improvement in physical status for 3, 3, 6, and 7.5 months. Seven patients retained or regained a normal activity status, and 4/5 patients with significant liver pain experienced complete pain relief subsequent to treatment. Seven patients died at 3 to 18 months (8.5 months median). All responders to therapy died of brain metastases, and liver disease progressed only during the latter phases of their illness.

Five additional patients were treated with IV-DTIC plus hyperthermia because the percutaneous infusion catheter could not be placed into the hepatic artery. In this group of patients, there were no responders and all patients were dead of progressive liver disease by 4.5 months.

The response rate, survival and quality of life for the patients treated with combined therapy has been very encouraging. Whether or not benefit from localized hyperthermia will prove to be superior to that of the infused DTIC alone [71] for patients with metastases to liver will require more investigation. A prospective randomized trial comparing IA-DTIC with and without hyperthermia is currently underway at our institution.

7.5. Colon carcinoma

Because of the poor prognosis for patients with liver metastases from colon carcinoma who are treated with conventional intravenous 5-FU, Dr. Kenneth Ramming of the UCLA Division of Surgical Oncology devised a unique therapy plan. After the distal hepatic artery is ligated, a continuous infusion of 5-FU administered through the proximal hepatic artery is combined with monthly hyperthermia treatments. The rationale for the therapy plan was based on several recent findings. Because liver metastases generally receive their blood supply from the hepatic artery, interruption of the arterial flow alone could cause some degree of tumor necrosis. Moreover, since effective hyperthermia of many solid tumors appears to be dependent on reduced tumor blood flow [18], interruption of the arterial supply could impair the tumor's ability to dissipate heat and induce increased independent tumor temperatures. Direct infusion of chemotherapy also could increase the extracellular drug gradient at the site of the tumor with less systemic drug toxicity. Even though hyperthermia appeared to be tumoricidal as a single agent it might increase intracellular uptake of drug in the target tissue. A pilot study of the thermochemotherapy approach showed no increase in toxicity over drug alone and achieved several encouraging responses.

A prospective randomized trial is now underway to evaluate combined thermochemotherapy for colon metastases in liver. The role of hepatic artery ligation and infusion therapy is being compared to conventional IV-5-FU administration. Of 11 patients initially treated with 5-FU and hepatic hyperthermia, one had complete response at 13 months follow-up, one had partial response at 9 months, and seven patients had no progression of disease for 3 to 8 months (5 months median) [73]. Although it is too early to determine the contribution of infusion therapy, these preliminary results suggest that adjuvant hyperthermia may be of significant potential benefit for these patients.

7.6. Gastric and pancreatic carcinoma

Curative resection can be accomplished in less than 15% of patients who are explored for pancreatic carcinoma. Their median survival was 6 months with regional disease, 3 months with distant intraabdominal disease and 2.5 months with hepatic metastases [74]. Nearly two-thirds of patients with gastric carcinoma have unresectable disease and a median survival of 3 months and, of those resected, less than one-third will be alive at 5 years [75]. Recently, combinations of 5-FU, adriamycin, and Mitomycin-C (FAM) have produced a 40% response rate for pancreatic carcinoma and a 55% response rate for gastric carcinoma, associated with an enhanced quality of life for responders [76]. Although these results have been encouraging, they are far from optimal.

Therefore, we started a Phase I study to evaluate thermochemotherapy for these and other refractory gastrointestinal cancers. One patient with an unresectable gastric cancer that required twice weekly blood transfusions was treated with FAM plus hyperthermia monthly and was rendered symptom free for 1 year. Unfortunately, the patient died from a rare blood dyscrasia caused by the drugs. However, another patient with metastatic gastric carcinoma in liver was treated with infused IA-FAM with hyperthermia and achieved a complete response at 4 months of follow-up with no increase in drug toxicity. One patient with an unresectable pancreatic carcinoma and liver metastases who required intrathecal morphine for control of pain was treated with IA-FAM, via the celiac artery, combined with regional upper-abdominal hyperthermia. After two monthly courses of therapy, the patient was pain free with stable disease but had subsequent disease progression on the intravenous combined therapy. One patient with an undifferentiated hepatic neoplasm who had failed FAM and is-platinum infusion therapy was treated with IA-cis-platinum plus heat and had no progression of disease at 5 months follow-up.

Although these results are anecdotal, responses suggest that further combined thermochemotherapy trials are needed, particularly those that are combined with infusion therapy.

Once hyperthermia therapy is optimized, it may be possible to achieve responses at lower drug doses, which, in turn, may reduce drug toxicity and prolong the duration of therapy. It may also be possible to reinstitute use of previously less effective drugs with the expectation of enhanced activity due to hyperthermia.

References

1. Busch W: Uber den Eingluss, welchen heftigere Erysepeln zuweilen auf organisierte Neubeldungers ausuben. Verhanal d Naturh Verd Pruess Rheinl u Westphal, Bonn 23: 28–30, 1866.
2. Coley WB: The treatment of malignant tumors by repeated inoculations of erysipelas, with a report of ten original cases. Am J Med Sc 105: 487–511, 1893.
3. Nagelschmidt F: Lehrbuch der diathermie, aufe III, 1926.
4. Westermark N: The effect of heat upon rat tumors. Skand Arch Physiol 52: 257–322, 1927.
5. Warren SL: Preliminary study of the effect of artificial fever upon hopeless tumor cases. Am J Roentgenol Radium Ther 33: 75–87, 1935.
6. Crile G: Selective destruction of cancers after exposure to heat. Ann Surg 156: 404–407, 1962.
7. Cavaliere R, Ciocatto EC, Giovanella BC, *et al.*: Selective heat sensitivity of cancer cells. Biochemical and clinical studies. Cancer 20: 1351–1381, 1967.
8. Dickson JA, Suzanger M: 'In vitro' sensitivity screening system for human cancers to drugs and hyperthermia (42° C). Br J Cancer 28: 81–85, 1973.
9. Mondovi B, Strom R, Rotilio G, *et al.*: The biochemical mechanism of selective heat sensitivity of cancer cells. I. Studies on cellular respiration. Eur J Cancer 5: 129–136, 1969.
10. Mondovi B, Finazzi-Agro A, Rotilio G, *et al.*: The biochemical mechanism of selective heat sensitivity of cancer cells. II. Studies on nucleic acids and protein synthesis. Eur J Cancer 5: 137–147, 1969.
11. Strom R, Santoro AS, Crifo C, *et al.*: The biochemical mechanism of selective heat sensitivity of cancer cells. IV. Inhibition of RNA synthesis. Eur J Cancer 9: 103–112,1973.
12. Hahn, GM: Thermochemotherapy: Interactions between hyperthermia and chemotherapeutic agents. Proc Intl Symp on Cancer Ther by Hyperthermia, Drugs, and Radiation. J Natl Cancer Inst (Special Suppl), in press.
13. Strom R: Ricerche sul meccanismo d'azione del calore sui tumori. Atti Soc Ital Cancer V Nat Cong, vol 7, part 2, pp 49–60, 1970.
14. Turano C, Ferraro A, Strom R, *et al.*: The biochemical mechanism of selective heat sensitivity of

cancer cells. III. Studies on lysosomes. Eur J Cancer 6: 67–72, 1970.

15. Hardy JD, Stolwijk JAJ, Hammel HT: Skin temperatures and cutaneous pain during warm water immersion. J Appl Physiol 20: 1014–1021, 1965.

16. Overgaard K, Overgaard J: Investigations on the possibility of a thermic tumor therapy. Eur J Cancer 8: 65–78, 1972.

17. Dickson JA: Hyperthermia and laboratory animal systems. Chairman's address. In: Proc Intl Symp on Cancer Therapy by Hyperthermia and Radiation, Washington, D.C., Am Coll Rad Press, 1975, p 105–106.

18. Storm FK, Elliott RS, Harrison WH, et al.: Normal tissue and solid tumor effects of hyperthermia in animal models and clinical trials. Cancer Res 39: 2245–2251, 1979.

19. Giovanella BC, Morgan AC, Stehlin JS, et al.: Selective lethal effect of supranormal temperatures on mouse sarcoma cells. Cancer Res 33: 2568–2578, 1973.

20. Mantyla MJ: Regional blood flow in human tumors. Cancer Res 39: 2304–2306, 1979.

21. Le Veen HH, Wapnick S, Piccone V, et al.: Tumor eradication by radio-frequency therapy. Response in 21 patients. JAMA 235: 2198–2200, 1976.

22. Madden JL, Kandalaft S: Electrocoagulation in the treatment of cancer of the rectum; a continuing study. Ann Surg 174: 530–540, 1971.

23. Wanebo HJ, Quan SH: Failures of electrocoagulation of primary carcinoma of the rectum. Surg Gynecol Obstet 138: 174–176, 1974.

24. Doss JD: Use of RF fields to produce hyperthermia in animal tumors. In: Proc Intl Symp on Cancer Therapy by Hyperthermia and Radiation. Washington, DC, Am Coll Rad Press, 1975, p 226–227.

25. Sternhagen CJ, Doss JD, Day PW, et al.: Clinical use of radio-frequency current in oral cavity carcinomas and metastatic malignancies with continuous temperature control and monitoring. In: Cancer Therapy by Hyperthermia and Radiation, Streffer C (ed), Baltimore, Urband & Schwarzenberg, 1978, p 331–334.

26. Manning MR, Cetas TC, Miller RC, et al.: Clinical hyperthermia: Results of a Phase I trial employing hyperthermia alone or in combination with external beam or interstitial radiotherapy. Cancer 49: 205–216, 1982.

27. Rand RW, Snyder M, Elliott D, et al.: Selective radio-frequency heating of ferrosilicone occluded tissue: A preliminary report. Bulletin L.A. Neurol Soc 41: 154–159, 1976; personal communication, 1981.

28. Schwan HP: Electromagnetic and ultrasonic induction of hyperthermia in tissuelike substances. Rad Environ Biophys 17: 189–203, 1980.

29. Lele PP: Hyperthermia by ultrasound. In: Proc Intl Symp on Cancer Therapy by Hyperthermia and Radiation. Washington, DC, Am Coll Rad Press, 1975, p 168–178.

30. Lele PP: Induction of deep, local hyperthermia by ultrasound and electromagnetic fields – Problems and choices. Rad Environ Biophys 17: 205–217, 1980; personal communication, 1981.

31. Marmor JB, Hahn G: Clinical studies with ultrasound for the induction of localized hyperthermia. Proc Third Intl Symp on Cancer Therapy by Hyperthermia, Drugs and Radiation. J Natl Cancer Inst (Special Suppl.), in press.

32. Guy AW: Physical aspects of the electromagnetic heating of tissue volume. In: Proc Intl Symp on Cancer Therapy by Hyperthermia and Radiation. Washington, D.C., Am Coll Rad Press, 1975, p 179–192.

33. Robinson JE Cheung AY, Samaras GM: Microwave phase array: personal communication, 1980.

34. Storm FK, Morton DL, Kaiser LR, et al.: Clinical radio-frequency hyperthermia: A review. Proc Third Intl Symp on Cancer Therapy by Hyperthermia, Drugs and Radiation. J Natl Cancer Inst (Special Suppl.), in press.

35. Le Veen HH, Ahmed N, Piccone VA: RF therapy: Clinical experience. Ann NY Acad Sci 335: 362–371, 1980.

382

36. Kim JH, Hahn EW: Clinical and biological studies of localized hyperthermia. Cancer Res 39: 2258–2261, 1979.
37. Elliott RS, Harrison WH, Storm FK: Hyperthermia: electromagnetic heating of deep-seated tumors. IEEE Trans BME: 29: 61–64, 1982.
38. Storm FK, Harrison WH, Elliott RS, *et al.*: Thermal distribution of magnetic-loop induction hyperthermia in phantoms and animals: Effect of the living state and velocity of heating. Int J Rad Oncol Biol Phys 8: 865–871, 1982.
39. Pettigrew RT, Galt JM, Ludgate CM, *et al.*: Circulatory and biochemical effects of whole body hyperthermia. Br J Surg 61: 727–730, 1974.
40. Pettigrew RT, Galt JM, Ludgate CM, Smith AN: Clinical effects of whole body hyperthermia in advanced malignancy. Br Med J 4: 679–682, 1974.
41. Bull JM, Less DE, Schuette WA, *et al.*: Whole-body hyperthermia – now a feasible addition to cancer treatment. Proc Am Soc Clin Oncol 19: 405, 1978.
42. Larkin JM, Edwards WS, Smith DE, Clark PJ: Systemic thermotheraphy: Description of a method and physiologic tolerance in clinical subjects. Cancer 40: 3155–3159, 1977.
43. Parks LC, Minaberry D, Smith DP, *et al.*: Treatment of far-advanced bronchogenic carcinoma by extracorporeally induced systemic hyperthermia. J Thorac Cardiovasc Surg 78: 883–892, 1979.
44. Kim JH, Hahn EW, Tokita N: Combination hyperthermia and radiation therapy for cutaneous malignant melanoma. Cancer 41: 2143–2148, 1978.
45. Storm FK, Harrison WH, Morton DL: Human hyperthermic therapy: Relationship between tumor type and capacity to induce hyperthermia by radio frequency. Am J Surg 138: 170–174, 1979.
46. Baker HW, Snedecor PA, Goss JC, *et al.*: Regional hyperthermia for cancer. Am J Surg 143: 586–590, 1982.
47. Dickson JA, Shah SA, Waggoh D: Tumor eradication in the rabbit by radiofrequency heating. Cancer Res 37: 2162–2169, 1977.
48. Joines WT, U R, Noell TK, *et al.*: Techniques and results of using microwaves and x-rays for the treatment of tumors in man. Proc Intl Symp on the Biol Effects of Electromagnetic Waves (Abstract S-7), p 160, 1977.
49. Luk KH, Phillips TL, Holse RM: Hyperthermia in cancer therapy. Western J Med 132: 179–185, 1980.
50. Storm FK, Elliott RS, Harrison WH, *et al.*: Hyperthermia therapy for human neoplasms: Thermal death time. Cancer 46: 1849–1854, 1980.
51. Guy AW, Lehmann JF, Stonebridge JB: Therapeutic applications of electromagnetic power. Proc IEEE 62: 55–75, 1974.
52. Stehlin JS, Giovanella BC, Ipolyi PD: Results of hyperthermic perfusion for melanoma of the extremities. Surg Gynecol Obstet 14: 339–346, 1975.
53. Storm FK, Sparks FC, Morton DL: Treatment for melanoma of the lower extremity with intralesional injection of bacille Calmette-Guerin and hyperthermic perfusion. Surg Gynecol Obstet 149: 17–21, 1979.
54. Goldenberg DM, Langer M: Direct and abscopal antitumor action of local hyperthermia. Z Naturforsch 26: 359–361, 1971.
55. Marmor JB, Hahn N, Hahn GM: Tumor cure and cell survival after localized radio-frequency heating. Cancer Res 37: 879–883, 1977.
56. Dickson J, Shah S: Immune parameters. In: Hyperthermia in Cancer Therapy, Storm FK (ed). Boston, GK Hall & Co, 1982, in press.
57. Herman TS, Gerner EW, Magun BE, *et al.*: Rate of heating as a determinant of hyperthermic toxicity. Cancer Res 41: 3519–3524, 1981.
58. Storm FK, Elliott RS, Harrison WH, *et al.*: Radio-frequency hyperthermia of advanced human sarcomas. J Surg Oncol 17: 91–98, 1981.
59. Selawry OS, Carlson JC, Moore GE: Tumor response to ionizing rays at elevated temperatures.

Am J Roent 80: 833–839, 1958.

60. Gerweck LE, Gillette EL, Dewey WC: Killing of Chinese hamster cells in vitro by heating under hypoxic or aerobic conditions. Eur J Cancer 10: 691–693, 1974.

61. Gerner EW, Connor WG, Boone MLM, *et al.*: The potential of localized heating as an adjunct to radiation therapy. Radiology 116: 433–439, 1975.

62. Ben-Hur E, Elkin MM, Bronk BV: Thermally enhanced radio response of cultured Chinese hamster cells: Inhibition of repair of sublethal damage and enhancement of lethal damage. Radiat Res 58: 38–51, 1974.

63. Hornback NB, Shupe RE, Shidnia H, *et al.*: Preliminary clinical results of 433 MHz microwave therapy and radiation therapy on patients with advanced cancer. Cancer 40: 2854–2863, 1977.

64. Abe M, Hiraoka M, Takahashi M, *et al.*: Clinical experience with microwave and radio-frequency thermo-therapy in the treatment of advanced cancer. In: Proc Third Intl Symp on Cancer Ther by Hyperthermia, Drugs and Radiation (Abstract T-III-1), p 116, 1980.

65. Bicher HI, Sandhu TS, Hetzle FW: Hyperthermia fractionation protocol: Preliminary results of a clinical trial. In: Proc Third Intl Symp on Cancer Ther by Hyperthermia, Drugs and Radiation (Abstract T-III-6), p 118, 1980.

66. Johnson HA, Pvelec M: Thermal enhancement of thio-tepa toxicity. J Natl Cancer Inst 50: 903–910, 1973.

67. Muckle DS, Dickson JA: Hyperthermia (42° C) as an adjuvant to radiotherapy and chemotherapy in the treatment of the allogeneic VX2 carcinoma in the rabbit. Br J Cancer 27: 307–315, 1973.

68. Hahn GM, Braun J, Har-Kedar I: Thermochemotherapy: Surgery between hyperthermia (42–43° C) and adriamycin (or bleomycin) in mammalian cell inactivation. Proc Natl Acad Sci USA 72: 937–940, 1975.

69. Mann BD, Storm FK, Kern DH, Giuliano A, Morton DL: Predictive value of the clonogenic assay in the treatment of melanoma with DTIC and DTIC + hyperthermia. Proc Am Soc of Clin Oncol 17: 432, 1981.

70. Ramming KP, Sparks FC, Eilber FR, Morton DL: Management of hepatic metastases. Sem Oncol 4: 71–80, 1977.

71. Einhorn LH, McBride CM, Luce JK, *et al.*: Intraarterial infusion therapy with imidazole carboxamide for malignant melanoma. Cancer 32: 749–755, 1973.

72. Storm FK, Kaiser LR, Goodnight JE, *et al.*: Thermo-chemotherapy for melanoma metastases in liver. Cancer 49: 1423–1428, 1982.

73. Ramming KP: Personal communication. Department of Surgery, Division of Oncology, UCLA School of Medicine, 1982.

74. Die-Goyanes A, Pack GT, Bowden L: Cancer of the body and tail of the pancreas. Rev Surg 28: 153–159, 1971.

75. Lawrence W: End results and prognosis. In: McNeer Neoplasms of the Stomach, Lippincott, Philadelphia, 1967, p 484.

76. Bitram JD, Desseer RK, Koxloff MF, *et al.*: Treatment of metastatic pancreatic and gastric adenocarcinoma with 5-fluorouracil adriamycin and mitomycin-C (FAM). Cancer Treat Rep 63: 2049–2051, 1979.

77. Parks L, Smith G: Systemic hyperthermia by the extracorporeal technique. In: Hyperthermia in Cancer Therapy, Storm FK (ed). Boston GK Hall & Co, 1982, in press.

Index